OUTLINE OF ORTHOPAEDICS

John Crawford Adams
MD (London), MS (London), FRCS (England)
Honorary Consulting Orthopaedic Surgeon, St Mary's Hospital, London, UK; Honorary Civil Consultant in Orthopaedic Surgery, Royal Air Force; Formerly Production Editor, Journal of Bone and Joint Surgery.

David L. Hamblen
PhD, FRCS (England), FRCS (Edinburgh), FRCS (Glasgow)
Professor of Orthopaedic Surgery, University of Glasgow, Glasgow, UK.

TWELFTH EDITION

CHURCHILL
LIVINGSTONE

EDINBURGH HONG KONG LONDON MADRID MELBOURNE NEW YORK AND TOKYO 1995

CHURCHILL LIVINGSTONE

Medical Division of Pearson Professional Limited

Distributed in the United States of America by Churchill
Livingstone Inc., 650 Avenue of the Americas, New York,
N.Y. 10011, and by associated companies, branches and
representatives throughout the world.

2006407 1

First edition 1956
Second edition 1958
Third edition 1960
Fourth edition 1961
Fifth edition 1964
Sixth edition 1967
Seventh edition 1971

Eighth edition 1976
Ninth edition 1981
Tenth edition 1986
Eleventh edition 1990
Twelfth edition 1995
Reprinted 1996

ISBN 0 443 05149 6

British Library Cataloguing in Publication Data
A catalogue record for this book is available from the British Library.

Library of Congress Cataloging in Publication Data
A catalog record for this book is available from the Library of Congress.

The
publisher's
policy is to use
**paper manufactured
from sustainable forests**

Produced by Longman Singapore Publishers (Pte) Ltd.
Printed in Singapore

Contents

Prefaces

PREFACE TO THE TWELFTH EDITION

The publication of the 11th edition marked a new era for this book, with a change to dual authorship and a new format. The adoption of a slightly increased page size, which has allowed improvements in layout and clarity of the illustrations, has proved popular and is therefore continued for this new Edition.

Where necessary, the material has been slightly expanded to take account of recent advances, particularly in imaging techniques, endoscopic procedures, and skeletal tumours. Corresponding deletion of obsolete material has enabled us to keep the length of the book virtually within its previous bounds. In some sections the illustrations have been improved or replaced by more representative examples. The list of references has been updated.

J.C.A.
D.L.H.

PREFACE TO THE ELEVENTH EDITION

The 11th edition sees *Outline of Orthopaedics* in a slightly altered format. The page size has been increased slightly but the book is correspondingly slimmer. We were agreed that there should be a decrease rather than an increase in the length of the text, and this has been achieved by the deletion of obsolete material. There is however some overall enlargement from the inclusion of additional illustrations.

Despite the rejuvenation of the book, all that was best in the previous editions has been retained, including the logical classification of orthopaedic conditions, the concise descriptions, and above all the clear instructions for clinical examination of the limbs and spine, so vital for the examination candidate, and helpful in guiding the clinician towards correct diagnosis.

The book is still intended primarily for the undergraduate medical student, but it has also proved useful for postgraduates studying for the higher examinations in surgery, for general practitioners, and for physiotherapists and orthopaedic nurses. For the benefit of the harrassed undergraduate, detail that is not essential reading has been set in small type, but it is there for any student—undergraduate or postgraduate—who wishes to pursue a subject in greater depth. An enlarged and updated list of references is provided as a source for further reading.

J.C.A.

D.L.H.

NOTE ON TERMINOLOGY

The anatomical nomenclature used in this book conforms to that recommended by the International Anatomical Nomenclature Committee and approved at the Eighth International Congress of Anatomists at Wiesbaden in 1965. This nomenclature, which differs only in minor respects from the earlier Birmingham revision of the Basle nomenclature, has been adopted at most schools of anatomy and it is to be hoped that it will become the standard terminology acceptable to anatomists and surgeons alike.

The recommended method of recording and expressing joint movement conforms to that laid down by the American Academy of Orthopaedic Surgeons in the booklet *Joint Motion* published by the Academy in 1965 and revised recently, and approved by most of the Orthopaedic Associations of the English-speaking world. The guiding principle of the method is that for any joint the extended 'anatomical position' is regarded as zero degrees, and movement at the joint is measured from this starting position. For example, in the knee the straight position is described as zero degrees and the fully flexed position is expressed as (say) 145 degrees of flexion; likewise at the elbow. At the ankle the anatomical position, with the foot at a right angle to the leg, is the zero position, from which plantarflexion and dorsiflexion (extension) are measured.

The Academy booklet also gives figures for the normal range of movement at each joint. In some instances these do not accord with authors' experience and they have not always been followed in this text. Individual variations are common, so that any statement of the normal must necessarily be imprecise.

Introduction

HISTORICAL NOTE
The orthopaedic surgeon today is concerned with diseases and injuries of the trunk and limbs. His field is not confined to the bones and joints; it includes in addition the muscles, tendons, ligaments, bursae, nerves, and blood vessels. He is not concerned with injuries of the skull, which fall within the province of the neurosurgeon; or with injuries of the jaws, which are the responsibility of the facio-maxillary or dental surgeon.

The term orthopaedic is derived from the Greek words ορθος (straight) and παις (child). It was originally applied to the art of correcting deformities by Nicolas Andry, a French physician, who in 1741 published a book entitled *Orthopaedia: Or the Art of Correcting and Preventing Deformities in Children: By such Means, as may easily be put in Practice by Parents themselves, and all such as are Employed in Educating Children.*

In Andry's time orthopaedic surgery in the form known today did not exist. Surgery was still primitive. Indeed, except for sporadic attempts by ingenious individuals, it is probable that little real progress had been made since the days of Hippocrates, who lived in about 400 BC.

That is not to say that surgeons were unintelligent or that they lacked a capacity for careful study and research. Early writings prove that many of them were shrewd observers, and from the time of John Hunter (1728–1793) onwards this was increasingly true. Take, for example, the words of Sir Astley Cooper (1768–1848) in his *Treatise on Dislocations and Fractures of the Joints*: 'Nothing is known in our profession by guess; and I do not believe, that from the first dawn of medical science to the present moment, a single correct idea has ever emanated from conjecture. It is right, therefore, that those who are studying their profession should be aware that there is no short road to knowledge; that observations on the diseased living, examinations of the dead, and experiments upon living animals are the only sources of true knowledge; and that inductions from these are the sole basis of legitimate theory.'

The enthusiasm and the capacity for study were there. The real obstacle to progress was the lack of the essential facilities that we now take so much for granted—anaesthesia, asepsis, powerful microscopes, and x-rays. Any surgical operation that could not be completed within a few minutes was out of the question when the patient's consciousness could be clouded only by intoxication or exsanguination. And when every major operation was inevitably followed by suppuration which often proved fatal, it is small wonder that operations were seldom advised except in an attempt to save life.

Fig. 1
A seventeenth century amputation scene.
(From Fabricus: *Opera*, 1646.)

Thus orthopaedic surgery, until relatively recent times, was confined largely to the correction of deformities by rather crude pieces of apparatus, to the reduction of fractures and dislocations by powerful traction, and to amputation of limbs (Fig. 1).

LANDMARKS OF SURGERY IN THE NINETEENTH CENTURY
Fundamental advances in surgery were in fact dependent upon the development of other branches of science and of industry which provided, for instance, the high-powered microscope and the x-ray tube. It is therefore not surprising that, after centuries of stagnation, the facilities that were lacking were all made available within the span of a single life-time, at the period of the Industrial Revolution.

The first epoch-making advance was the introduction of anaesthesia. The credit for this should be given jointly to Crawford Long, of Athens, Georgia, who was the first to use ether in 1842 but delayed publication of his observations for seven years; and to W. T. G. Morton, of Boston, Massachusetts, whose use of ether anaesthesia was reported in 1846.

A few years later Louis Pasteur (1822–1895), working in Paris and equipped at last with an adequate microscope, was carrying out his fundamental research on bacteria as a cause of disease. Then in 1867 Joseph Lister (1827–1912), working in Glasgow, Scotland, on the basis of Pasteur's work introduced his antiseptic surgical technique which allowed the surgeon, for the first time in history, to look for primary healing of his operation wounds. Finally, in 1895, came Roentgen's report from Würzburg in Germany of his discovery of x-rays, which within a short time were put to practical use in surgical diagnosis.

THE EMERGENCE OF ORTHOPAEDICS AS A DISTINCT SPECIALITY

Thus at the dawn of the twentieth century the stage was set for the phenomenally rapid evolution of surgery that has been witnessed by many still alive today. With the consequent widening of the scope of surgical practice orthopaedic surgery, at first encompassed by the general surgeon, began to branch off as a distinct science and art; but it was not until after the First World War that it came to be widely recognised as a separate speciality.

In Great Britain many of the fundamental principles of orthopaedics had been propounded, just before the twentieth century began, by Hugh Owen Thomas[1] (1834–1891) of Liverpool. Thomas was not primarily concerned with operative surgery but rather with manipulative surgery and with conservative methods such as rest and splintage, and it was left to his nephew, Sir Robert Jones (1857–1933) to set orthopaedic surgery upon the sound foundation that it now enjoys. During and after the First World War Robert Jones trained many of the surgeons, British and American, who were among the first to devote their professional lives entirely to the practice of orthopaedics.

THE FUTURE

Advance has continued apace in recent decades. Of particular importance has been the development of joint replacement surgery in the treatment of arthritis. The results have been spectacular in the case of the hip, and only slightly less impressive in the knee. This has been a revolution indeed. Another has been the development of microsurgical techniques, allowing the anastomosis or repair of very small blood vessels and nerves and thus facilitating the transfer of living tissue—whether skin or bone or nerve—

[1]Thomas's name is remembered in the widely used Thomas's knee splint and in Thomas's test for fixed flexion at the hip.

from one site to another, and even the replantation of severed parts. A third important advance has been in the field of arthroscopy and arthroscopic surgery—a major boon to patients, not least because time spent in hospital has been substantially reduced.

At the same time orthopaedic surgeons—particularly in Western countries—have seen the virtual elimination of many diseases that were formerly prevalent—notably tuberculosis, poliomyelitis, tertiary syphilis and rickets. For these benefits research in disciplines other than orthopaedic surgery has been responsible; and it is necessary to recognise that future fundamental developments also are more likely to come from advances in immunology, microbiology, genetics or microsurgery than from the orthopaedic surgeon's laboratory.

It thus behoves present aspirants to orthopaedic surgery—particularly those with an academic bent—to familiarise themselves at an early stage of their training with research techniques and developments in at least one or two of these newer disciplines. For the rest, now that the great surge of discovery has slowed, the aim must be to consolidate the knowledge gained and to develop an ever more sound judgement, so that in devising treatment for our patients we do the right thing at the right time. 'Get it right first time' should be the slogan. This is still quite a challenge; a challenge that adds to the fascination of orthopaedic surgery.

References and bibliography, page 403.

PART ONE

CLINICAL METHODS

In this part guidance is given on the correct line of approach to an orthopaedic problem, with particular reference to diagnosis and treatment.

As in all branches of medicine and surgery, proficiency in diagnosis can be acquired only from long experience. There is no short cut to a familiarity with physical signs or to skill in radiographic interpretation. Nevertheless the inexperienced surgeon who tackles the problem methodically step by step will often give a better account of himself than his more experienced colleague who makes a 'snap' diagnosis after no more than a cursory investigation.

In the choice of treatment the development of a sound judgement is also largely a matter of experience. Yet more than that is needed. Other essential qualities are common sense and a sympathetic appreciation of human problems. There are surgeons who never acquire a sound judgement, however long their apprenticeship. Others seem to have a natural aptitude that quickly matures under proper guidance and training.

1. Diagnosis of orthopaedic disorders

As in other fields of medicine and surgery, diagnosis of orthopaedic disorders depends first upon an accurate determination of all the abnormal features from: 1) the history; 2) clinical examination; 3) radiographic examination and other methods of imaging; and 4) special investigations. Secondly, it depends upon a correct interpretation of the findings.

HISTORY

In the diagnosis of orthopaedic conditions the history is often of first importance. In cases of torn meniscus in the knee, for instance, the clinical diagnosis sometimes depends upon the history alone. Except in the most obvious conditions, a detailed history is always required.

First the exact nature of the patient's complaint is determined. Then the development of the symptoms is traced step by step from their earliest beginning up to the time of the consultation. The patient's own views on the cause of the symptoms are always worth recording: often they prove to be correct. Enquiry is made into activities that have been found to improve the symptoms or to make them worse, and into the effect of any previous treatment. Facts that often have an important bearing on the condition are the age and present occupation of the patient, his previous occupations, his hobbies and recreational activities, and previous injuries.

When a full history of the local symptoms has been obtained, do not omit to enquire whether there have been symptoms in other parts of the body, and whether the general health is affected. Ask also about previous illnesses.

Finally, in cases that seem trivial, a tactful enquiry as to why the patient decided to seek advice, and to what extent he is worried by his disability, will often give a valuable clue to the underlying problem. It should be remembered that very often a patient seeks advice not because he is handicapped by his disability (which is often insignificant) but because he fears the development of some serious disease such as cancer, paralysis, or progressive crippling deformity.

CLINICAL EXAMINATION

The part complained of is examined according to a rigid routine which should become habitual. If this is done, familiarity with the routine will ensure that no step in the examination is forgotten. Accuracy of observation is essential: it can be acquired only by much practice and by diligent attention to detail.

The examination of the part complained of does not complete the clinical examination. It sometimes happens that symptoms felt in one part have their origin in another. For example, pain in the leg is often caused by a lesion in the spine, and pain in the knee may have its origin in the hip. The possibility of a distant lesion must therefore be considered and an examination made of any region under suspicion.

Finally, localised symptoms may be the first or only manifestation of a generalised or widespread disorder. A brief examination is therefore made of the rest of the body with this possibility in mind.

Thus the clinical examination may be considered under three headings:
1) examination of the part complained of;
2) investigation of possible sources of referred symptoms;
3) general examination of the body as a whole.

1. EXAMINATION OF THE PART COMPLAINED OF

The following description of the steps in the clinical examination is intended only as a guide. The technique of examination will naturally be varied according to individual preference. Nevertheless, it is useful to stick to a particular routine, for a familiarity with it will ensure that no step in the examination is forgotten.

Exposure for examination

It is essential that the part to be examined should be adequately exposed and in a good light. Many mistakes are made simply because the student or practitioner does not insist upon the removal of enough clothes to allow proper examination. When a limb is being examined the sound limb should always be exposed for comparison.

Inspection

Inspection should be carried out systematically, with attention to the following four points. 1) **The bones**: Observe the general alignment and position of the parts to detect any deformity, shortening, or unusual posture. 2) **The soft tissues**: Observe the soft-tissue contours, comparing the two sides. Note any visible evidence of general or local swelling, or of muscle wasting. 3) **Colour and texture of the skin**: Look for redness, cyanosis, pigmentation, shininess, loss of hair, adventitious tufts of hair or other changes. 4) **Scars or sinuses**: If a scar is present, determine from its appearance whether it was caused by operation (linear scar with suture marks), injury (irregular scar), or suppuration (broad, adherent, puckered scar).

Palpation

Again there are four points to consider. 1) **Skin temperature**: By careful comparison of the two sides judge whether there is an area of increased warmth or of unusual coldness. An increase of local temperature denotes increased vascularity. The usual cause is an inflammatory reaction; but it should be remembered that a rapidly growing tumour may also bring about marked local hyperaemia, with increase in skin warmth. 2) **The bones**: The general shape and outline of the bones are investigated. Feel in particular for thickening, abnormal prominence, or disturbed relationship of the normal landmarks. 3) **The soft tissues**: Direct particular attention to the muscles (are they in spasm, or wasted?), to the joint tissues (is the synovial membrane thickened, or the joint distended with fluid?), and to the detection of any local swelling (? cyst; ? tumour) or general swelling of the part. 4) **Local tenderness**: The exact site of any local tenderness should be mapped out and an attempt made to relate it to a particular anatomical structure.

> **Determining the cause of a diffuse joint swelling**. The question often arises: what is the cause of a diffuse swelling of a joint? The answer can be supplied after careful palpation. For practical purposes a *diffuse* swelling of the joint as a whole can have only three causes: 1) thickening of the bone end; 2) fluid within the joint; and 3) thickening of the synovial membrane. In some cases two or all three causes may be combined, but they can always be differentiated by palpation. *Bony thickening* is detected by deep palpation through the soft tissues, the bone outlines being compared on the two sides. A *fluid effusion* generally gives a clear sense of fluctuation between the two hands. *Synovial thickening* gives a characteristic boggy sensation—rather as if a layer of soft sponge-rubber had been placed between the skin and the bone. It is nearly always accompanied by a well marked increase of local warmth, for the synovium is a very vascular membrane.

Measurements

Measurement of limb length is often necessary, especially in the lower limbs, where discrepancy between the two sides is important. Measurement of the circumference of a limb segment on the two sides provides an index of muscle wasting, soft-tissue swelling or bony thickening. Details will be given in the chapters on individual regions.

Estimation of fixed deformity

Fixed deformity exists when a joint cannot be placed in the neutral (anatomical) position. Its causes are described on page 39. The degree of fixed deformity at a joint is determined by bringing the joint as near as it will come to the neutral position and then measuring the angle by which it falls short.[1]

---

[1]Explanation is needed of the commonly used terms *valgus* and *varus*, which are often confusing to students. In valgus deformity the distal part of a member is deviated laterally (outwards) in relation to the proximal part. Thus, for example, in hallux valgus the toe is deviated outwards in relation to the foot; and in genu valgum the lower leg is deviated outwards in relation to the thigh. Varus deformity is the opposite: the distal part of a member is deviated medially (inwards) in relation to the proximal part (examples—cubitus varus and genu varum).

Movements

In the examination of joint movements information must be obtained on the following points: 1) What is the range of active movement? 2) Is passive movement greater than active? 3) Is movement painful? 4) Is movement accompanied by crepitation?

In measuring the range of movement it is important to know what is the normal. With some joints the normal varies considerably from patient to patient; as, for instance, at the metacarpo-phalangeal joint of the thumb: so it is wise always to use the unaffected limb for comparison. Restriction of movement in all directions suggests some form of arthritis, whereas selective limitation of movement in some directions with free movement in others is more suggestive of a mechanical derangement.

Except in two sets of circumstances passive movement will usually be found equal to the active. The passive range will exceed the active only in the following circumstances: 1) when the muscles responsible for the movement are paralysed; and 2) when the muscles or their tendons are torn, severed or unduly slack.

Stability

The stability of a joint depends partly upon the integrity of its articulating surfaces and partly upon intact ligaments. When a joint is unstable there is abnormal mobility—for instance, lateral mobility in a hinge joint. It is important, when testing for abnormal mobility, to ensure that the muscles controlling the joint are relaxed; for a muscle in strong contraction can often conceal ligamentous instability.

Power

The power of the muscles responsible for each movement of a joint is determined by instructing the patient to move the joint against the resistance of the examiner. With careful comparison of the two sides it is possible to detect gross impairment of power. By general convention, the strength of a muscle is recorded according to the Medical Research Council grading as follows: 0 = no contraction; 1 = a flicker of contraction; 2 = slight power, sufficient to move the joint only with gravity eliminated; 3 = power sufficient to move the joint against gravity; 4 = power to move the joint against gravity plus added resistance; 5 = normal power.

In the occasional instances when more precise information is required muscle strength can be measured against weights, spring balances, or deflection bars.

Sensibility

It is necessary to test sensibility both to light touch and to pin prick throughout the whole of the affected area. In unilateral affections the opposite side should be similarly tested. The precise area of any blunting or loss of sensibility should be carefully mapped out, and from a knowledge of the cutaneous distribution of the peripheral nerves the particular nerve or nerves affected may be identified and the root value established.

Peripheral circulation

Symptoms in a limb may be associated with impairment of the arterial circulation. Time should therefore be spent in assessing the state of the circulation by examination of the colour and temperature of the skin, the texture of the skin and nails, and the arterial pulses; and by such special investigations as may be necessary. This examination is particularly important in the case of the lower limb. Further details are given on page 359.

Reflexes

As part of the neurological examination the appropriate deep and superficial reflexes must be tested. Details will be given in the sections on individual regions of the body.

Tests of function

It is necessary next to test the function of the part under examination. How much does the disorder affect the part in its fulfilment of everyday activities? Methods of determining this vary according to the part affected. To take the lower limb as an example, the best test of function is to observe the patient standing, walking, running, and jumping. Special tests are required to investigate certain functions—for example, the Trendelenburg test for abductor efficiency at the hip (p. 289).

2. INVESTIGATION OF POSSIBLE SOURCES OF REFERRED SYMPTOMS

When the source of the symptoms is still in doubt after careful examination of the part complained of, attention must be directed to possible extrinsic disorders with referred symptoms. This will entail examination of such other regions of the body as might be responsible. For instance, in a case of pain in the shoulder it might be necessary to examine the neck for evidence of a lesion interfering with the brachial plexus, and the thorax and abdomen for evidence of diaphragmatic irritation, because either of these conditions may be a cause of shoulder pain. Again, in a case of pain in the thigh the examination will often have to include a study of the spine, abdomen, pelvis and genito-urinary system as well as a local examination of the hip and thigh.

3. GENERAL EXAMINATION

The mistake is sometimes made of confining the attention to the patient's immediate symptoms and failing to assess the patient as a whole. It should be made a rule in every case, however trivial it may seem, to form an opinion not only of the patient's general physical condition but also of his psychological outlook. In simple and straightforward cases this general survey may legitimately be brief and rapid, but it should never be omitted.

DIAGNOSTIC IMAGING

Until recent years radiography was the only method by which bone and other relatively dense tissues could be shown as a visual image contrasting with adjacent less dense tissues. This is no longer the case, for technical developments have led to alternative methods of imaging. These include: 1) ultrasound scanning; 2) radioisotope scanning; 3) x-ray computerised tomography (CT scanning); and 4) magnetic resonance imaging (MRI).

RADIOGRAPHIC EXAMINATION

Plain radiography

The correct interpretation of radiographs becomes easier if the films are examined methodically according to a standard routine. In this way abnormalities are far less likely to be missed than they are if one simply gazes

Fig. 2   Fig. 3

To show the importance of assessing bone density in the study of radiographs. The two hands were exposed simultaneously on the same film. The hand in Figure 2 is the hand of a normal person. That in Figure 3 is the hand of a patient with osteomalacia complicating idiopathic steatorrhoea. Note the marked general rarefaction of the bones.

hopefully but haphazardly into the viewing box. The following routine is suggested. 1) Take all the films out of the packet and place them on a flat surface. (Films are surprisingly 'slippery' and will slide away if placed even on a gentle slope.) 2) Set each film or set of films in turn in the anatomical position on a viewing box: simply to hold the films up against the light is to invite mistakes. 3) Note what part of the body is shown and by which projections the films have been made. 4) Stand back from the viewing box to assess the *general density* of the bones (Figs 2 and 3): judge from experience whether the density seems normal, or whether it is reduced (rarefaction[2]) or increased (sclerosis). 5) Look more closely for any *local changes of density*. 6) Examine the *cortex* of each bone: run the eye round the outline of the bone, looking for breaks in the continuity of the cortex, and for irregularities or areas of erosion; then examine the substance of the cortex for thickening, thinning, alteration of texture, or new bone formation. 7) Examine the *medulla* of each bone: look for alterations of texture and for areas of destruction or sclerosis. 8) Examine the *joints*: look for narrowing of the so-called joint space (more correctly, the cartilage space), for erosion, irregularity or roughening of the joint surfaces, for peripheral new bone formation (osteophytes) (Fig. 4), and for loose bodies.

Fig. 4   **Fig. 5**

Figure 4—Osteoarthritis of hip. The characteristic features of osteoarthritis are well shown—namely narrowing of the cartilage space, subchondral sclerosis and osteophytes at the joint margin. Figure 5—It is important to study the soft-tissue areas as well as the bones. The shadow between the metacarpal heads in this radiograph is a calcified deposit. It might at first be mistaken for a displaced fragment of bone, but it is distinguished from bone by the fact that it is homogeneous and lacks the trabecular pattern that is characteristic of bone.

9) Examine the *soft tissues* so far as they are shown: look for areas of ossification or calcification (Fig. 5), for relatively dense shadows that might denote an abscess or other fluid collection or a solid mass of tissue (Fig. 6), and for areas of relative transradiancy that might denote the presence of gas or fat.

---

[2]The term rarefaction is used here to include osteoporosis and osteomalacia. Pathologically, *osteoporosis* implies increased porosity of bone from attenuation of its trabeculae: the matrix is deficient as well as the bone salts. In *osteomalacia*, which is distinct pathologically, the matrix remains but its mineralisation is deficient, the trabeculae being composed largely of osteoid tissue. Radiologically, there is nothing to distinguish osteoporosis from osteomalacia: in both states the bone looks 'thin'. For this radiological appearance the all-embracing term *rarefaction* is the most appropriate.

The mistake is often made, when an abnormality has been discovered, of disregarding the rest of the film. It should never be forgotten that two or more separate abnormalities may be present on one film: the routine

Fig. 6
Faint fusiform shadowing about the thoracic vertebral column, representing an abscess in a case of tuberculosis of the spine.

method of inspection should always be completed regardless of any lesion already discovered. Plenty of time should be spent on the examination of radiographs, and the trap of jumping to hasty conclusions before the films have been properly examined should be avoided at all costs.

Special radiographic techniques

In the routine radiography of most parts of the body plain antero-posterior and lateral films are all that are required. In cases of difficulty special techniques will give more complete information than the plain films alone. These include tomography, contrast radiography and cineradiography.

Tomography. By moving film and x-ray tube in opposite directions during the exposure the structures in the plane corresponding to the axis of movement remain in sharp definition, whereas the structures superficial and deep to that plane are blurred and thus concealed by the movement. By this technique the parts can be shown, as it were, in serial 'slices' cut at varying depths from the surface. Tomography is particularly useful in regions such as the spine where, in plain films, the part to be studied is often obscured by overlapping shadows.

The special scanning technique known as computerised tomography is described separately on page 17.

Contrast radiography. In this technique a water-soluble, absorbable radio-opaque fluid is injected into cavities or tissue spaces before the

Fig. 7
Radiculograph showing central herniation of a lumbar intervertebral disc at
the L.4–5 level. The column of radio-opaque fluid is compressed and there
is failure to fill the L.5 nerve root sheaths on both sides.

Fig. 8
Arteriography provides clear evidence about the state of the arterial tree.
This example shows occlusion of the right common iliac artery at its
origin from the aorta.

radiographs are taken, thereby defining clearly the limits and outline of the space. In some techniques air can be used as the contrast medium instead of, or as well as, a radio-opaque fluid. Methods in common use are: *myelography*, in which the spinal theca is outlined, now largely superseded in the lumbar region by *radiculography* (Fig. 7), which allows visualisation of the nerve sleeves as well as the spinal theca itself; *arthrography*, to outline the cavity of a joint; *arteriography* or *angiography*, to show the arterial tree (Fig. 8); *venography*, to show the network of veins; *lymphangiography*, to show the lymphatic network; and *sinography*, to define the course and ramifications of a sinus. The injection of contrast medium can also be combined with the newer imaging techniques such as computerised tomography (CT scanning).

In recent years important advances have been made in the techniques of contrast radiography. Thus in *digital subtraction angiography* a computerised technique allows overlapping shadows to be removed, so that the clarity of the arterial network is enhanced. This allows an adequate arterial image to be obtained from the injection of contrast medium into a vein—a much safer invasion than the intra-arterial injection formerly required.

Interventional radiology. In another advance, improved radiological techniques allow a cannula, inserted into a superficial artery, to be guided into a particular vessel or branch which may be positively identified by the injection of contrast medium locally through the cannula. This is important, for instance, in effecting embolisation for tumour or angioma, or for trans-luminal angioplasty (dilation of an atheromatous artery by a distensible balloon).

Cineradiography. By linking a cine camera or video-tape recorder to the x-ray image intensifier a moving picture of a joint can be obtained and stored for future reference. This technique is often helpful in showing the pattern of joint movement, especially in the spinal column. Thus it may show more reliably than any other method whether a particular spinal joint is mobile or immobile—for instance after attempted surgical fusion.

ULTRASOUND SCANNING

In this technique the part under investigation is scanned by ultrasound waves, and the echoes received are analysed and displayed as an image. The production of a clear image depends upon there being a sharp contrast in density between the part under study and the surrounding tissues. The applications of ultrasound scanning to orthopaedic surgery are not yet clearly defined: it has been used for detecting a rupture of muscle or tendon, for measuring the diameter of the spinal canal (Porter, Wicks and Ottewell 1978), for detecting the position of the femoral head in new-born babies (Williams 1980), and for the detection of major foetal abnormalities in the first half of pregnancy. Ultrasound also has an established and important place in the measurement of peripheral blood flow (see p. 361).

Ultrasound techniques have the merit of being entirely harmless to the patient; but on the other hand the achievement of reliable results depends to a considerable extent upon the skill of the operator.

Fig. 9

Plain radiograph of lower lumbar spine and pelvis, with (below) a technetium-labelled isotope bone scan of the same patient showing multiple metastatic deposits from a breast carcinoma, not yet visible in the plain radiograph.

RADIOISOTOPE SCANNING

Radioisotope scanning (scintigraphy; radionuclide scanning) of bone is now widely used in orthopaedic practice (Hughes 1980; Galasko and Weber 1984). For routine studies the bone-seeking radioisotope now commonly used is a compound of ^{99m}technetium with diphosphonate, which is injected intravenously: the emitted rays are charted with a gamma camera or a whole body rectilinear scanner. There is immediate diffusion of isotope into the bone matrix from the blood: thus an increased uptake of isotope locally in the skeleton denotes hyperaemia of the bone. Within about two hours isotope is also taken up by bone-forming cells, increased uptake thus denoting increased osteogenic activity (Fig. 9).

Radioisotope bone scanning is of value in the early detection of skeletal metastases and in the diagnosis of infections of bone or joint, primary bone tumours, osteoid osteoma, stress fractures and certain other lesions (Fig. 9).

X-RAY COMPUTERISED TOMOGRAPHY

In computer-assisted x-ray tomography (CT scanning) the part of the body under investigation is scanned from many angles by an x-ray tube and detector system. With a computer a cross-sectional image of the part of the

Fig. 10
Computerised tomographic scan through the pelvis, which is represented in transverse section viewed from below. Note on the right side (left of picture) that the wing of the ilium has been expanded and partly replaced by a large cyst.

trunk or limb under study is reconstructed and displayed on an oscilloscope, variations of tissue density being shown. Clear images are produced, especially where there is sharp variation in density between the tissue under review and the surrounding tissue. CT scanning, with its ability to show changes in bone and soft tissue that cannot be picked up in plain

Fig. 11

Image made by x-ray computerised tomography, showing 'cuts' of both mid-thighs. Note the extensive zone of reduced density around the femur in the right-hand picture. This represents a haemangioma involving the quadriceps muscle. This scan illustrates the value of computerised tomography in revealing the extent of deep-seated lesions. The scan on the left is normal.

radiographs, has many applications in orthopaedic surgery, particularly in the study of the spinal column and spinal canal, and of the pelvis and its contents (Fig. 10). It is also relevant to certain problems in the limbs (Fig. 11).

MAGNETIC RESONANCE IMAGING
(Nuclear magnetic resonance scanning)

Magnetic resonance imaging (MRI) provides a further method of imaging which offers great promise for the future. The technique depends on the

Fig. 12
Magnetic resonance scan showing sarcoma of tibia. The extent of the invasion of the soft tissues is clearly shown.

magnetic behaviour of the nuclei of hydrogen atoms (protons) in the tissues. When the part of the body under investigation is placed in a magnetic field, the nuclei of the atoms line up in the direction of the field. Being then subjected to a burst of radio-frequency electro-magnetic radiation, they assume a new orientation. Upon cessation of the radiation they revert to the initial state, at the same time emitting radio-frequency signals which are analysed and converted into a two-dimensional image.

Nuclear magnetic resonance imaging provides images of tissue slices broadly resembling those produced by CT scanning (Fig. 12), though with different gradations of contrast between the various tissues—for instance, it can differentiate white from grey matter in the brain. It has the advantage over radiological techniques that x-rays are not used: it should therefore be entirely safe. Its applications to orthopaedic surgery are important in many situations, especially in the study of the spinal column and the related soft tissues, and in the assessment of the extent of invasion by tumours.

Fig. 13   **Fig. 14**

Computerised tomography and magnetic resonance imaging compared, in the delineation of a sarcoma invading the vastus lateralis muscle of the right thigh. Figure 13—Computerised tomographic scan, showing the thigh in transverse section. Figure 14—Magnetic resonance scan, showing the area in longitudinal section.

Choice of imaging technique

With a variety of imaging techniques now available, it is not always easy to decide which method is the most appropriate in particular circumstances. Plain radiography still has the widest application, being used routinely where bone or joint is concerned; and contrast radiography is a refinement of it that is unlikely to be displaced. The newer methods described above should thus be regarded as complementary to plain radiography rather than as a substitute for it.

Ultrasound scanning is clearly attractive because it does not cause discomfort to the patient and is relatively inexpensive; but it has so far found fewer applications in orthopaedic work than in other branches of surgery, largely because bone forms a barrier to the waves.

Radioisotope scanning probably finds its main usefulness in the early detection of bone metastases and in the demonstration of inflammatory processes in bones or joints.

Computerised tomography and magnetic resonance imaging are expensive and at present not universally available, but both can provide information that cannot be gained by any other technique—for instance in the early detection of pulmonary metastases and in the delineation of soft-tissue masses in the trunk, pelvis or limbs (Figs 13 and 14). Magnetic resonance imaging is particularly useful in its ability to delineate lesions—for instance prolapse of an intervertebral disc—that cannot otherwise be demonstrated except by an invasive technique.

OTHER INVESTIGATIONS

More often than not the diagnosis can be established without the aid of special investigations. In any case the possibilities should be narrowed down to as few as possible before such investigations are ordered. If doubt then exists, appropriate tests are ordered to support or weaken each possible diagnosis.

Tests commonly employed in orthopaedic diagnosis include haematological studies; biochemical tests upon urine, faeces, plasma and cerebrospinal fluid; serological and bacteriological tests; electrical tests; arthroscopy; and histological examination of specimens excised at biopsy or at definitive operation. Further description is required here only of electrical tests and arthroscopy. Biopsy is considered on page 35.

Electrical tests (electrodiagnosis)
The two most common electrodiagnostic techniques used in orthopaedic practice are nerve conduction tests and electromyography.

Nerve conduction tests are used to determine whether or not a nerve is able to transmit an electrical impulse. The principle is to apply a stimulating electrode over a point on the nerve trunk distal to the lesion, and to observe whether or not the muscles supplied by the nerve will contract in response to the stimulus. The nerves in the sound limb are examined first, to determine the threshold of current required to cause a muscle contraction. If in the affected limb a current at least twice as great as the threshold fails to produce a muscle contraction, nerve conduction is absent. A nerve conduction test provides a simple method of determining whether or not a clinical paralysis is due to a complete lesion of the nerve, which has resulted in degeneration of its myelin sheath. If nerve conduction is present the lesion cannot be complete and myelin degeneration has not occurred.

Nerve conduction tests may also be used to measure motor conduction velocity in the peripheral nerve, and the principle can also be applied to afferent sensory testing. A slowing in the velocity of conduction may indicate the site of an incomplete lesion in the nerve trunk, such as may occur in compression neuropathy. Using stimulating electrodes, applied both proximal and distal to the suspected lesion, the latent period before the appearance of the muscle action potentials is measured. The difference in conduction time and the distance between the electrodes provide a measurement of velocity, which can be compared with the normal side, or with normal values (40–70 m/s).

The measurement of sensory nerve conduction is technically more difficult, but has found a recent clinical application in spinal cord monitoring. Surface electrodes are used to provide repetitive peripheral stimulations during spinal surgery so that recordings of central cortical responses can be used to detect any interference with cord function.

Electromyography. In this technique the electrical changes occurring in a muscle are picked up by a needle or surface electrode, suitably amplified and studied in the form of sound through a loud speaker, or as a tracing on an oscillograph. Normal muscle is electrically 'silent' at rest, but on voluntary contraction shows increasing electrical discharges in the form of triphasic action potentials, as more motor units are recruited into activity. Partly denervated or totally denervated muscle shows only spontaneous contractions of individual fibres (fibrillation potentials). Repeated testing at intervals can be used to detect evidence of re-innervation, as small polyphasic motor unit action potentials reappear and spontaneous fibrillation disappears. The motor unit action potentials gradually increase in duration and amplitude, but do not return to a normal pattern until remyelination of the nerve is complete. Electromyography may show diagnostic changes in some types of myopathy, as well as in anterior horn cell disease such as poliomyelitis and motor neurone disease.

Arthroscopy

In recent years the technique of direct inspection of the interior of a joint through a fine telescope introduced through a cannula has become highly developed. Indeed it is relied upon almost routinely in the diagnosis of mechanical derangements within the knee and also in the study of many non-traumatic affections of doubtful nature. The use of arthroscopy is still confined mainly to the knee (see p. 330), but it has also been applied to other joints, particularly to the shoulder.

INTERPRETATION OF THE FINDINGS

When the study of the patient is complete the abnormal findings elicited from the history, clinical examination, diagnostic imaging, and appropriate special investigations should be assembled together to form a composite clinical picture. This can then be matched against the recognised disorders of the region under consideration. It is comforting to remember that the number of disorders that commonly affect a particular region is limited. Often the number is not large. Theoretically, therefore, if all the possibilities are listed and thereafter confirmed or eliminated one by one the correct diagnosis must always be revealed.

This is, of course, an over-simplification. In practice diagnosis is not as simple as that. But it is nevertheless true that if the problem is tackled logically, step by step, in the manner described, a correct conclusion can be formed in the great majority of cases. The only essentials are a capacity for painstaking enquiry, with strict attention to detail, accurate observation, and a working knowledge of the salient features of the common disorders.

Psychogenic or stress disorders

This heading is included to issue a word of warning. When the cause of a patient's symptoms remains obscure despite a thorough investigation there is a prevalent tendency to discount the genuineness of the symptoms and to ascribe them to 'functional' or 'psychogenic' factors, or simply to stress. This must be deplored as a dangerous policy that has led on many occasions to the overlooking of a serious organic disease.

Just because we fail to discover the cause of a particular symptom it by no means follows that the symptom is imaginary or psychogenic; it usually means only that we are not sufficiently skilled in diagnosis. Admittedly, true hysterical disorders are encountered from time to time in orthopaedic practice, but they are few and far between. Much more often a long-continued organic pain leads to a distracted state of mind that is wrongly interpreted as a hysterical manifestation. It is far safer to err on the side of disregarding possible psychogenic factors than to overlook an organic lesion on the supposition that the symptoms are imaginary.

References and bibliography, page 403.

2. Treatment of orthopaedic disorders

Orthopaedic treatment falls into three categories: 1) No treatment—simply reassurance or advice; 2) non-operative treatment; 3) operative treatment. In every case these three possibilities of treatment should be considered one by one in the order given. At least half of the patients attending orthopaedic out-patient clinics (excluding cases of fracture) do not require treatment: all that they need is reassurance and advice. In many cases the sole reason for the patient's attendance is that he fears that he may have cancer, tuberculosis, impending paralysis or other serious disease. If he can be reassured that there is no evidence of serious disease he goes away satisfied, and his symptoms immediately become less disturbing.

If active treatment seems to be required it is a good general principle that whenever practicable a trial should be given first to non-operative measures; though obviously there are occasions when early or indeed immediate operation must be advised. Most orthopaedic operations fall into the category of 'luxury' rather than life-saving procedures. Consequently the patient should seldom be persuaded to submit himself to operation: rather should he have to persuade the surgeon to undertake it. When one is undecided whether to advise conservative treatment or operation it is wise always to err on the side of non-intervention.

METHODS OF NON-OPERATIVE TREATMENT

Rest

Since the days of H. O. Thomas (p. 3), who emphasised its value in diseases of the spine and limbs, rest has been one of the mainstays of orthopaedic treatment. Complete rest demands recumbency in bed or immobilisation of the diseased part in plaster. But by 'rest' the orthopaedic surgeon does not necessarily mean complete inactivity or immobility. Often he means no more than 'relative rest', implying simply a reduction of accustomed activity and avoidance of strain. Indeed complete rest is required much less often now than it was in the past, because diseases for which rest was previously important, such as poliomyelitis or tuberculosis, can now be prevented or are more readily amenable to specific remedies such as antibacterial agents. Complete rest after operations, formerly favoured, has given place in most cases to the earliest possible resumption of activity.

Support

Rest and support often go together; but there are occasions when support is needed but not rest—for example, to stabilise a joint rendered insecure by muscle paralysis, or to prevent the development of deformity. When support is to be temporary it can be provided by a cast or splint made from plaster of Paris or from one of the newer splinting materials. When it is to be prolonged or permanent an individually made surgical appliance, or orthosis, is required. Examples in common use are steel-reinforced lumbar corsets, spinal braces, cervical collars, wrist supports, walking calipers, below-knee steels with ankle straps, and devices to control drop foot (Figs 106–108, p. 135).

Physiotherapy

Physiotherapy in its various forms occupies an important place in the non-operative—and in the post-operative—treatment of orthopaedic disabilities. Being easily prescribed, and entailing no trouble to the surgeon, it is no doubt often misused with the result that much treatment is given that can have no beneficial effect, except perhaps psychologically. Enlightened teaching and a more scientific basis to practice has helped to produce an awareness among physiotherapists of the hazards as well as the merits of their art. This has led to a correct emphasis being placed upon the value in many conditions of active rather than of passive treatment: in other words, of helping the patient to help himself. This approach is particularly rewarding in the rehabilitation of patients after injury or after operation, and in diseases such as poliomyelitis, cerebral palsy, hemiplegia, and peripheral nerve palsies.

When it is used, physiotherapy should be pursued thoroughly. Half-hearted treatment at infrequent intervals is unlikely to be helpful. Ideally it should be practised daily and the patient should also be taught to treat himself whenever possible. In addition to exercise regimes, physiotherapists now have a wide range of electrophysical techniques available for the treatment of both acute and chronic disorders of the musculoskeletal system.

Active exercises. Exercise may be given for three purposes: 1) to mobilise joints; 2) to strengthen muscles; and 3) to improve coordination or balance. In mobilising exercises the patient's active efforts to move the joint may be assisted by gentle pressure by the physiotherapist's hand (assisted active exercises). In muscle-strengthening exercises the patient is encouraged to contract the weakened muscles against the resistance of weights or springs, the resistance being increased as the muscles gain power. Exercises to improve coordination are of particular importance in cerebral palsy.

Hydrotherapy. Hydrotherapy is a valuable way of allowing active pain-free movements of all joints in warm water. The warmth and buoyancy of the water relieve muscle spasm and thus help to reduce pain. Thus hydrotherapy may be particularly useful in the treatment of rheumatoid polyarthritis.

Passive joint movements. The chief use of passive movements, or 'mobilisation', is to preserve full mobility when the patient is unable to move the joint actively—that is, when the muscles are paralysed or severed. They are important in poliomyelitis and after nerve injuries—especially to preserve mobility in the hand. Recently the use of machines to provide continuous passive motion of joints after operation or injury has become popular to minimise complications and encourage healing of articular cartilage.

Certain movements that are not under the control of the patient may also be used passively for treatment purposes—notably distraction, which is commonly employed, for instance, in the treatment of prolapsed cervical disc and of certain other painful conditions of the spinal column (see also manipulation p. 25).

Electrical stimulation of muscles. If a muscle has its nerve supply intact electrical stimulation is of little importance in increasing muscle strength: active exercises are generally much more effective. Nevertheless, electrotherapy does sometimes have a place when used in conjunction with exercises—for example, in improving the function of the intrinsic muscles of the foot, in restoring activity to a quadriceps muscle that has been inhibited after operation on the knee, or in re-education after a tendon transfer operation. Since the nerve supply is intact the muscle may be stimulated through its motor nerve by 'faradism' (that is, by shocks of short duration (1 ms at 50 Hz) induced by an electronic stimulator).

If the muscle is denervated (for instance, after a peripheral nerve injury) it may be stimulated electrically while recovery of nerve function is awaited, in order to retard the process of fibrosis that occurs after about two years in any denervated muscle. Such a muscle can be stimulated only by 'galvanism'—that is, by shocks of relatively long duration (100–1000 ms at frequency of 5–1.5 Hz) which stimulate the muscle fibres directly, not through its motor nerve. There is nothing to be gained from prescribing this treatment if recovery of nerve function within two years cannot be hoped for.

Electrophysical agents. These may be used to alter the local temperature in the tissues by up to 10°C, either by the direct application of heating or cooling agents, or by inducing an increase in temperature with electromagnetic waves.

Local heat can be easily applied to the superficial tissues with hot packs, infra-red lamps and paraffin wax baths. The heat results in vasodilation, reduced muscle spasm, and decreased pain. Heating effects can also be induced in deeper tissues, including joints, by the use of *short-wave* and *microwave diathermy*. The technique has the additional benefit of stimulating circulatory mechanisms and is particularly useful for joint disorders including muscle and tendon tears, haematoma, bursitis, and synovitis.

Ultrasound waves at about 10^6 Hz can be projected as a beam from a transducer to induce a heating effect in deep tissues. They may also produce benefit from their mechanical and chemical effects on collagen and proteoglycans. Ultrasound is frequently used to reduce post-traumatic haematoma, oedema, and adhesions of joints and their associated soft tissues.

Cryotherapy by the application of ice or cold packs may also be used to produce vasoconstriction and to block pain pathways in the treatment of acute traumatic and inflammatory swelling.

Interferential therapy and *transcutaneous nerve stimulation* are now gaining popularity for the treatment of chronic and intractable pain, particularly when this is of sympathetic origin, such as causalgia and reflex sympathetic dystrophy. The interference effect uses two differing medium frequency alternating currents applied simultaneously through two electrodes to induce a current at the site of their interaction in the deep tissues. Transcutaneous nerve stimulation uses direct current pulses of adjustable frequency to stimulate the larger sensory nerve fibres selectively and thereby to set up a gate control mechanism blocking the activity of the small fibres which conduct pain signals.

Local injections

The indications for local injections fall into two groups: 1) osteoarthritis or rheumatoid arthritis, in which the substance (usually hydrocortisone with or without a local anaesthetic solution) is injected directly into the affected joint with rigid aseptic precautions; and 2) extra-articular lesions of the type often ascribed (for want of more precise knowledge) to chronic strain, as exemplified by tennis elbow, tendonitis about the shoulder, and certain types of back pain. The response depends upon the nature of the basic lesion: permanent relief is often gained in extra-articular lesions such as tennis elbow, but in arthritis the benefit is often no more than temporary, and repeated injections are seldom to be recommended.

Drugs

Drugs have rather a small place in orthopaedic practice. Those used may be placed in seven categories: 1) antibacterial agents; 2) analgesics; 3) sedatives; 4) anti-inflammatory drugs; 5) hormone-like drugs; 6) specific drugs; and 7) cytotoxic drugs.

Antibacterial agents are of immense importance in infective lesions, especially in acute osteomyelitis and acute pyogenic arthritis. To be successful treatment must be begun very early. These drugs are also of definite value in certain chronic infections, notably in tuberculosis.

Analgesics should be used as little as possible. Many orthopaedic disorders are prolonged for many weeks or months, and it is undesirable to prescribe any but the mildest analgesics continuously over long periods, except for incurable malignant disease.

Sedatives may be given if needed to promote sleep, but as with analgesics the rule should be to prescribe no more than is really necessary.

Anti-inflammatory drugs are those that damp down the excessive inflammatory response that may occur especially in rheumatoid arthritis and related disorders, by inhibiting prostaglandin formation. Non-steroidal anti-inflammatory drugs are generally to be preferred—especially in the first instance—and they are a mainstay in the treatment of rheumatoid arthritis. Many of these drugs also have an analgesic action. The powerful steroids cortisone, prednisone and their analogues should be used with extreme caution and indeed should be avoided altogether whenever possible, because through their side effects they may sometimes do more harm than good.

Hormone-like drugs include the corticosteroids noted above, and sex hormones or analogues used for the prevention of osteoporosis in post-menopausal women and for the control of certain metastatic tumours such as hormone-dependent breast and prostatic tumours.

Specific drugs work well in certain special diseases. Examples are vitamin C for scurvy, vitamin D for rickets and salicylates for the arthritis of rheumatic fever.

Cytotoxic drugs form the basis of chemotherapy for malignant tumours. These anti-cancer drugs include cyclophosphamide, melphelan, vincristine and amethopterin. They have serious side effects and are used only under expert supervision.

Manipulation

Treatment by manipulation is practised widely by orthopaedic surgeons and by others in allied professions. Strictly, the term might legitimately be used to include the passive movements, or 'mobilisations', that form part of the daily activities of a physiotherapy department and which have already been referred to above; but it is used here in a more restricted sense, to describe passive movements of joints, bones or soft tissues carried out by the surgeon—with or without an anaesthetic, and often forcefully—as a deliberate step in treatment.

The subject will be considered under three general headings: 1) manipulation for correction of deformity; 2) manipulation to improve the range of movements at a stiff joints; and 3) manipulation for relief of chronic pain in or about a joint.

Manipulation for correction of deformity. In this category manipulation has its most obvious application in the reduction of fractures and dislocations. It is also used to overcome deformity from contracted or short soft tissues—as, for example, in congenital club foot. Yet another simple example is the forcible subcutaneous rupture and dispersal of a ganglion over the dorsum of the wrist.

Technique. An anaesthetic may or may not be required, according to the nature of the condition that is being treated. In many instances—as in manipulation for a fracture or dislocation—the aim is to secure full reduction at the one sitting; but in resistant deformities such as club foot repeated manipulation may be required at intervals of a week or so, a little further improvement being gained each time.

Subsequent management. After manipulation for a deformity that is liable to recur—as in most cases of displaced fracture and in chronic deformities of joints—the limb is usually immobilised on a splint or in plaster to maintain the correction. In cases of resistant deformity gradual yielding of the soft tissue allows re-application of the splint in a more favourable position each time it is changed.

Manipulation for joint stiffness. The type of case mainly concerned here is that in which a joint shows serious limitation of movement after an acute injury—usually a fracture of a limb bone. 'Frozen' shoulder (periarthritis) in its non-active stage may also be included in this category. In such cases the stiffness is caused by adhesions either within the joint itself or, more often, in the soft tissues about or near the joint. Forcible manipulation by the surgeon is not required very often for stiffness of this type, because it will usually respond gradually to treatment by active exercises under the care of a physiotherapist, combined with increasing use of the limb.

The joint that is most amenable to manipulation is the knee. The shoulder and the joints of the foot may also respond. Manipulation of the elbow and of the joints of the hand may increase the stiffness and should not be attempted.

Technique. Muscular relaxation should be secured by anaesthesia, supplemented if necessary by a relaxant drug. Great force should not be used: it is better to gain slight improvement by moderate force and then to repeat the manipulation after an interval. Excessive force may fracture a bone; or it may cause fresh bleeding within the joint, thereby aggravating the stiffness.

Subsequent management. Manipulation for joint stiffness should always be followed by intensive active exercises designed to retain the increased range of movement.

Manipulation for relief of chronic pain. In this third category of case treatment by manipulation is somewhat empirical, because in many instances it is impossible to determine precisely the nature of the underlying pathology, and consequently the way in which manipulation acts is a matter of conjecture. Manipulation is used in such cases simply because previous experience has proved that it is often successful.

The painful conditions that respond best to manipulation are chronic strains, especially of the tarsal joints, the joints of the spinal column, and the sacro-iliac joints. A chronic strain may be the consequence of an acute injury that has not been followed by complete resolution, or it may be caused by long-continued mechanical overstrain. It is generally surmised that adhesions are present that prevent the extremes of joint movement (even though a restriction of movement may not be obvious clinically), that these adhesions are painful when stretched, and that the effect of manipulation is to rupture them. An alternative explanation that is advanced in certain cases is that there is a minor displacement of the joint surfaces or of an intra-articular structure (even though this can seldom be demonstrated radiologically), and that the effect of manipulation is to restore normal apposition.

Technique. Manipulation for relief of pain from chronic strain consists in putting the affected joint or joints forcibly through a full range of movement, usually while the patient is fully relaxed under an anaesthetic but sometimes without an anaesthetic. Steady longitudinal distraction of the joint is often a useful preliminary to the forcing of the extreme range.

Subsequent management. The manipulation should usually be followed by physiotherapy to maintain the function of the joint. It may be repeated after an interval if initial improvement does not progress to complete cure.

Dangers and safeguards in treatment by manipulation. Manipulation may do harm if it is undertaken for the stiffness of inflammatory arthritis in an active stage, or if a tumour or other destructive disease exists close to the joint. It is also inadvisable in cases of acute back pain due to prolapsed intervertebral disc, because it may cause further extrusion of disc material. This emphasises the importance of careful clinical and radiological examination—supplemented when necessary by other investigations such as determination of the erythrocyte sedimentation rate, radioisotope scanning, radiculography or magnetic resonance imaging—before treatment is begun. It must be emphasised again that manipulation is of no value for stiffness of the metacarpo-phalangeal joints and interphalangeal joints of the hand.

During the manipulation itself care must be taken to avoid disasters such as the fracture of a bone or massive displacement of an intervertebral disc. It is well known that a fracture—especially of the patella or humerus—may be caused easily by injudicious manipulations. This risk is greatly increased if the bone is already weak from the osteoporosis of disuse or from other rarefying disease.

Radiotherapy

Radiotherapy—by x-rays or by the gamma rays of radio-active substances—may be used for certain benign conditions or for malignant disease. Because of its possible ill effects—particularly the risk of inducing malignant change—it should be advised only with caution for benign lesions, but its use may rarely be justified in the treatment of recalcitrant ankylosing spondylitis and in cases of giant-cell tumour of bone that are unsuitable for local excision. In malignant disease radiotherapy is occasionally curative but more often palliative. In conditions such as malignant bone tumours, for which a tumour dose in the range of 5000–6000 centiGray may be required, only the penetrating rays produced by a super-voltage x-ray plant or by a radio-active cobalt unit should be used. With such apparatus a high dose can be delivered to the tumour with the least possible damage to the skin.

OPERATIVE TREATMENT

The chief essential of any operation is that it should not make the patient worse than he was before he submitted to it. This is so obvious that the statement may sound almost absurd. Yet it is unfortunately true that a disturbing number of operations carried out for orthopaedic conditions do in fact cause more harm than good for one reason or another. Hence the selection of cases for operation, the choice of the most appropriate operation in given circumstances, the technical performance of the operation, and the post-operative management are matters of the highest importance, and they call for a high degree of judgment and skill. Herein lies much of the fascination of orthopaedic surgery.

A detailed account of operative techniques is unnecessary here. All that is required is a brief mention of the more important operations.

Synovectomy

Synovectomy is the operation for removal of the inflamed lining of a joint, while leaving the capsule intact. It may be of value in some types of chronic infective arthritis as well as in early rheumatoid arthritis. Because of the difficulty in gaining anatomical access, it is necessarily a subtotal procedure; but it may nevertheless afford worthwhile relief by reducing local pain and swelling. There is no clear evidence that it protects the articular cartilage from further damage; but the removal of a large part of this invasive granulation tissue or pannus may be of benefit by reducing the production of proteolytic enzymes.

Osteotomy

Osteotomy is the operation of cutting a bone or creating a surgical fracture (from the Greek words οστεον = bone, and τομο = cut). It has almost supplanted *osteoclasis* (forcible bending or incomplete breaking of a bone), which formerly was often used to correct deformities of the long bones in children with rickets and which may still be suitable occasionally for that purpose.

Indications. The general indications for osteotomy are as follows: 1) to correct excessive angulation, bowing or rotation of a long bone; 2) to permit angulation of a bone in order to compensate for mal-alignment at a joint; 3) to permit elongation or shortening of a bone in the lower limb in order to correct a discrepancy of length between the two sides. In addition, there are certain special indications for osteotomy at the upper end of the femur, as follows: 4) to improve stability at the hip by altering the line of weight transmission (abduction osteotomy, p. 301); and 5) to relieve the pain of an osteoarthritic hip (displacement osteotomy, p. 310).

Technique. If the bone is relatively soft (as in children) it may be divided simply with an osteotome or, in the case of a thin bone, by bone-cutting forceps. The strong cortex of the major long bones in an adult is not easily divided in that way because it tends to splinter; so most surgeons weaken the bone by making multiple drill holes before applying the osteotome, or, alternatively, they use a powered saw or a high-speed dental burr. When the bone has been divided and the necessary correction made it is often convenient to fix the fragments with a plate, nail-plate, or medullary nail: this may allow external splintage to be dispensed with. If internal fixation is not used the fragments may be immobilised by an external fixator; or they may be held in position by a suitable splint or plaster until union has occurred.

Arthrodesis

The operation of arthrodesis, or joint fusion, is still widely used, though since the advent of reliable techniques of joint reconstruction, or arthroplasty, it is used less frequently than in the past for the major limb joints. The disability from a single stiff joint is usually slight, and patients readily adapt themselves to it. Even when two or three joints are fused function may be surprisingly good, depending upon the particular joints affected.

Fig. 15	**Fig. 16**
Three methods of arthrodesis of the shoulder. 1. Intra-articular arthrodesis with fixation by a nail. 2. Extra-articular arthrodesis: acromion turned down into a slot in the greater tuberosity. 3. Extra-articular arthrodesis: strut graft between humerus and scapula. Combinations of the methods may be used.	Three methods of arthrodesis of the hip. 1. Intra-articular arthrodesis with fixation by a nail. 2. Extra-articular arthrodesis by ilio-femoral graft. 3. Extra-articular arthrodesis by ischio-femoral graft. The methods may be combined.

Indications. Arthrodesis is indicated mainly in the following conditions: 1) advanced osteoarthritis or rheumatoid arthritis with disabling pain, especially when confined to a single joint; 2) quiescent tuberculous arthritis with destruction of the joint surfaces, to eliminate risk of recrudescence and to prevent deformity; 3) instability from muscle paralysis, as after poliomyelitis; 4) for permanent correction of deformity, as in hammer toe.

Methods of arthrodesis. Arthrodesis may be intra-articular or extra-articular, or the two may be combined. In *intra-articular* arthrodesis the joint is opened and the bone ends are displayed. The articular cartilage (or what remains of it) is removed so that raw bone is exposed. The joint is placed in the desired position and immobilised, usually by metallic internal fixation as well as by a plaster-of-Paris splint, until clinical tests and radiographs show sound bony fusion.

In *extra-articular* arthrodesis the joint itself is left undisturbed (though it may be immobilised by a nail or screw), but it is 'by-passed' by securing bone-to-bone fusion outside the joint, usually through the medium of a bone graft. The method is applicable mainly to the spine, shoulder, and hip. It has a theoretical advantage in cases of infective joint disease, because any risk of reactivating or disseminating the infection by opening the joint is avoided.

Examples of methods of arthrodesing the shoulder and hip are illustrated in Figures 15 and 16.

Position for arthrodesis. The best position for arthrodesis should not be regarded as rigidly established for each joint: variations may be appropriate and desirable in individual cases—for instance, to conform to the requirements of the patient's work. The following is only a general guide. *Shoulder:* 30 degrees of abduction and flexion, with 40 degrees of medial rotation. *Elbow:* If only one elbow is affected, 75 degrees of flexion from the fully extended position (or according to the requirements of the patient's work). If both elbows are affected, one should be in flexion 10 degrees above the right angle and the other about 20 degrees below the right angle. If forearm rotation is lost the most useful position of the forearm is in 10 degrees of pronation. *Wrist:* Extended 20 degrees. *Metacarpo-phalangeal joints:* Flexed 35 degrees. *Interphalangeal joints:* Semiflexed. *Hip:* About 15 degrees of flexion; no abduction or adduction. *Knee:* About 20 degrees of flexion. *Ankle:* In men, right angle; in women, 15–25 degrees of plantarflexion, according to accustomed height of heel. *Metatarso-phalangeal joint of big toe:* Slight extension, depending upon the accustomed height of shoe heel.

Arthroplasty

Arthroplasty is the operation for construction of a new movable joint. It is not applicable to every joint: in practice, its use is mainly confined to the hip, the knee, the shoulder, the elbow, certain joints in the hand, and the metatarso-phalangeal joints in the foot.

Indications. The indications for arthroplasty vary with the particular joint affected and the degree of disability. Broadly, it has a use in the following conditions: 1) advanced osteoarthritis or rheumatoid arthritis with disabling pain, especially in the hip, knee, shoulder, elbow, hand and metatarso-phalangeal joints; 2) quiescent destructive tuberculous arthritis especially of the elbow or hip; 3) for the correction of certain types of deformity (especially hallux valgus); 4) certain ununited fractures of the neck of the femur. It will be realised that in several of these conditions arthroplasty is an alternative to arthrodesis.

Methods of arthroplasty. Three methods are in general use: 1) excision arthroplasty; 2) half-joint replacement arthroplasty; and 3) total replacement arthroplasty. Each has its merits, disadvantages and special applications.

Excision arthroplasty. In this method one or both of the articular ends of the bones are simply excised, so that a gap is created between them (Fig. 17). The gap fills with fibrous tissue, or a pad of muscle or other soft tissue may be sewn in between the bones. By virtue of its flexibility the interposed tissue allows a reasonable range of movement, but the joint often lacks stability. Excision arthroplasty is used most commonly at the metatarso-phalangeal joint of the big toe, in the treatment of hallux valgus and hallux rigidus (Keller's operation). It is also commonly used at the hip, usually as a salvage operation after failed replacement arthroplasty. It is used occasionally at the elbow, the shoulder, and certain of the small joints of the hands and feet.

Half-joint replacement arthroplasty (hemi-arthroplasty). In half-joint replacement arthroplasty only one of the articulating surfaces is removed and replaced by a prosthesis of similar shape. The prosthesis is usually made from metal. When appropriate it may be fixed into the recipient bone with acrylic filling compound or 'cement'. The opposing, normal articulating surface is left undisturbed. The technique has its main application at the hip, where prosthetic replacement of the head and neck of the femur is commonly practised for femoral neck fracture in the elderly (Fig. 18). It has rather a limited use elsewhere, examples being the replacement of the head of the radius after certain types of fracture, and replacement of the lunate bone in Kienböck's disease.

Fig. 17   **Fig. 18**   **Fig. 19**

Three methods of arthroplasty, as exemplified at the hip. Figure 17—Excision arthroplasty. Note the interposed soft tissue. Figure 18—Half-joint replacement arthroplasty: the femoral head is replaced by a metal prosthesis. Figure 19—Total replacement arthroplasty. The femoral head is replaced by a metal prosthesis and the acetabulum by a plastic socket. Both components may be held in place by acrylic filling compound or 'cement'.

Total replacement arthroplasty. In this technique both of the opposed articulating surfaces are excised and replaced by prosthetic components (Fig. 19). In the larger joints one of the components is usually of metal and the other of high density polyethylene, and it is usual for both components to be held in place by acrylic 'cement'. In small joints such as the metacarpo-phalangeal joints a flexible one-piece prosthesis made from silicone rubber may be used.

Total replacement arthroplasty has proved very successful at the hip and to a lesser extent at the knee. It has been extended, so far with only moderate success, to many other joints including the shoulder, elbow, ankle, metacarpo-phalangeal joints and metatarso-phalangeal joints. A disadvantage—which applies also to half-joint replacement arthroplasty—is that there is a tendency for the prosthesis to work loose after a variable time that cannot be predicted. A well fitted replacement joint may, however, give good service for many years, especially in the case of the hip.

Bone grafting operations

Bone grafts are usually obtained from another part of the patient's body (autogenous grafts or autografts). If it is impracticable or undesirable to take bone from the patient's own body, grafts from another human subject may be used (allografts, homogenous grafts or homografts). These must be stored frozen under aseptic conditions until they have been proved to be free from transmissible infection, including HIV and other dangerous viral infections. For bone from living donors (mainly femoral heads removed during hip replacement operations) this necessitates retesting after six to nine months to ensure that the donor was not incubating infectious disease at the time of removal of the bone. Cadaveric bone sterilised by irradiation is sometimes used and is increasingly available from large tissue banks. Grafts obtained from animals (xenografts, heterogenous grafts or hetero-grafts) may be applicable if they are specially treated to reduce their antigenic properties. At some centres limited use is still made of such bone (chiefly bovine) prepared commercially in sterile packs, but it has been shown to be far inferior to the patient's own bone and cannot be relied upon to become incorporated with the host bone.

Figs 20 and 21
Examples of bone grafting techniques. Figure 20—Cortical slab graft held by four screws, as used to bridge an ununited fracture. Figure 21—Cancellous grafts used to fill a cavity in a bone.

Fig. 20   **Fig. 21**

Bone transferred as a free autograft from one site to another does not survive wholly in a living state. For the most part the bone cells die, although a proportion may possibly survive, especially in cancellous bone. The purpose of the graft—as of allografts and heterografts—is mainly to serve as a scaffolding or temporary bridge upon which new bone is laid down. It also provides an osteogenic stimulus to the host cells from the bone morphogenic proteins released from the non-cellular bone matrix. Thus the whole of a graft is eventually replaced by new living bone. This process of replacement is dependent upon adequate revascularisation of the graft; so a graft that lies in a highly vascular bed is more likely to succeed than one that is surrounded by relatively ischaemic tissue.

With refinements in the technique of microvascular surgery it is now possible to transfer bone with its soft-tissue coverings on a vascular pedicle to a distant recipient site, with immediate anastomosis of its nutrient vessels to those in the new bed. Such living grafts are found to become incorporated rapidly. This recent advance in grafting technique is valuable in major reconstructive procedures after extensive loss of bone and soft tissue.

Indications. Bone grafts are used mainly in three types of case: 1) in cases of ununited fracture, to promote union; 2) in arthrodesis of joints, either to supplement an intra-articular arthrodesis or to promote extra-articular fusion (see p. 29); 3) to fill a defect or cavity in a bone.

> **Technique.** Autogenous bone for grafting may be obtained as a solid slab, or it may be used in the form of multiple slivers or strips, or of small chips.
> *Slab grafts.* A slab graft is usually obtained from strong cortical bone: the subcutaneous part of the tibia is a common site. The graft is fixed to the recipient bone either by screws or by inlaying. Such a graft serves as an internal splint as well as providing a framework for the growth of new bone (Fig. 20).
> *Strip grafts.* Sliver or strip grafts are generally obtained from spongy cancellous bone— especially from the crest of the ilium. They are used commonly for ununited fractures. They are laid about the fracture, deep to the periosteum, and are held in place by suture of the soft tissues over them (Phemister 1947).
> *Chip grafts.* These also are preferably obtained from cancellous bone. They serve the same purposes as sliver grafts but are smaller pieces of bone. The chips are packed firmly into, or around, the recipient bone and are held in place simply by suture of the soft tissues over them (Fig. 21).

Tendon transfer operations

In the operation of tendon transfer, or tendon transplant, the insertion of a healthy functioning muscle is moved to a new site, so that the muscle henceforth has a different action. In this way the function of a paralysed or severed muscle can be taken over by one that is intact. In properly selected cases there need be no noticeable loss of power in the former sphere of action of the transferred muscle, because there is often considerable duplication or overlap in the function of individual muscles. Thus a tendon of flexor digitorum superficialis may be transferred to a new site without appreciably impairing the power of finger flexion, which can be adequately controlled by the flexor profundus. Similarly the extensor indicis can be spared for a new function without seriously interfering with the power of extension of the index finger (Fig. 22).

Indications. Tendon transfers have their main application in three groups of conditions: 1) in cases of muscle paralysis, to restore or improve active control of a joint by re-routing a healthy muscle to act in place of a paralysed one; 2) in cases of deformity from muscle imbalance, to maintain correction by switching healthy muscles to restore proper balance; and 3) in cases of ruptured or cut tendon, when direct suture of the ends is impracticable.

> **Technique.** The tendon to be transferred is divided at an appropriate point, re-routed in the direction of its new action, and secured to its new insertion. If it is to be inserted into bone it is passed through a drill hole and held by suturing back on itself or by suturing to the periosteum or soft tissues on the deep aspect of the bone. If it is to be united to a tendon stump the junction may be secured by end-to-end suture or, preferably, by interlacing the tendons one through the other and transfixing them with mattress sutures.
> **Examples.** 1) In a case of paralysis of the radial nerve, with loss of active extension of the wrist, fingers and thumb, function may be restored by the following tendon transfers:

pronator teres is transferred to extensor carpi radialis brevis; flexor carpi ulnaris is transferred to extensor digitorum and extensor pollicis longus; and palmaris longus is transferred to abductor pollicis longus. 2) In a case of congenital talipes equino-varus (p. 372) transfer of the tendon of the tibialis anterior or tibialis posterior to the outer side of the foot will help to

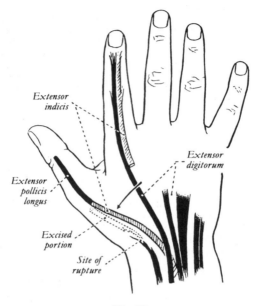

Extensor indicis

Extensor digitorum

Extensor pollicis longus

Excised portion

Site of rupture

Fig. 22

Transfer of extensor indicis to replace a ruptured extensor pollicis longus. This transfer is to be preferred to direct suture when the ends of the ruptured tendon are frayed.

prevent recurrence of the deformity. 3) In a case of rupture of the extensor pollicis longus, with extensive fraying of the tendon, direct repair may be impracticable. Function may be restored by transfer of the extensor indicis to the extensor pollicis longus (Fig. 22).

Tendon grafting operations

In tendon grafting a length of free tendon is used to bridge a gap between the severed ends of the recipient tendon.

Indications. The chief use of free tendon grafts is in the reconstruction of flexor tendons severed and adherent in the fibrous digital sheaths of the hand (p. 275).

> **Technique.** The free tendon graft is usually obtained from the palmaris longus or from one of the toe extensors at the dorsum of the foot. The original, adherent tendon is removed. Proximally, the graft is joined to the recipient tendon by sutures of stainless steel wire. Distally, it may be secured to the distal stump of the recipient tendon or it may be attached directly to bone through a drill hole.

Equalisation of leg length

If a patient's legs are of markedly unequal length, as in certain cases of congenital anomaly, previous poliomyelitis, or damage to a growth epiphysis, the discrepancy may be reduced or eliminated by operation. The methods available are: 1) leg lengthening; 2) leg shortening; and 3) arrest of epiphysial growth.

Leg lengthening is suitable mainly for children. It is achieved by dividing the appropriate bone (usually the tibia, sometimes the femur) and then gradually elongating the limb in a special screw-distraction apparatus at the rate of about 2 millimetres a day. A maximum of about 5 centimetres may be gained. The procedure is time-consuming and trying for the patient, and should be reserved for carefully selected cases in which the discrepancy in length is marked. A more recent innovation is the technique of bone transport, in which a length of the diaphysis is moved slowly downwards to fill a gap, while new bone forms to fill in the space created by its advancement. These techniques have been facilitated by the introduction of the ring frame distractor of Ilizarov, which allows correction of angulation as well as lengthening.

Leg shortening, by removing an appropriate length from the shaft of the longer femur or tibia, is less hazardous but not to be undertaken lightly because it disturbs a limb that was previously normal. In a patient who is fairly tall, and especially in adults, it is often preferable to leg lengthening.

Arrest of epiphysial growth (on the longer side) is applicable only to children with considerable growth still to come. It entails either destruction, or bridging by bone grafts or by metal staples, of the lower femoral epiphysis or of the upper tibial epiphysis, or both. The correction to be expected depends upon the amount of growth still to come from the corresponding epiphysis of the opposite (shorter) leg, which depends in turn upon the age at which the operation is undertaken, and upon the nature of the abnormality that is responsible for the shortening.

Biopsy

Biopsy is the operation of taking a specimen of living tissue for histological, electron-microscopic or other examination in order to elucidate the nature of a disease. Very often it is done as a final step in the diagnosis and staging of a tumour. Two techniques of biopsy are available: 1) needle biopsy, in which a core of tissue is extracted by a special hollow needle; and 2) open biopsy. Except in certain situations open biopsy is usually to be preferred despite a theoretically greater risk of tumour dissemination, because it is more likely to yield a representative specimen. Nevertheless needle biopsy has an important place, and with improvements in technique its application has been widened, though diagnostic accuracy still does not exceed 70 per cent.

The main essentials in a biopsy operation are: 1) that an adequate and representative piece of tissue be obtained; and 2) that the incision be so placed that it does not prejudice the success of a subsequent operation for total eradication of the tumour—especially in malignant disease. The scar must be so placed that it is conveniently included in the block of tissue to be excised.

References and bibliography, page 403.

PART TWO

GENERAL SURVEY OF ORTHOPAEDIC DISORDERS

This part, comprising six chapters, is devoted to a broad preliminary review of the field of orthopaedics. The main groups of disorders will be described without a detailed consideration of their local manifestations. Against this general background the features of the common disorders as they affect each particular region will be discussed in the subsequent chapters.

Recent injuries of the limbs and spine form a subject of separate study, and are dealt with in the companion volume to this work, *Outline of Fractures and Joint Injuries*.

CLASSIFICATION OF ORTHOPAEDIC DISORDERS
Most orthopaedic disorders fall within the following groups:

Deformities
  Congenital deformities
  Acquired deformities

General affections of the skeleton
  Bone dysplasias
  Inborn errors of metabolism
  Metabolic bone disease
  Endocrine disorders

Local affections of bone
  Infections of bone
  Tumours of bone
  Osteochondritis
  Cystic change
  Osteoid osteoma

Affections of soft tissue
  Inflammatory lesions of soft tissue
  Tumours of soft tissue

Affections of joints
  Arthritis
  Dislocation and subluxation
  Internal derangements

Neurological disorders
  Poliomyelitis
  Cerebral palsy
  Spina bifida
  Peripheral nerve lesions

3. Deformities

Deformities may be congenital or acquired, and they may reflect an underlying abnormality of bone, joint or soft tissue.

CONGENITAL DEFORMITIES

Congenital deformities or malformations, by definition, are attributable to faulty development and are present at birth, though they may not be recognised until later. They vary from severe malformations that are incompatible with life and may be found in still-born infants, to minor abnormalities of structure that have no practical significance. Incidence varies in different countries and among different races: in Britain probably 2 or 3 per cent of infants are born with some significant developmental abnormality, but only about half of these affect the musculo-skeletal system. Some of the better known anomalies are summarised in Table 1 (p. 40).

Causes

An abnormality of development may be caused by: 1) genetic abnormality; 2) environmental abnormality; or 3) combined genetic and environmental abnormalities. Studies of families and twins have helped geneticists to determine the influence of genetic and environmental factors, alone or combined, in the causation of many of the recognised malformations.

Genetic causes include mutation of a whole chromosome, as in Down's syndrome (mongolism), and mutation of a small part of a chromosome or of a single gene, as in achondroplasia. The defect is not necessarily always inherited from an affected parent: it may arise from a fresh mutation in the germ cell.

Environmental causes are not well understood. Experiments in animals have shown that many different types of environmental influence—dietetic, hormonal, chemical, physical or infective—may cause abnormalities of development, and the system of the body that is mainly affected depends upon the timing of the environmental 'insult'. But except for a few specific agents acting early in pregnancy there is no conclusive evidence that similar influences are important causes of malformations in man. The specific agents whose influence in man is well attested include radiation, the virus of rubella, and certain drugs (notably aminopterin and thalidomide).

Combined genetic and environmental factors seem to be the usual cause of the more common congenital malformations in man, on the evidence of twin and family studies. It is thought probable that developing embryos react differently to environmental influences: some have a natural resistance whereas others are susceptible. A malformation is therefore likely to arise when an environmental 'insult' is inflicted upon cells that have a genetically determined lack of resistance to it.

Practical significance

Many of the recognised congenital abnormalities of the musculo-skeletal system have little practical importance, either because they are very rare or because there is little that can be done for them: these will not all be considered further in this book. There are others, however, that present major problems to the orthopaedic surgeon and may demand energetic treatment. These include congenital dislocation of the hip (p. 292), congenital club foot (p. 372), spina bifida (p. 138), congenital scoliosis (p. 171), osteogenesis imperfecta (p. 47) and cervical rib (p. 159).

Inborn predisposition to disease in adults

It is well recognised that, quite apart from the overt congenital anomalies discussed above, there exists in some patients a genetically determined predisposition to abnormalities developing in later life. Examples of ortho-paedic conditions to which a susceptibility may exist include certain types of osteoarthritis (especially of the hips), ankylosing spondylitis, gouty arthritis, rheumatic fever, idiopathic scoliosis, osteochondritis dissecans, and Dupuytren's contracture.

ACQUIRED DEFORMITIES

Acquired deformities may be classified in two groups: those in which deformity arises at a joint, and those in which it arises in a bone.

DEFORMITY ARISING AT A JOINT

Deformity may be said to exist at a joint when the joint cannot be placed voluntarily in the neutral anatomical position.

Causes

The causes of deformity arising at a joint may be summarised under the following headings (Fig. 23): 1) dislocation or subluxation; 2) muscle imbalance; 3) tethering or contracture of muscles or tendons; 4) contracture of soft tissues; 5) arthritis; 6) posture; 7) unknown causes.

   Dislocation or subluxation. This is usually caused by injury, but it may occur as a congenital deformity, or it may follow disease of the joint (pathological dislocation).

   Muscle imbalance. Unbalanced action of muscles upon a joint may hold it continuously in a particular arc of its range. In time, secondary contractures occur in the dominant muscles or in the soft tissues, preventing the joint from returning to the neutral position (Fig. 23 (2)). The two

Table I
Some of the better known congenital deformities or anomalies of orthopaedic interest, with
their salient clinical features
(When a fuller description appears elsewhere in this book the relevant page number is given. Conditions not
thus designated are either so rare or of such little importance to the student that further description is
unnecessary.)

Name of deformity or anomaly	Clinical or pathological features
Generalised	
Osteogenesis imperfecta (fragilitas ossium) (p. 47)	Fragile soft bones, easily broken or deformed. Often blue sclerotics. Joint laxity. Otosclerosis.
Diaphysial aclasis (multiple exostoses) (p. 48)	Cartilage–capped bony outgrowths from metaphyses. Deficient remodelling. Stunted growth.
Dyschondroplasia (multiple chondromatosis; Ollier's disease (p. 49)	Masses of cartilage in metaphyses of long bones. Impaired growth. Deformity. Often unilateral.
Achondroplasia (chondro-dystrophy) (p. 47)	Short-limb dwarfing from defective growth of long bones. Trident hand. Large head.
Osteopetrosis (Albers-Schönberg disease; 'marble bones')	Hard dense bones, but with increased liability to fracture. Anaemia from obliteration of medulla.
Gargoylism (Hurler's syndrome)	Dwarfing. Kyphosis from deformed vertebrae. Corneal opacity. Large liver and spleen. Mental deficiency.
Cranio-cleido dysostosis (p. 55)	Impaired ossification of skull. Deficient clavicles. Often deficient symphysis pubis.
Arthrogryposis multiplex congenita (amyoplasia congenita)	Stiff deformed limb joints from defective development of muscles, usually secondary to nerve cell deficiency though a type due to primary dysplasia of muscle is also recognised. Hips often dislocated. Club feet.
Pseudohypertrophic muscular dystrophy	Genetic transmission to boys through female carriers. Progressive muscle weakness evident at age 3–6 years. Raised urinary creatine phosphokinase: carriers may thus be identified. The defect may be diagnosed in early pregnancy, when abortion may be advised.
Fibrodysplasia ossificans progressiva (p. 54)	Ectopic ossification, often beginning in trunk but extending to limbs. Short great toe.
Familial hypophosphataemia (p. 59)	Rachitic bone changes corrected only by massive doses of vitamin D. Hypophosphataemia not responsive to vitamin D.
Cystinosis (renal tubular rickets) (p. 60)	Rachitic rarefied bones with consequent deformity. Hypophosphataemia. Glycosuria; amino-aciduria.
Neurofibromatosis (Recklinghausen's disease) (p. 54)	*Café au lait* areas or spots. Cutaneous fibromata. Neurofibromata on cranial or peripheral nerves. Often scoliosis. Occasionally, overgrowth of bone.
Haemophilia (p. 125)	Prolonged blood clotting time from deficiency of Factor VIII. Bleeding into joints or soft tissue.
Gaucher's disease (p. 55)	Deposition of kerasin in reticulum cells, causing cyst-like appearance in bones, and large liver and spleen.
Down's syndrome (mongolism)	Mental and physical impairment from trisomy of chromosome 21, giving 47 instead of 46 chromosomes.

Table I—*contd.*

Name of deformity or anomaly	Clinical or pathological features
Trunk and spine	
Congenital short neck (Klippel-Feil syndrome (p. 150)	Short stiff neck with low hair-line. Fused or deformed cervical vertebrae.
Congenital high scapula (Sprengel's shoulder) (p. 150)	Scapula tethered high up, usually only on one side. Scapular movement impaired.
Cervical rib (p. 159)	Often symptomless. Vascular symptoms (partial ischaemia) or nerve symptoms (paraesthesiae, lower trunk paresis).
Hemivertebra (congenital scoliosis) (p. 171)	Defective development of vertebra (and often of adjacent structures) on one side. Scoliosis.
Spina bifida (spinal dysraphism) (p. 138)	Spina bifida occulta, meningocele or myelocele. Often leg deformities from paralysis or muscle imbalance. Often incontinence. Often associated hydrocephalus. Diagnosable in early pregnancy from excess of alpha fetal protein in urine and amniotic fluid.
Limbs	
Congenital arterio-venous fistula	Hypertrophy and lengthening of limb. Bruit.
Congenital amputation	Part or whole of one or more limbs absent.
Phocomelia	Aplasia of proximal part of limb, the distal part being present ('seal-limb'). Diagnosable in pregnancy by ultrasonography.
Constriction rings	Limb or digit constricted as if by a tight string. May be associated with syndactyly.
Absence of radius (radial club hand)	Hand deviated laterally from lack of normal support by radius. Thumb often absent.
Absence of thumb	Thumb alone may be absent, but other deformities may co-exist.
Absence of proximal arm muscles	Trapezius, deltoid, sternomastoid or pectoralis major absent.
Radio-ulnar synostosis	Forearm bones fused at proximal ends, preventing rotation.
Madelung's deformity (dyschondrosteosis) (p. 255)	Head of ulna dislocated dorsally from lower end of radius. Radius bowed.
Syndactyly	Webbing of two or more digits.
Polydactyly	More than five digits.
Ectrodactyly	Lobster-claw appearance of hand, with pincer grip.
Congenital dislocation of hip (p. 292)	Neonatal: diagnostic click obtainable. Later infancy: shortening; limited abduction. Radiographs diagnostic.
Congenital coxa vara (p. 321)	Defective ossification of femoral neck, with reduced neck-shaft angle.
Congenital short femur	Proximal end of femur deficient or rudimentary. Thigh short.
Absence of fibula	Leg under-developed on outer side. Foot small and everted; lateral two or three digital rays may be absent.
Congenital club foot (p. 372)	Foot inverted and plantarflexed (equino-varus), or everted and dorsiflexed (calcaneo-valgus).
Congenital curled toe (p. 396)	Lateral angulation of one or more toes. Toe may lie over or under adjacent toe.

fundamental causes of muscle imbalance are: 1) weakness or paralysis of muscles; and 2) spasticity of muscles. Thus equinus deformity at the ankle may follow paralysis of the dorsiflexor muscles (for instance, in poliomyelitis) because the action of the plantarflexors and of gravity is unopposed. Or a similar deformity may be caused by spasticity of the calf muscles, which overpower their antagonists. This occurs commonly in cerebral palsy (p. 136).

Fig. 23

Seven causes of deformity arising at a joint. 1. Dislocation. 2. Muscle imbalance. 3. Tethering of muscle or tendon. 4. Soft-tissue contracture. 5. Arthritis. 6. Posture. 7. Idiopathic (cause unknown).

Tethering or contracture of muscles or tendons. If something happens to muscles or tendons that prevents their normal to-and-fro gliding, or their elongation and retraction, the joint may be held in a position of deformity. Thus a muscle or tendon may be tethered to the surrounding tissues in consequence of local infection or injury (Fig. 23 (3)). An example is the anchoring of a flexor tendon of a finger within its fibrous sheath as a result of suppurative tenosynovitis, with consequent flexion deformity at the interphalangeal joints. Or a muscle may lose its elasticity and contractile power from impairment of its blood supply. An important example is Volkmann's ischaemic contracture of the forearm flexor muscles (p. 250) from occlusion of the brachial artery or from increased intra-compartmental pressure, with consequent flexion deformity of the wrist and fingers.

Contracture of soft tissues. Apart from any disturbance of the muscles, contracture of soft tissues alone can account for joint deformity. An example is the common condition of Dupuytren's contracture (p. 272), in which the thickened and contracted palmar aponeurosis pulls the metacarpo-phalangeal and proximal interphalangeal joints of one or more fingers into flexion. Similarly, a flexion deformity of the knee or elbow, or indeed of any joint, may occur from contracture of the scarred skin after burns of the flexor surface of the limb (Fig. 23 (4)).

Arthritis. The various types of arthritis will be discussed in a later chapter. Any type of arthritis may lead to joint deformity. In some cases the joint is firmly fixed in a deformed position by bony or fibrous ankylosis. In other instances the joint retains some movement but is prevented from reaching the neutral position. Thus flexion and adduction deformity is common in osteoarthritis of the hip, flexion deformity is common in arthritis of the knee, and the deformity of ulnar deviation of the fingers (Fig. 214, p. 257) is a well known feature of rheumatoid arthritis of the metacarpo-phalangeal joints.

Posture. The habitual adoption of a deformed position of a joint often leads in time to permanent deformity. A common example is the lateral deviation of the great toe at the metatarso-phalangeal joint—hallux valgus—so common in women who cramp their feet into narrow pointed shoes (Fig. 23 (6)). Another postural deformity that is still seen occasionally—though it should never be allowed to occur—is fixed flexion of the knees in a patient confined to bed for a long time with the knees bent over a pillow.

Unknown causes. In some cases deformity occurs at a joint for no apparent reason. Thus many children develop knock-knee deformity between the ages of 3 and 5 years without demonstrable cause. It is usually unimportant because it tends to correct itself spontaneously. Another common and more serious example is the inversion deformity of the foot known as talipes equino-varus or congenital club foot. A more sinister deformity that is equally ill explained is the idiopathic scoliosis of adolescents (p. 172).

DEFORMITY ARISING IN A BONE

Deformity exists in a bone when it is out of its normal anatomical alignment.

Causes

There are three causes of deformity arising in bone: 1) fracture; 2) bending; and 3) uneven epiphysial growth (Figs 24–26).

Fracture. This is by far the most common cause. Unless a fracture is reduced so that the fragments are perfectly aligned deformity will result. Examples are the genu valgum (knock knee) that is often the consequence of compression fractures of the lateral condyle of the tibia, the cubitus valgus that may follow displaced fractures of the lateral condyle of the humerus, and the common 'dinner-fork' deformity of an unreduced fracture of the lower end of the radius.

Bending of softened bone. Many unrelated conditions can cause softening of bone, with liability to bending and consequent deformity. They are mostly generalised disorders in which several or all of the bones are affected. The following are examples. *Metabolic disorders*: rickets, osteomalacia. *Endocrine disturbances*: parathyroid osteodystrophy, Cushing's syndrome. *Affections of unknown cause*: Paget's disease (osteitis deformans), fibrous dysplasia of bone, senile osteoporosis. The main features of these disorders will be described in a later chapter.

Fig. 24   **Fig. 25**   **Fig. 26**

Three causes of deformity arising in a bone. Figure 24—Fracture. Figure 25—Bending of softened bone. Figure 26—Uneven epiphysial growth.

Uneven growth of bone. In children any disturbance of the growing epiphysial cartilage (growth plate) may lead to uneven growth and consequent deformity. The usual effect of interference with a growing epiphysial cartilage is that its growth is retarded; occasionally it is accelerated. Deformity will follow only if the growing cartilage is affected more in one part than another, or if the interference with growth affects only one bone of a pair, as in the forearm or leg (Fig. 26). The most frequent causes of retarded epiphysial growth are: 1) crushing fracture involving the epiphysial growth plate; 2) infection of the cartilage, usually from adjacent osteomyelitis or joint infection; 3) enchondroma (a benign tumour) adjacent to the cartilage, as in Ollier's disease (multiple enchondromatosis (p. 49). In the relatively uncommon cases in which epiphysial growth is accelerated the usual cause is local hyperaemia induced by an adjacent focus of infection or by a vascular tumour such as a haemangioma.

Treatment of deformities

Each deformity must be considered as an individual problem. Many do not require treatment, or are not amenable to it. In other cases an attempt may be made to correct or improve the deformity. One or more of the following methods may be used in appropriate cases: 1) manipulative correction and retention in a plaster or splint (example—for displaced fracture); 2) gradual correction by prolonged traction (example—for deformity in certain types of arthritis); 3) division or excision of contracted or tethered soft tissues (examples—for Dupuytren's contracture or scarring from burns); 4) osteotomy or osteoclasis (examples—for deformity from rickets or mal-united fracture); 5) arthrodesis (example—for scoliosis); 6) selective retardation of epiphysial growth (in children) (example—for deformity from uneven epiphysial growth).

References and bibliography, page 403.

4. General affections of the skeleton

A large number of general affections of the skeleton have been described. Even an incomplete description could occupy a large volume. Fortunately many of these affections are so rare that it is unnecessary for the student to concern himself with them. Most of the others require only brief consideration. Clearly, many of the affections to be described have a congenital basis and many of them cause deformity; so there is inevitably some overlap between this chapter and Chapter 3.

CLASSIFICATION

The following classification is based on that of Wynne-Davies and Fairbank (1976).

Bone dysplasias and malformations

Achondroplasia
Osteogenesis imperfecta
Diaphysial aclasis
Dyschondroplasia (Ollier's disease)
Paget's disease
Polyostotic fibrous dysplasia
Neurofibromatosis
Fibrodysplasia ossificans progressiva
Cranio-cleido dysostosis

Inborn errors of metabolism

Gaucher's disease
Histiocytosis X

Metabolic bone disease

Hyperparathyroidism
Nutritional rickets
Other forms of rickets
Nutritional osteomalacia
Other forms of osteomalacia
Vitamin C deficiency

Endocrine disorders

Senile osteoporosis
Hypopituitarism
Gigantism
Acromegaly
Hypothyroidism
Glucocorticoid excess

BONE DYSPLASIAS

ACHONDROPLASIA

Achondroplasia is a congenital affection in which there is marked shortness of the limbs, with consequent dwarfing. It is of autosomal dominant inheritance but many cases arise from a fresh gene mutation.

Fig. 27
Achondroplasia, showing the typical features in a child. The dwarfing is due to shortness of the limbs, especially in their proximal segments; development of the trunk is but little impaired. Note the 'trident' hands.

Pathology. There is a failure of normal ossification in the long bones, which may be only half their normal length. Growth of the trunk is only slightly impaired.

Clinical features. Achondroplasia is apparent at birth, the child being strikingly dwarfed, with very short limbs that are out of proportion to the trunk: shortness is especially marked in the proximal segments of the limbs (Fig. 27). Adult achondroplasts are seldom more than 130 centimetres (4 feet 3 inches) in height. The hands are short and broad, the central three digits being divergent and of almost equal length ('trident' hand). The head is slightly larger than normal, with a bulging forehead and depressed nasal bridge. There is marked lumbar lordosis, often with thoracic kyphosis, which may occasionally lead to compression of the spinal cord. There is no mental impairment and life expectancy is usually normal.

Radiographic features. Apart from striking shortness of the limbs, there are characteristic changes in the pelvis, the inlet being widened from side to side but narrowed in the antero-posterior diameter, with notably small greater sciatic notches. The spinal canal is also narrowed in the antero-posterior diameter. The calvarium of the skull is large, but the base short.

Treatment. With improved techniques of leg lengthening, there may be increasing scope in the future for worthwhile gain in stature.

OSTEOGENESIS IMPERFECTA
(Fragilitas ossium)

Osteogenesis imperfecta is a congenital and inheritable disorder—or more probably a heterogeneous group of disorders—in which the bones are abnormally soft and brittle, on account of defective collagen formation. In addition to the bones, other collagen-containing tissues such as teeth, skin, tendons and ligaments may be abnormal. It is usually transmitted as an autosomal dominant, but in a severe variant of the disease the parents are normal and a fresh gene mutation or autosomal recessive inheritance is postulated.

Fig. 28
Recent and old fractures of the bones of the upper limbs in an infant with osteogenesis imperfecta (fragilitas ossium).

Clinical features. In the worst cases, which occur sporadically rather than from inheritance and probably represent a distinct entity, the child is born with multiple fractures and does not survive. In the less severe examples fractures occur after birth, often from trivial violence. As many as fifty or more may be sustained in the first few years of life. The fractures unite readily, but in the more severe cases marked deformity often develops, either from malunion or from bending of the soft bones (Fig. 28), and such patients may be badly crippled. In the milder cases there is a tendency for fractures to occur less frequently in later life.

Additional features, not always present, are a deep blue coloration of the sclerotics of the eyes, deafness from otosclerosis (which becomes worse in later life), and ligamentous laxity.

Treatment. Fractures are generally treated in the ordinary way, but in a severe case intramedullary nailing of affected long bones should be considered as a means of preventing crippling deformity and permitting earlier resumption of activity (Sofield 1959). Newer techniques have been developed with telescoping rods, to obviate the need for multiple operations (Nicholas and James 1990). Protective appliances, such as walking calipers, may be required in older children and adults.

DIAPHYSIAL ACLASIS
(Multiple hereditary exostoses)

This is a congenital affection characterised by the formation of multiple exostoses (osteochondromata) at the metaphysial regions of the long bones. It is transmitted by a dominant mutant gene.

Pathology. The fault is in the epiphysial cartilage plate. Nests of cartilage cells become displaced and give rise to bony outgrowths, which are capped by proliferating cartilage.

Growth of the exostoses usually ceases at skeletal maturity. These exostoses, or osteo-chondromata, constitute one type of benign bone tumour (p. 82). The number of out-growths varies; often there are between ten and twenty, of varying size. In severe cases the process of remodelling by which a bone attains its normal adult shape is impaired, and there may be marked deformity, with reduction of longitudinal growth and consequent shortness of stature. Rarely, malignant change in the cartilaginous cap of one of the tumours leads to the development of a chondrosarcoma.

Fig. 29   **Fig. 30**

Diaphysial aclasis (multiple exostoses). Figure 29 shows stunting of the upper end of the femur due to failure of the remodelling process that accompanies normal growth. Defective remodelling is a characteristic feature of the disease in its more severe forms. Figure 30 shows typical exostoses (osteochondromata) projecting from femur and tibia. Such outgrowths are always directed away from the end of the bone.

Clinical features. Usually the only symptoms and signs are those caused by the local swellings, or by their pressure effects. The patient is often of short stature, and there may be marked deformity of the limbs. Malignant change is suggested by rapid enlargement of one of the swellings.

Radiographs show the bony outgrowths. In severe cases the bones are broad and ill modelled (Figs 29 and 30).

Treatment. An outgrowth that is causing trouble should be excised.

DYSCHONDROPLASIA

(Multiple enchondromatosis; Ollier's disease)

In dyschondroplasia masses of unossified cartilage persist within the metaphyses of certain long bones, and the growth of the bone is retarded. The condition becomes evident in childhood, but the cause is unknown. In contrast with diaphysial aclasis, heredity plays no part.

Pathology. The fault is in the epiphysial cartilage plate. In this respect dyschondroplasia resembles diaphysial aclasis, but the two conditions are otherwise distinct. Nests of cartilage cells are displaced from the epiphysial plate into the metaphysis, where they persist as enchondromata.

Any bone formed in cartilage may be affected. The more rapidly growing ends of the femur and tibia (that is, the ends near the knee) and the small long bones of the hands and feet are particularly common sites. There is a tendency for the disorder to affect one side of the body predominantly, or even exclusively. When a major long bone is affected interference with growth at the epiphysial cartilage adjacent to the lesion may lead to serious shortening and distortion of the bone (Fig. 31). When skeletal growth ceases the masses of cartilage may ossify. Rarely one of the tumours undergoes malignant change, to become a chondrosarcoma (p. 89).

| Fig. 31 | Fig. 32 |

Multiple enchondromatosis (Ollier's disease). Figure 31—Masses of proliferating cartilage occupy the metaphyses of one tibia. Growth is retarded and uneven. The normal tibia is shown for comparison. Figure 32—Multiple enchondromata in the metacarpals and phalanges.

Clinical and radiographic features. A limb affected by dyschondroplasia is usually short and may be markedly deformed. The hands may be grotesquely enlarged by multiple cartilaginous swellings or outgrowths. *Radiographs* show multiple areas of transradiance in the affected bones (Figs 31 and 32).

Treatment. Osteotomy may be required to correct deformities resulting from uneven growth of bone. If there is marked discrepancy in the length of the lower limbs a leg equalisation procedure (p. 34) may be advisable. Lesions in the hand may be curetted and packed with bone chips.

PAGET'S DISEASE
(Osteitis deformans)

Paget's disease of bone is a slowly progressive disorder of one or several bones. Affected bones are thickened and spongy, and show a tendency to bend. The disease is one of the commonest general affections of the skeleton. The cause is unknown. It has been suggested that infection with a slow virus of the paramyxovirus family may be responsible, on the evidence

Fig. 33
Paget's disease. Half pelvis, side by side with a normal one shown for comparison. Note the coarse trabeculae and slight distortion of the softened pelvic ring, with deepening of the acetabulum.

Fig. 34
Paget's disease. Tibia, showing bending, coarsening of trabeculae, and thickened cortex which, however, is not sharply demarcated from the medulla.

Fig. 35
The typical appearance of a patient with widespread Paget's disease. Note the bowing of the legs and shortening of the trunk from collapse of softened vertebrae. The head was also enlarged.

Fig. 34

Fig. 35

of inclusion bodies that have been found consistently in the osteoclasts of affected bones (Harvey 1984; Singer and Mills 1985).

Pathology. The basic abnormality is thought to be defective function of osteoclasts, with consequent irregular bone resorption and increase of bone turnover. The bones most commonly affected are the pelvis, vertebrae, femur, tibia, and skull. The disease may be confined to a single bone at first, but it often spreads to involve other bones later. The cortex of the bone loses its normal compact density and becomes spongy. At the same time the cortex is widened by the formation of new bone on both its outer and inner surfaces. The whole bone is thus thickened, but the usual sharp distinction between cortex and medulla is lost. The marrow spaces are filled with fibrous tissue. Whereas the bone is soft and vascular at first, in the later stages there is a tendency for it to become denser and very hard.

In the spongy state the softened bones are liable to bend. Pathological fracture may occur. In rare instances osteosarcoma develops in the diseased bone.

Clinical features. The affection seldom begins before the age of 40, but a childhood form is recognised. Often there are no symptoms, the condition being discovered incidentally during routine radiographic examination. When long bones are affected pain is sometimes complained of, but it is by no means an invariable feature. Bending of the softened long bones leads to deformity, usually in the form of anterior and lateral bowing of the femur or tibia (Fig. 35). Thickening may be obvious clinically, especially in the case of the tibia or the skull. Thus if the patient wears a hat he may notice that he requires progressively larger sizes. More importantly, bone thickening may also cause constriction of foramina in the skull, with risk of damage to a nerve—for instance the optic nerve or the auditory nerve.

Imaging. The main *radiographic* features (Figs 33 and 34) are: 1) thickening of the bone, mainly from widening of the cortex; 2) diminished density of the cortex, which loses its compact appearance and assumes a spongy or honeycombed texture; 3) marked coarsening of the bone trabeculae; 4) in the later stages a general increase of density of the affected bones. The long bones are often shown to be bowed, the pelvis may be deformed, the vertebrae may be compressed and the vault of the skull thickened. *Radio-isotope scanning* with ^{99m}technetium shows markedly increased uptake in the affected bones.

Investigations. The alkaline phosphatase content of the plasma is increased, often to a high level if several bones are affected. Urinary hydroxyproline is increased, reflecting the increased resorption of bone matrix.

Complications. The important complications are pathological fracture, compression of cranial nerves and, occasionally, osteosarcoma.

Treatment. Very often treatment is not required because the disability is negligible. Treatment is needed mainly for bone pain and for complications. Two drugs are known to affect the outcome—calcitonin and biphosphonates.

Both drugs inhibit bone resorption. They reduce bone turnover, with lowering of plasma alkaline phosphatase, and both are effective in relieving bone pain in a high proportion of cases. Treatment must, however, be prolonged. Unlike calcitonin, which must be injected (though nasal spray and suppository forms are being tried), a biphosphonate compound may be taken by mouth. Moreover its benefit often persists for up to six months after the drug has been discontinued; so it is the preferred drug in the first instance, on the basis of cost and ease of administration.

POLYOSTOTIC FIBROUS DYSPLASIA

Replacement of bone by fibrous tissue forms a conspicuous part of several unrelated bone diseases. In two conditions in particular, fibrous replacement is the predominant change. In one of these—parathyroid osteodystrophy—the changes are associated with hyperparathyroidism (p. 57). In the other, now to be described, there is fibrous replacement without any evidence of excessive parathyroid secretion.

Figs 36 and 37
Polyostotic fibrous dysplasia affecting the radius (Fig. 36) and the tibia (Fig. 37). Parts of the skeleton are replaced by fibrous tissue, giving in places a 'ground-glass' appearance. Unlike hyperparathyroidism, this disorder is not associated with any known endocrine dysfunction.

Fig. 36   **Fig. 37**

Polyostotic fibrous dysplasia, then, is a condition in which parts of several bones are replaced by masses of fibrous tissue, but in which there is no evidence of hyperparathyroidism. The condition is rare and the cause is unknown. There is no evidence to suggest a genetic basis.

Pathology. The number of bones involved varies from two or three to twelve or more. The major long bones are those mainly affected—especially the femur. The skull and mandible are also commonly involved. Affected bones are liable to bend or break.

Clinical features. The onset is in childhood but the condition is often not recognised until adult life. The main features are deformity, from bending or local enlargement of bone, and pathological fracture. The disease progresses for years and may lead to severe crippling.

Radiographs of the affected bones show well defined transradiant areas which often have a characteristic homogeneous or 'ground-glass' appearance: these changes may be localised and patchy rather than uniform. The lesions are in the shaft and metaphyses rather than the epiphyses. When the lesion is extensive the cortex is expanded and thin, and the bone is bent. Sometimes the lesion has a honeycombed appearance (Figs 36 and 37).

Investigations. There is no consistent biochemical abnormality of the blood. In a few cases the plasma alkaline phosphatase has been raised.

ALBRIGHT'S SYNDROME
The bone lesions of polyostotic fibrous dysplasia sometimes occur in association with patchy pigmentation of the skin and, in females, sexual precocity. This combination of clinical features is known as Albright's syndrome.

NEUROFIBROMATOSIS

(von Recklinghausen's disease)

This is a congenital inheritable affection characterised by pigmented areas on the skin, cutaneous fibromata, and multiple neurofibromata in the course of the cranial or peripheral nerves. It is ascribed to a dominant mutant gene.

Pathology. The neurofibromata consist of connective tissue arranged in whorls, with a few nerve fibres.

Clinical features. Skin lesions are seldom present at birth but often develop in early childhood. They consist of multiple '*café au lait*' areas, and of small fibromata which may be flat or raised. Neurofibromata may occur on any of the cranial or peripheral nerves, and important pressure effects may occur, including compression of the spinal cord.

The orthopaedic significance of neurofibromatosis lies mainly in the liability to scoliosis and to neurological disturbances in the limbs. There may also be pathological fracture—usually of the tibia in infants, due to fibrous infiltration of the bone (congenital pseudarthrosis).

Scoliosis. Why scoliosis should occur is unknown: but it is a common complication and it sometimes progresses to an angulation so severe that the function of the spinal cord is impaired.

Neurological disturbances. There may be impairment of function of cranial or peripheral nerves in consequence of neurofibromata lying in the course of nerve trunks. Various manifestations are observed, depending upon the site of the tumour. For instance, a tumour of a nerve root within the spinal canal may compress the spinal cord and give the typical picture of a spinal cord tumour. Or it may compress the cauda equina or an individual nerve trunk, with consequent radiating pain and impairment of function of the involved nerve. Thus neurofibromatosis enters into the differential diagnosis of brachial pain and sciatica.

Imaging. *Plain radiographs* may show erosion of a bone where a neurofibroma lies in contact with it. *CT or MR scanning* may be helpful in outlining the extent of a bulky neurofibroma.

Diagnosis. The pigmented spots or areas, and cutaneous fibromata, afford important clues to the diagnosis. A positive family history is important corroborative evidence.

Complications. Occasionally a neurofibroma may undergo malignant change, to become a fibrosarcoma.

Treatment. A neurofibroma that is causing trouble should be excised.

FIBRODYSPLASIA OSSIFICANS PROGRESSIVA

(Myositis ossificans progressiva)

Fibrodysplasia ossificans progressiva is a congenital affection characterised by the formation of masses of bone in the soft tissues, with consequent progressive impairment of movement of the underlying joint or joints. It is often associated with shortness of the great toe or of other digits (microdactyly). It is probably of autosomal dominant inheritance but genetic transmission is rare because death usually occurs before the age of parenthood. Thus a fresh gene mutation must usually be postulated.

Pathology.[1] The ectopic bone is formed by metaplasia of connective-tissue cells, not from displaced osteoblasts.

Clinical features. Changes usually appear first in early childhood. Swellings develop in the region of the neck and trunk. At first soft and perhaps transient, they later give place to hard masses of bone which lie in the course of muscles, ligaments and fasciae. Movements of the spine and ribs, and later of the limb joints, are reduced progressively until in the worst cases there may be total immobility. In most cases the great toe is congenitally short; the thumbs or other digits may also be short.

Radiographs show the plates of bone in the soft tissues.

Progress. After many years increasing rigidity renders the patient bedridden. No curative treatment is known. Systemic treatment by biphosphonates after excision of bony bars may retard their regeneration, but the eventual fatal outcome seems unlikely to be influenced significantly.

CRANIO-CLEIDO DYSOSTOSIS
(Cleido-cranio dysplasia)

In this dysplasia the most striking features are enlargement of the frontal and parietal regions of the head with delayed ossification and delayed fusion of the skull bones, and absence or partial absence of the clavicles. Other bones may also show less striking anomalies. The disorder is of autosomal dominant inheritance.

Clinical features. The disorder usually becomes apparent in early childhood. The head is somewhat larger than normal, with bulging frontal and parietal regions. The clavicles are either absent or rudimentary, in consequence of which the two shoulders can be approximated anteriorly—a characteristic feature. Life expectancy is normal.

Radiographs in childhood show delayed fusion of the skull bones, with Wormian bones in the suture lines; absence of the clavicles either in whole or in the lateral parts; and delayed ossification of the pelvic bones with wide symphysis pubis.

INBORN ERRORS OF METABOLISM

GAUCHER'S DISEASE

Gaucher's disease is one of the group of lysosomal storage diseases included under the generic title *mucopolysaccharidoses* or *sphingolipidoses*. It is a rare lipoid storage disease of autosomal recessive inheritance, in which the enzyme beta-glucosidase is deficient and gluco-cerebroside accumulates in reticulo-endothelial cells of the spleen, liver, bone marrow and other tissues.

---

[1]This disease, formerly known as myositis ossificans progressiva, must not be confused with post-traumatic myositis ossificans. The two conditions are entirely distinct. Post-traumatic 'myositis ossificans' is misnamed: it is nothing more than ossification within a subperiostial haematoma.

Clinical features. Symptoms usually appear first in adult life. There is enlargement of the spleen and liver. There may be a feeling of weakness due to anaemia, but often the general health is good. Skeletal involvement, which takes the form of infiltration and replacement of bone by masses of lipoid-laden reticulo-endothelial cells (Gaucher cells) brings a risk of pathological fracture. Bone pain or joint pain is a common feature.

Radiographs show irregular cyst-like spaces in some of the bones, sometimes with expansion of the cortex, especially of the femur, the lower end of which may appear flask-shaped. Avascular necrosis of the head of the femur or the head of the humerus, with consequent disorganisation of the corresponding joint, is also common.

Investigations. Bone marrow biopsy usually yields typical Gaucher cells.

Treatment. Splenectomy relieves local discomfort but it does not influence the chronic course of the disease.

HISTIOCYTOSIS X
(Skeletal granulomatosis)

The title histiocytosis X comprises a group of diseases characterised by proliferation of histiocytes and storage within them of cholesterol. The three clinical entities to be briefly described are: 1) eosinophilic granuloma; 2) Hand-Schüller-Christian disease; and 3) Letterer-Siwe disease. All occur mostly in children or young adults.

EOSINOPHILIC GRANULOMA

In eosinophilic granuloma the bone lesion is usually solitary. It consists of brownish granulation tissue containing abundant histiocytes and eosinophils, with leucocytes and giant cells. Often there are no symptoms, but there may be local pain, or occasionally a pathological fracture.

Radiologically the lesion is seen as a clear-cut hole in the bone—usually a rib, skull bone, vertebra, pelvic bone, femur or humerus. An affected vertebral body may collapse, becoming compressed into a thin wafer (see Calvé's vertebral compression, p. 189). Examination of the blood usually fails to show any abnormality.

Eosinophilic granuloma may simulate a bone cyst, a primary or metastatic bone tumour, or tuberculosis. If multiple, it resembles Hand-Schüller-Christian disease.

Treatment. The lesion often heals spontaneously. Surgical curettage may accelerate healing. Radiotherapy has sometimes been given but it is now widely regarded as unnecessary.

HAND-SCHÜLLER-CHRISTIAN DISEASE

In this condition there is proliferation of reticulo-endothelial cells to form multiple lesions, often in the skull but also in other bones. The yellowish deposits consist of granulation tissue with abundant histiocytes, many of which contain cholesterol esters and from their vacuolated appearance are known as foam cells.

Radiologically the lesions appear as punched-out areas, without any surrounding reaction. The areas of destruction are often large. The occasional occurrence of diabetes insipidus and exophthalmos is explained by the presence of lesions in the base of the skull, involving the hypophysis and orbits. There may be other manifestations of pituitary dysfunction, such as retarded growth. The disease progresses very slowly but is often fatal eventually.

Treatment. Radiotherapy may cause the lesions to regress, but the long-term prognosis is poor.

LETTERER-SIWE DISEASE

This is the most serious form of non-lipoid granulomatosis or histiocytosis X. It begins in early childhood and progresses rapidly, usually with fatal outcome. Granulomatous deposits occur not only in bone but also in lymph glands, spleen and liver, which may show enlargement clinically. Radiologically the skeletal lesions resemble those of Hand-Schüller-Christian disease.

METABOLIC BONE DISEASE

HYPERPARATHYROIDISM
(Parathyroid osteodystrophy; generalised osteitis fibrosa cystica;
von Recklinghausen's disease)

The characteristic features of hyperparathyroidism are lassitude, dyspepsia, generalised osteoporosis, and cystic changes in some of the bones.

Cause. It is caused by excessive parathyroid secretion, usually from an adenoma of one of the parathyroid glands.

Pathology. The excessive secretion of parathormone causes generalised absorption of bone, the calcium from which is liberated into the blood, whence it is excreted in excessive quantities in the urine. The bone becomes spongy and the cortices are thin. Cystic changes often develop in one or more of the long bones: from their macroscopic appearance these are commonly referred to as brown cysts. A consequence of the increased excretion of calcium is that the kidneys frequently contain calculi.

Clinical features. The patient is adult. There are pains in the bones, indigestion, and weakness. There may also be deformity from bending of softened bone, or a pathological fracture.

Fig. 40

Figs 38–40

Hyperparathyroidism. Figures 38 and 39—Radiographs showing the typical changes in the long bones: diffuse osteoporosis with marked thinning of the cortex and scattered fibrocystic changes (pathologically, 'brown' cysts). Figure 40—The skull is fuzzy and finely mottled.

Fig. 38   **Fig. 39**

Radiographic features. Radiographs show rarefaction of the whole skeleton. The loss of density may be marked, and the cortices very thin. An early sign is irregular subperiosteal cortical erosion in the phalanges of the fingers. Scattered cystic changes may be present in the long bones (Figs 38 and 39). The skull shows a uniform fine granular mottling, sometimes with small translucent cyst-like areas (Fig. 40). Radiographs of the renal tracts often show nephrolithiasis.

Investigations. The plasma calcium is increased but the plasma inorganic phosphate is diminished. Excretion of calcium and phosphate in the urine is increased.

Diagnosis. This is from other causes of diffuse or generalised rarefaction of bone. These are summarised in Table III (p. 64).

Treatment. The causative parathyroid tumour should be located and removed.

NUTRITIONAL RICKETS

In rickets there is defective calcification of *growing* bone[1] in consequence of a disturbed calcium-phosphorus metabolism. With the general improvement in economic conditions infantile rickets has become rare in Western countries. There is, however, a relatively higher incidence among immigrants from the West Indies and from Asia.

Cause. Nutritional rickets is caused by a deficiency of vitamin D in the diet and by inadequate exposure to sunlight, which promotes the synthesis of vitamin D in the body.

Fig. 41
Rickets. Note the typical widening and 'cupping' of the metaphyses of the radius and ulna. The depth of the epiphysial cartilage is increased, and the general density of the bones is reduced.

Pathology. Vitamin D promotes the absorption of calcium and phosphorus from the intestine. Its deficiency therefore leads to inadequate absorption of calcium and phosphorus. The level of calcium in the blood can then be maintained only at the expense of the skeletal calcium. Proliferating osteoid tissue in the growing epiphyses thus remains

---

[1]When similar influences act on mature adult bone the condition is known as osteomalacia.

uncalcified, and there is a general softening of the bones already formed (Fig. 41).

Clinical features. The ordinary nutritional rickets usually occurs in children about one year old. The general health is impaired. The predominant signs are a large head, retarded skeletal growth, enlarged epiphyses, curvature of long bones, and deformity of the chest, which may show a transverse sulcus. In a typical case these signs produce an easily recognised clinical picture.

Radiographic features. There is a general loss of density of the skeleton with thinning of the cortices. The most striking changes, however, are in the growing epiphyses. The vertical depth of the epiphysial lines is increased, the epiphyses are widened laterally, and the ends of the shafts are hollowed out or 'cupped' (Fig. 41). Bending of the bones may be obvious.

Investigations. The plasma phosphate level is usually decreased. The plasma calcium is normal. The alkaline phosphatase is increased, often markedly: its level gives some indication of the severity of the disease and of the response to treatment. Measurement of the serum levels of 25-hydroxyvitamin D is a useful guide to diagnosis and treatment.

Diagnosis. If rickets is suspected an antero-posterior radiograph of a wrist should be obtained. The radiographic features are diagnostic of rickets, but biochemical examinations are required to indicate its type (Table II, p. 61).

Treatment. Nutritional rickets responds well to vitamin D in ordinary doses. Severe bony deformity persisting after vitamin therapy should be corrected by osteotomy or osteoclasis.

OTHER FORMS OF RICKETS

The characteristic epiphysial changes seen in nutritional rickets occur in a number of other diseases, the primary factor responsible for the disordered calcium-phosphate metabolism being different in each type. Four types will be described: familial hypophosphataemia, cystinosis, uraemic osteo-dystrophy, and coeliac (gluten-induced) rickets.

FAMILIAL HYPOPHOSPHATAEMIA
(Chronic phosphate diabetes; vitamin-resistant rickets)
Familial hypophosphataemia is a hereditary disorder transmitted by an X-linked dominant gene. The nature of the primary defect is uncertain: it may be a failure of normal reabsorption of phosphate by the renal tubules, or it may be a fault in the absorption of calcium from the intestine. Bone changes, which are like those of nutritional rickets, may become manifest soon after the first year of life. The characteristic biochemical features are: normal plasma calcium, low plasma phosphate level *not corrected by vitamin D*, increased alkaline phosphatase, and excess of phosphate in the urine (Table II, p. 61). Relatives who are clinically unaffected may nevertheless show hypophosphataemia.

Treatment. Vitamin D in high doses should be combined with the administration of phosphates. Treatment on these lines corrects the bone changes but does not restore the plasma phosphate to a normal level. Improved results have been achieved by the use of a synthetic vitamin D analogue, 1α-hydroxyvitamin D3. Surgical correction of residual deformities may be required.

CYSTINOSIS
(Fanconi syndrome; renal tubular rickets with glycosuria and amino-aciduria)
In cystinosis (Fanconi syndrome) rachitic changes in the bones are associated with renal glycosuria and amino-aciduria. The primary defect, a congenital fault transmitted by a recessive mutant gene, is a failure of the proximal renal tubules to reabsorb phosphate, glucose, and certain amino acids in the normal way. The excessive loss of phosphates in the urine leads to depletion of the bone phosphate. Onset may be later in childhood than that of nutritional rickets, but the bone changes are the same. The characteristic biochemical features are: normal plasma calcium; low plasma phosphate; increased alkaline phosphatase; and excess of phosphate in the urine, which also contains glucose and certain amino acids (Table II, p. 61).

Treatment. The intake of calcium, phosphate, and vitamin D should be increased. Alkalis (sodium citrate) should be given to combat the associated acidosis.

RELATED DISORDERS
A number of similar disorders from renal tubular defects are recognised. In all of them there is deficient reabsorption of phosphate, but they differ in the extent to which other functions of the tubules are impaired.

URAEMIC OSTEODYSTROPHY
(Renal osteodystrophy; renal (glomerular) rickets; renal dwarfism)
In uraemic osteodystrophy general skeletal changes are associated with chronic renal impairment. The skeletal changes often become manifest between the ages of 5 and 10 years.

Pathology. The renal impairment may be due to congenital cystic changes, to ureteric obstruction with hydronephrosis, or to chronic nephritis. The mechanism by which the renal

Fig. 42
Rachitic changes in the epiphyses of a renal dwarf aged 14 years. There was diffuse rarefaction of the skeleton, with multiple deformities from bending of softened bones.

deficiency leads to rachitic changes in the skeleton is uncertain, and probably complex. One factor may be that impaired excretion of phosphorus by the kidneys leads to retention of phosphorus in the blood, and its excretion in the intestine. There it forms an insoluble compound with calcium, which in consequence is not absorbed in proper amounts.

The skeletal changes consist in deficient epiphysial growth and multiple deformities from bone softening. The parathyroid glands are hypertrophied, probably as a secondary effect.

Clinical features. The child is dwarfed and deformed. There are symptoms of renal impairment, such as excessive thirst and sallow complexion. The common skeletal deformities are coxa vara, genu valgum, and severe valgus deformity of the feet.

Radiographs show epiphysial changes that are generally similar to those of nutritional rickets (Fig. 42).

Table II

Summary of the biochemical changes in the various forms of rickets and osteomalacia

	Primary fault and mechanism	Plasma calcium	Plasma inorganic phosphate	Urine	Stools
Nutritional rickets (children) Nutritional osteomalacia (adults)	Deficiency of vitamin D in diet → impaired absorption of calcium and phosphorus	Normal	Low	Normal	Normal
Familial hypophosphataemia	Inherited fault: impaired reabsorption of phosphates by renal tubules → excessive excretion of phosphates in urine	Normal	Low	Excess of phosphate	Normal
Cystinosis (Fanconi syndrome)	Impaired reabsorption of phosphates, glucose and some amino acids by renal tubules → excessive excretion of phosphates, etc. in urine	Normal	Low	Glucose Amino acids Excess of phosphate	Normal
Uraemic osteodystrophy	Mechanism uncertain. Possibly impaired glomerular function → retention of phosphorus → excretion in bowel → combination with calcium preventing its normal absorption	Low	High	Albumin	Normal
Coeliac rickets (children) Idiopathic steatorrhoea (adults)	Digestive deficiency → impaired absorption of vitamin D and calcium	Low	Normal	Normal	Excess of fat

NOTE: The plasma alkaline phosphatase is increased in all types of rickets in the active stage. It is an index of activity rather than of type.

Investigations. The biochemical changes are characteristic (Table II). The plasma phosphate is markedly increased. The plasma calcium is low. The blood urea is raised, often to a high figure. Albumin is usually present in the urine.

Prognosis. Unless the renal lesion is remediable gradual progression is likely, with poor prognosis.

Treatment. This should be directed primarily against the underlying renal condition. The diet should be supplemented with calcium and vitamin D.

COELIAC (GLUTEN-INDUCED) RICKETS

Coeliac disease (gluten-induced enteropathy) is a digestive disorder characterised by malabsorption and consequently by an excess of fat in the stools. Before a knowledge was gained of how to control the disease it was often complicated by rachitic changes in the bones. Such changes will now be seen only in neglected cases.

The primary fault is a susceptibility of the villi of the small intestine to atrophy under the influence of gluten, the protein fraction of flour. This villous atrophy leads to deficient absorption of fats and of fat-soluble vitamin D.

The disease begins in infancy or early childhood. The general features are wasting, impaired growth, failure to gain weight, muscular hypotonia, distended abdomen, and loose offensive stools containing 40–80 per cent fat after drying (normal = 25 per cent). The skeletal changes, which do not develop for several years, are like those of nutritional rickets.

Investigations. The biochemical changes in the blood differ from those of nutritional rickets. The plasma calcium is low. The plasma phosphate is normal or low (Table II, p. 61). Diagnosis should be confirmed by jejunal biopsy effected by a swallowed capsule with a special cutting device.

Treatment. There is steady improvement in the calcification of the skeleton as the primary disorder is brought under control. The diet should be free from gluten and should contain an abundant supply of calcium and vitamin D.

NUTRITIONAL OSTEOMALACIA

Nutritional osteomalacia[1] is the adult counterpart of infantile (nutritional) rickets. It is regarded as rare except in certain Asiatic countries. Nevertheless it may be more common than is generally realised, especially in elderly women.

Cause and pathology. As in infantile rickets, there is a deficiency of vitamin D (and often of calcium) in the diet. In consequence the intestinal absorption of calcium and phosphorus is inadequate, and calcium is withdrawn from the bones to maintain a reasonable level in the blood. The bone trabeculae are not abnormally thin, but they are largely composed of poorly calcified osteoid tissue. There is an abundance of fibrous tissue in the marrow.

Clinical features. The main features are pain in the bones, and deformity. Because of the porosity of the bones fractures are common.

Radiographic features. There is rarefaction of the whole skeleton. The bone cortices are abnormally thin (Fig. 43). The long bones may be curved and the pelvis triradiate. Multiple spontaneous fractures (Looser's zones), seemingly ununited though possibly bridged by unmineralised osteoid tissue, may be shown in ribs, pelvic rami, or elsewhere. These are characteristic of osteomalacia and are not seen in osteoporosis.

Investigations. The plasma calcium is normal or low. Plasma phosphate

---

[1]The essential distinction between *osteoporosis* and *osteomalacia* was made in a footnote on page 12.

is low. Alkaline phosphatase is increased. The calcium balance is negative (Table II, p. 61). Serum levels of 25-hydroxyvitamin D will be low.

Diagnosis. Nutritional osteomalacia must be distinguished from other causes of diffuse rarefaction of bone (Table III, p. 64). In the elderly it may be mistaken for senile osteoporosis.

Treatment. Recalcification of the skeleton is induced by adequate diet and administration of vitamin D and calcium. Osteotomy may be required to correct deformity.

OTHER FORMS OF OSTEOMALACIA

Just as in children rachitic changes in the bones may occur from a number of different metabolic faults, so in adults osteomalacia may arise from causes other than purely nutritional. Such causes include advanced renal disease, and malabsorption syndromes such as chronic obstruction of the bile ducts, chronic pancreatic disease and idiopathic steatorrhoea. Of these, only idiopathic steatorrhoea will be described here, as an example.

Fig. 43

Demonstration of generalised rarefaction by radiography of one of the patient's hands side by side with a hand of a normal person (*left*) of the same sex and age. Note the obvious difference in bone density. A case of osteomalacia in a patient with idiopathic steatorrhoea.

IDIOPATHIC STEATORRHOEA

In most instances so-called idiopathic steatorrhoea is the adult counterpart of coeliac disease and may therefore be termed gluten-induced enteropathy. There is deficient absorption of fats, and consequently of the fat-soluble vitamin D and of calcium. Eventually, skeletal changes may occur which are identical with those of nutritional osteomalacia.

Clinical features. The disease may be unrecognised until a fracture occurs or a deformity becomes evident. *Radiographs* show rarefaction of bone (Fig. 43), with thinning of the cortices. *Investigations* (Table II, p. 61): The stools contain an excess of fat and of

Table III
Ten causes of diffuse rarefaction of bone

Cause	Diagnostic features
Osteoporosis	
Prolonged recumbency	History of confinement to bed for months or years.
Senile (idiopathic)	Post-menopausal. Spine predominantly affected. No biochemical change in blood.
Hyperparathyroidism	Diagnostic biochemical changes in blood: plasma calcium increased; plasma phosphate decreased.
Glucocorticoid excess (Cushing's syndrome)	Characteristic clinical features: obesity, hypertrichosis, hypertension, amenorrhoea in women.
Osteomalacia	
Rickets (all types)	Rachitic changes at growing epiphyses. Biochemical changes depend on type of rickets (Table II, p. 61).
Nutritional osteomalacia	Dietary deficiency apparent. Characteristic biochemical changes in blood: plasma calcium normal (or decreased); plasma phosphate decreased (Table II, p. 61).
Idiopathic steatorrhoea	Excess of fat in faeces. Blood changes: plasma calcium decreased; plasma phosphate normal (Table II, p. 61)
Tumour	
Multiple myeloma	Usually multiple circumscribed lesions, but may be diffuse. Bence-Jones proteose often present in urine. Marrow biopsy shows excess of plasma cells.
Diffuse carcinomatosis	Primary tumour demonstrable.
Leukaemia	Blood examination and marrow biopsy show excess of immature white cells.

calcium. The plasma calcium is low. The plasma phosphate is normal. The urinary excretion of calcium is low. Jejunal biopsy may show villous atrophy.

Treatment. In cases ascribed to the influence of gluten, a gluten-free diet, supplemented with calcium and vitamin D, should be ordered.

VITAMIN C DEFICIENCY

(Infantile scurvy)

Scurvy is a haemorrhagic disease caused by a deficiency of vitamin C (ascorbic acid) in the diet. It is rare in Western countries, especially in adults.

Pathology. The most striking changes are in the long bones. There is a lack of osteoblastic activity in the epiphysial growth cartilage (growth plate). Haemorrhage, beginning at the epiphysial cartilage, extends beneath the periosteum, which may be raised from the bone throughout its whole length. Haemorrhages also occur from other sites, especially from the gums or within the orbit.

Clinical features. Scurvy affects infants during the second six months of life if the diet is deficient in fresh milk or other sources of vitamin C. The onset is rapid, with loss of use of a limb because of pain (pseudoparalysis). The limb is swollen and exquisitely tender over the affected bone or bones. The gums are often spongy and bleed, and there may be a 'black' eye.

Radiographic features. Plain radiographs show a dense line at the junction between metaphysis and epiphysial cartilage, with a clear band of rarefaction on the diaphysial side (Fig. 44). Later there is ossification in the subperiosteal haematoma, as a result of which the bone is often markedly thickened (Fig. 45).

Figs 44 and 45
Infantile scurvy. Figure 44—Early active stage. Note the clear zone in the metaphysis, indicating arrest of osteoblastic activity, and the dense zone adjacent to the epiphysial cartilage. Figure 45—Later stage, showing well marked ossification in the subperiosteal haematoma.

Fig. 44   Fig. 45

Investigations. Ascorbic acid is deficient in the plasma.

Diagnosis. The skeletal features of scurvy in infants resemble those of syphilitic metaphysitis, which, however, occurs at an earlier age—namely during the first six months of life. Other distinctive features are the positive Wassermann reaction in syphilis and bleeding from the gums in scurvy. Scurvy may also be confused clinically with acute osteomyelitis. Deficiency of plasma ascorbic acid is diagnostic.

Treatment. The disease responds readily to the administration of vitamin C.

ENDOCRINE DISORDERS

SENILE OSTEOPOROSIS
(Idiopathic osteoporosis; post-menopausal osteoporosis)

This condition is characterised by diffuse osteoporosis of unknown cause. It affects the elderly, especially post-menopausal women, but it may be seen also in patients of middle age. It may possibly have an endocrine basis.

Pathology. The whole skeleton is affected, but the changes in the spine are more obvious than those elsewhere. The cortices of the vertebrae are thinner than normal, and the bone is rarefied throughout from thinning of the individual trabeculae and widening of the vascular canals. In other words there is a reduction of total bone mass. Compression fracture of one or more of the vertebral bodies is liable to occur from only trivial violence. Even without fracture the thoracic vertebrae tend gradually to become wedge-shaped so that the spine bends forward to produce a rounded kyphosis. The long bones—particularly the upper end of the femur and the lower end of the radius—are also prone to fracture easily.

Fig. 46

Figs 46 and 47
Senile osteoporosis. Note the rounded kyphosis and the shortened trunk with transverse furrow across the abdomen. The radiograph (Fig. 47) shows marked loss of density, with thinning of the cortices. The intervertebral discs are ballooned into the concave vertebral surfaces. Several vertebral bodies have collapsed. Differential diagnosis was from parathyroid osteodystrophy, osteomalacia, myelomatosis, diffuse carcinomatous deposits, and leukaemia.

Fig. 47

Clinical features. The patient is often a woman of over 60. The osteoporosis may be symptomless and may be found only by chance. In other cases there is pain in the back. The pain occurs in two forms—a mild generalised ache, and a sharper pain of sudden onset, denoting a compression fracture. Examination reveals a rounded kyphosis in the thoracic region. If a vertebral body has collapsed there may be a more angular kyphosis with prominence of a spinous process in the thoracic or thoracolumbar region. The trunk is shortened and there is a transverse furrow across the abdomen (Fig. 46).

Radiographic features. The striking feature is the reduced density of the vertebral bodies, which become concave at their upper and lower surfaces from pressure of the intervertebral discs. Often there is wedging of one or more of the vertebral bodies from compression fracture (Fig. 47). Other parts of the skeleton are also rarefied, but less obviously.

Investigations. The biochemistry of the blood is normal. Metabolic balance studies may show a negative calcium balance.

Diagnosis. Senile osteoporosis may be confused with other forms of diffuse rarefaction of bone, especially that caused by parathyroid osteodystrophy, glucocorticoid excess (Cushing's syndrome), osteomalacia of various types, carcinomatosis, myelomatosis, or leukaemia (Table III, p. 64). Diagnosis rests largely on the exclusion of these specific disorders.

Prevention. Hormone replacement therapy (HRT) with oestrogens, supplemented by progesterone for ten days of the month unless the patient has had a hysterectomy, is an important option in post-menopausal women.

Treatment. Once osteoporosis is established, treatment is rather unsatisfactory. It may be possible to restore the patient to positive calcium balance by high dosage calcium supplements to the diet, combined with calcitriol if malabsorption is present; but the gain is slow because of the slow turnover rate of bone tissue. Thus a dramatic improvement in the radiographic appearance cannot be expected.

A number of drugs have been used in trials to treat established osteoporosis in the older patient, particularly after vertebral or femoral neck fractures. These are selected for their ability to decrease osteoclastic bone resorption or to stimulate the formation of new bone by osteoblasts. At present the most promising inhibitors of bone resorption are biphosphonates, while fluoride and the peptide of parathyroid hormone may promote new bone formation.

HYPOPITUITARISM

Deficient secretion of the anterior lobe of the pituitary leads to various types of disturbance of skeletal growth, often with impairment of sexual development and sometimes with mental backwardness. The patient may be dwarfed, or on the other hand there may be good stature with marked obesity. The orthopaedic importance of this latter condition is that it may predispose to slipping of the upper femoral epiphyses in adolescents (p. 317)—as indeed may obesity from any cause.

GIGANTISM

In gigantism (one form of hyperpituitarism) skeletal overgrowth is caused by an excess of anterior pituitary hormone occurring before the growth epiphyses have fused.

Pathology. There is an eosinophilic adenoma of the anterior lobe of the pituitary. Excessive growth occurs at the epiphysial cartilages. Despite this overactivity, epiphysial fusion occurs at about the normal time.

Clinical features. The patient, usually a boy, may grow to a height of 7 feet or more, the main increase being in the limbs. Sexual development is often impaired and the mentality may be subnormal. Signs of acromegaly often develop later.

Diagnosis and treatment are as for acromegaly (see below).

ACROMEGALY

The primary fault is the same as in gigantism—namely, an excessive secretion of pituitary growth hormone—but it occurs after the epiphyses have fused. It is characterised by enlargement of the bones, especially of the hands, feet, skull, and mandible.

Pathology. As in gigantism, there is usually an acidophil adenoma of the anterior lobe of the pituitary. The enlargement of the bones is caused by deposition of new bone upon the surface of the original cortex.

Clinical features. The disease often begins in early adult life. The physical features become coarse and heavy, the skin is thickened, and the hands and feet slowly enlarge. At first strong, the patient often becomes weak and sluggish later. *Radiographs* show marked enlargement of the bones of the hands and feet, and especially of the mandible. The vertebral bodies are also enlarged, especially in the antero-posterior plane. The sella turcica of the skull may be expanded and eroded.

Diagnosis. This is made from the clinical appearance and by demonstration of excessive growth hormone excretion by radio-immunoassay.

Treatment. Early treatment—often by removal of the pituitary adenoma or sometimes by irradiation or by drug therapy—is important in preventing deterioration.

INFANTILE HYPOTHYROIDISM
(Cretinism)

Infantile hypothyroidism (cretinism) is characterised by dwarfism, with sexual and mental retardation. It is caused by congenital deficiency of thyroid secretion. From the orthopaedic viewpoint the important features are retarded growth of the limb bones, kyphosis, and distortion of the joint surfaces. Early diagnosis is important because marked improvement follows treatment with thyroid extract.

GLUCOCORTICOID EXCESS
(Cushing's syndrome)

This endocrine disorder is characterised by obesity, hypertrichosis, hypertension and, in women, amenorrhoea. It is induced by excessive secretion of adrenocortical hormones, caused either by a tumour of the adrenal cortex or by hyperplasia of the gland which may be secondary to a basophil adenoma of the pituitary. A similar condition may also be caused by prolonged administration of cortisone, prednisone, or related steroid drugs.

The orthopaedic significance of Cushing's syndrome lies in the fact that it is accompanied by generalised rarefaction of the skeleton, with liability to pathological fracture of porotic bone (Table III, p. 64).

References and bibliography, page 403.

5. Local affections of bone

The most important local disorders of bone are: 1) infection; 2) tumours; 3) osteochondritis; and 4) cystic changes.

INFECTIONS OF BONE

Infection of bone by pyogenic organisms is termed osteomyelitis.[1] It occurs in acute and chronic forms. The only other infections of bone with which the student in Western countries need concern himself are tuberculous infection and syphilitic infection.

ACUTE OSTEOMYELITIS
(Acute pyogenic infection of bone; acute osteitis)

Two distinct types of acute osteomyelitis must be considered: 1) haematogenous osteomyelitis, a disease mainly of childhood in which organisms reach the bone through the blood stream; and 2) osteomyelitis complicating open fracture or surgical operation, in which organisms gain entry directly through the wound. The two types are sufficiently distinct to require separate descriptions.

ACUTE HAEMATOGENOUS OSTEOMYELITIS

Acute haematogenous osteomyelitis is one of the important diseases of childhood. Only rare atypical cases occur in adults. Early diagnosis is especially important because a satisfactory outcome depends upon prompt and efficient treatment.

Cause. It is caused by infection of the bone with pyogenic organisms—usually the staphylococcus aureus, though a variety of other organisms are occasionally responsible, including salmonella. A minor injury to a bone may render it vulnerable to infection by organisms circulating in the blood.

---

[1]There is nothing to be gained by distinguishing between *osteitis* (inflammation of bone) and *osteomyelitis* (inflammation of bone and bone marrow). For practical purposes the two terms may be regarded as synonymous.

Pathology. Organisms reach the bone through the blood stream from a septic focus elsewhere in the body—for instance from a boil in the skin. In a rare atypical form in adults infection reaches the vertebral column through the spinal venous plexus from an infected intrapelvic lesion.

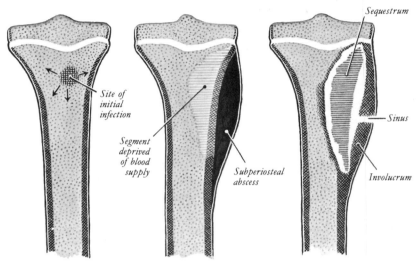

Fig. 48   Fig. 49   Fig. 50

The natural evolution of a focus of osteomyelitis. Figure 48—Initial lesion in the metaphysis. Figure 49—Pus has escaped to the surface of the bone and formed a subperiosteal abscess. Part of the bone has lost its blood supply from septic thrombosis of vessels. Figure 50—The devitalised area eventually separates as a sequestrum. Meanwhile new bone (involucrum) is formed beneath the stripped-up periosteum; it is perforated by sinuses through which pus escapes. This is the stage of chronic osteo-myelitis. With prompt treatment the disease can often be arrested at the stage shown in Figure 48.

In the usual childhood manifestation, the infection begins in the metaphysis of a long bone, which must be presumed to form a productive medium for bacterial growth (Fig. 48); thence it may spread to involve a large part of the bone. The organisms induce an acute inflammatory reaction, but the marshalling of the body's defensive forces is greatly handicapped in bone because its rigid structure does not allow swelling. Pus is formed and soon finds its way to the surface of the bone where it forms a subperiosteal abscess (Fig. 49); later the abscess may burst into the soft tissues and may eventually reach the surface to form a sinus.

Often the blood supply to a part of the bone is cut off by septic thrombosis of the vessels (Fig. 49). The ischaemic bone dies and eventually separates from the surrounding living bone as a sequestrum (Fig. 50). Meanwhile new bone is laid down beneath the stripped-up periosteum, forming an investing layer known as the involucrum (Fig. 50).

The epiphysial cartilage plate is a barrier to the spread of infection, but if the affected metaphysis lies partly within a joint cavity the joint is liable to become infected (acute pyogenic arthritis). Metaphyses that lie wholly or partly within a joint cavity include the upper metaphysis of the humerus, all the metaphyses at the elbow, and the upper and lower metaphyses of the femur (Fig. 51). Even when the joint is not infected it may swell from an effusion of clear fluid (sympathetic effusion).

Fig. 51
The metaphyses shown in black are wholly or partly intracapsular. Infection at one of these sites is liable to involve the adjacent joint, with consequent pyogenic arthritis.

With efficient treatment, the infection may be aborted in its earliest phase. But when it has progressed to the stage of septic thrombosis and death of bone it almost inevitably passes into a state of chronic osteomyelitis.

Clinical features. Except for rare exceptions acute haematogenous osteomyelitis is confined to children, especially boys. The bones most commonly affected are the tibia, the femur and the humerus. The onset is rapid. The child complains of feeling ill, and of severe pain over the affected bone. There may be a history of recent boils or of a minor injury.

On examination there is obvious constitutional illness with pyrexia. Locally there is exquisite tenderness over the affected bone. The area of tenderness is clearly circumscribed; it is usually near the end of the bone in the metaphysial region. The overlying skin is warmer than normal, and often the soft tissues are indurated; later a fluctuant abscess may be present. The neighbouring joint is sometimes distended with clear fluid, but a good range of movement is retained. (In the event of associated septic arthritis movement would be greatly restricted.)

Imaging. *Radiographic examination* in the early stage does not show any alteration from the normal (Fig. 53). Only after two or three weeks do visible changes appear, and they may never do so if efficient treatment is

Fig. 52
Osteomyelitis of the femur in an infant, three weeks after onset. Note new bone outlining the raised periosteum, and area of rarefaction in metaphysis and epiphysis. The infection spread to the knee joint.

Fig. 53 **Fig. 54**
Acute osteomyelitis of the ulna in a child. Figure 53—The initial film taken two days after the onset does not show any abnormality. Figure 54—Two weeks later a faint shadow along the radial side of the ulna denotes new bone formation beneath the raised periosteum.

started very early. The important changes are diffuse rarefaction of the metaphysial area and new bone outlining the raised periosteum (Figs 52 and 54).

Radioisotope scanning with ^{99m}technetium is reserved for the diagnosis of bone infection in the less clinically accessible sites such as the hip, pelvis and spine. Accumulation of isotope depends upon the rate of bone turnover and its vascularity, so that in the early stages of disease inadequate blood supply may result in a 'cold' lesion. More commonly, within a few hours or days of the onset of symptoms there is an increased uptake of isotope, giving a 'hot' scan at the site of the bone lesion. In the more obscure low-grade infections associated with prostheses and other surgical implants in bone, scanning with re-injected leucocytes labelled with ^{111m}indium may provide improved diagnostic accuracy.

Investigations. Blood culture may be positive in the incipient stage but this is not an invariable feature. Later there is a marked polymorphonuclear leucocytosis. The erythrocyte sedimentation rate is increased.

Diagnosis. Acute osteomyelitis is to be distinguished from pyogenic arthritis of the adjacent joint by the following features: 1) the point of greatest tenderness is over the bone rather than the joint; 2) a good range of joint movement is retained; and 3) although the joint may be distended with

Fig. 55
Two complications of osteomyelitis. Figure 55—Pyogenic arthritis, which led in this case to bony ankylosis. Figure 56—Arrest of epiphysial growth, with consequent shortening. The normal humerus is shown for comparison.

Fig. 56

fluid it does not contain pus (this may be confirmed by aspiration). Acute osteomyelitis may also be confused with poliomyelitis (which in the early stages is associated with limb pain), with rheumatic fever, and, in infants, with vitamin C deficiency (scurvy) (p. 64) or syphilitic metaphysitis (p. 78). Whenever possible the causative organism must be identified bacteriologically. It is important that blood for culture be taken before antibiotic therapy is commenced.

Complications. The important complications are: 1) septicaemia or pyaemia; 2) extension of infection to the adjacent joint with consequent pyogenic arthritis (Fig. 55); and 3) retardation of growth from damage to the epiphysial cartilage (Fig. 56). Acute osteomyelitis often passes into a state of chronic infection.

Treatment. Efficient treatment must be begun at the earliest possible moment.

General treatment. This is by rest in bed and systemic antibiotic therapy, started intravenously to ensure high blood levels. Initially, it is recommended that reliance be placed upon a combination of flucloxacillin and fusidic acid, or of flucloxacillin and ampicillin in children under 5; but as soon as the causative organism has been identified the antibiotic to which it is most sensitive should be ordered. Antibiotics should be continued for at least four weeks, even when the response has been rapid.

Local treatment. The question of operation and its timing is still controversial. Operation may be unnecessary if effective antibiotic treatment can be begun within twenty-four hours of the onset of symptoms, and this should always be the aim. But in practice diagnosis is not always so prompt, and in that event it seems wiser to undertake early operation, in order to release pus and to relieve pain, which is often severe. Release of pus may also reduce the risk of ischaemic bone necrosis; and furthermore it allows the organism to be identified and its sensitivity to antibiotics determined. An incision is made down to the bone and subperiosteal pus is evacuated. It is advisable—though not always essential—to make one or two drill holes through the cortex to improve medullary drainage. In most cases the wound may safely be sutured. Thereafter the limb is splinted until the infection is overcome.

OSTEOMYELITIS COMPLICATING OPEN FRACTURE OR SURGICAL OPERATION

When acute infection complicates open fracture or surgical operation the organisms are introduced directly through the wound. Any part of the bone may be affected, depending upon the site of injury. Suppuration and necrosis occur as in haematogenous osteomyelitis, but the pus discharges through the primary wound rather than collecting under the periosteum. The infection often becomes chronic.

Clinical features. This type of osteomyelitis may occur in children or in adults. The temperature fails to settle after the primary treatment of the wound or rises a few days later. Pain is not a prominent feature because pus is not contained under tension. Re-examination of the wound reveals a purulent discharge.

Radiographic features. In the early stages radiographs do not help significantly. Later there may be local rarefaction, and eventually sequestrum formation may be evident.

Treatment. The main principle of treatment is to secure free drainage through the wound, which may be enlarged if necessary for the purpose. Appropriate antibacterial drugs should be ordered. Later, any bone fragment that has sequestrated should be removed.

CHRONIC OSTEOMYELITIS
(Chronic pyogenic osteomyelitis)

Chronic osteomyelitis is nearly always a sequel to acute osteomyelitis. Occasionally infection is subacute or chronic from the beginning.

Cause. As with acute osteomyelitis, the staphylococcus is the usual causative organism, but streptococci, pneumococci, typhoid bacilli, or other bacteria may be responsible.

Pathology. It is commonest in the long bones. It is often confined to one end of the bone, but it may affect the whole length. The bone is thickened and generally denser than normal, though often honeycombed with granulation tissue, fibrous tissue or pus. Sequestra are commonly present within cavities in the bone. Often a sinus track leads to the skin surface: the sinus tends to heal and break down recurrently, but if a sequestrum is present it never heals permanently.

Fig. 57
Extensive chronic osteomyelitis of the tibia. The upper part of the shaft is thickened and shows patchy sclerosis. Two cavities are evident, each containing a sequestrum.

Clinical features. The main symptom is usually a purulent discharge from a sinus over the affected bone. In other cases pain is the predominant feature which brings the patient to the doctor. Discharge of pus may be continuous or intermittent. Reappearance of a sinus that has been healed for some time is heralded by local pain, pyrexia, and the formation of an abscess. This is termed a 'flare-up', or 'flare', of infection.

On examination the bone is palpably thickened, and there are nearly always a number of overlying scars or sinuses.

Imaging. *Radiographic examination*: The bone is thickened and shows irregular and patchy sclerosis which may give a honeycombed appearance. If a sequestrum is present it is seen as a dense loose fragment, with irregular but sharply demarcated edges, lying within a cavity in the bone (Fig. 57). *Radioisotope scanning* may show increased uptake in the vicinity of the lesion. In diffuse disease *CT scanning* may be of value for localisation of abscess cavities and sequestra, thus allowing accurate planning of operative treatment.

Complications. If the bone has been much weakened by disease pathological fracture may occur. Rarely, amyloid disease may complicate long-continued chronic osteomyelitis with persistent discharge of pus. Another rare complication in cases of many years' duration is the development of squamous celled carcinoma in a sinus.

Treatment. An acute flare-up of chronic osteomyelitis often subsides with rest and antibiotics. If an abscess forms outside the bone it must be drained. If there is a persistent and profuse discharge of pus a more extensive operation is advised. The aim should be to remove fragments of infected dead bone (sequestra) and to open up or 'saucerise' abscess cavities by chiselling away the overlying bone. Sometimes it is possible to obliterate a cavity with a flap of muscle, or to exteriorise it and line its walls directly with split-skin grafts.

Fig. 58
Brodie's abscess. The cavity in the tibia is surrounded by a zone of sclerosis.

BRODIE'S ABSCESS (Chronic bone abscess)
This is a special form of chronic osteomyelitis which arises insidiously, without a preceding acute attack. There is a localised abscess within the bone, often near the site of the metaphysis. A deep 'boring' pain is the predominant symptom. *Radiographically*, the lesion is seen as a circular or oval cavity surrounded by a zone of sclerosis (Fig. 58). The rest of the bone is normal. *Treatment* is by operation. The cavity is de-roofed and the pus evacuated. Whenever possible the cavity should be filled with a muscle flap to obliterate the dead space.

TUBERCULOUS INFECTION OF BONE

Tuberculous infection of bone is uncommon except in the vertebral bodies and in association with tuberculous infection of joints. Occasionally it occurs as an isolated lesion in a long bone or in a bone of the hand or foot.

Pathology. Tubercle bacilli reach the bone either through the blood stream or by direct extension from an adjacent focus of infection in joint or soft tissue. There is a typical tuberculous inflammatory reaction. Part of the bone is destroyed and replaced by granulation tissue. A tuberculous abscess is commonly formed; it tracks beneath the soft tissues or towards the surface of the body. With treatment there is a tendency to healing, with fibrosis.

Tuberculosis of a vertebra. The infection typically affects the vertebral body. It may arise initially in the bone (Fig. 59) or it may spread to the vertebra from the adjacent intervertebral disc. Tuberculous vertebral bodies collapse anteriorly but often retain their full depth behind, thereby becoming wedge-shaped (Fig. 60). An abscess usually tracks downwards along the vertebral column; it may also extend backwards towards the spinal canal, where it may interfere with the spinal cord.

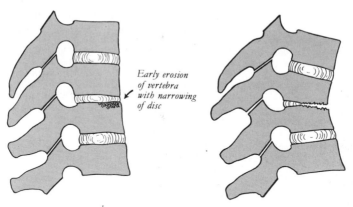

Early erosion of vertebra with narrowing of disc

Fig. 59   **Fig. 60**

Tuberculosis beginning in a vertebral body. The infection starts close to the anterior border and adjacent to an intervertebral disc (Fig. 59). It soon involves the disc and may spread to adjoining vertebrae. The bone destruction is most marked anteriorly; so the affected vertebral bodies become wedge-shaped (Fig. 60).

Fig. 61

Juxta-articular tuberculous focus in the neck of the femur. There is no sclerosis of the surrounding bone. If unchecked by treatment, such a focus of infection may spread to involve the joint.

Fig. 62

Tuberculous dactylitis. The affected phalanx has been 'distended' by destruction of the original cortex and the laying down of new cortical bone beneath the expanded periosteum.

Juxta-articular tuberculosis. The articular ends of bones are frequently eroded by tuberculosis beginning primarily in the joint. Less often there is an isolated focus of infection within the bone (Fig. 61). From such a lesion the infection may spread eventually to the neighbouring joint.

Bony tuberculosis in the hand or foot. The metacarpals or phalanges are the bones most commonly affected (tuberculous dactylitis). Characteristically the bone is enlarged by a fusiform swelling which at first represents thickened and raised periosteum. Later, much of the original bone is destroyed, but at the same time new bone is laid down beneath the expanded periosteum, giving the affected metacarpal or phalanx a 'distended' appearance (Fig. 62). Similar changes may affect a bone of the foot, or occasionally a long bone.

Clinical features. There is usually evidence of constitutional ill health. The local symptoms and signs depend upon the site of the infection. In general, pain is the initial symptom; and at most sites it is associated with obvious swelling and often with the formation of a 'cold' abscess. When the bone lesion is associated with tuberculous joint disease the joint symp-toms predominate (see sections on the individual joints).

Imaging. The typical *radiographic features* of tuberculous infection of bone are: 1) diffuse rarefaction around the site of infection; 2) erosion or 'eating away' of bone, leaving a fluffy, ill defined outline with no suggestion of a surrounding zone of sclerosis; and 3) in many cases a shadow in the soft tissues, denoting abscess formation. On *radioisotope scanning* there is increased uptake of isotope in the vicinity of the lesion.

Investigations. Except in the case of quite small lesions the erythrocyte sedimentation rate is raised. The Mantoux test is positive. Aspirated pus is yellow and creamy: only occasionally can organisms be identified by direct examination, but culture may prove its tuberculous nature. Biopsy of affected bone or surrounding soft tissue will show the histological features of tuberculosis.

Diagnosis. The diagnosis can often be presumed with fair certainty from a consideration of the history, clinical features, and radiographic findings. Features that lend support are a history of contact with tuberculosis, a positive Mantoux test (particularly in children), a raised erythrocyte sedimentation rate, and evidence of a tuberculous lesion elsewhere. The diagnosis can be proved only by identifying the causative organism or by demonstration of the typical histological features in excised fragments of tissue.

Treatment. In most instances tuberculosis of bone is associated with infection of a joint, and the treatment is mainly that of the joint lesion (tuberculous arthritis, p. 117). The treatment of an isolated tuberculous focus in bone is along similar lines, main reliance being placed upon a combination of antituberculous drugs, as outlined on page 120. Local collections of pus should be removed by aspiration or, sometimes, by operative drainage followed by immediate suture of the wound. Resolution is indicated by improvement in the general health and weight, decrease of erythrocyte sedimentation rate, and improved radiographic appearance.

SYPHILITIC INFECTION OF BONE

In Western countries syphilitic infection of bone is uncommon. But it is still common in some parts of the world, and it is important that the possibility of its occurrence should be borne constantly in mind. Bone changes are a late manifestation of acquired syphilis, but they may appear early in life in patients with congenital syphilis. Similar bone changes may occur in yaws, a related disease seen commonly in many tropical countries.

Syphilis of bone can take many forms. Only two will be described here: 1) syphilitic metaphysitis of infants; and 2) osteo-periostitis (combined osteitis and periostitis) in children or adults.

SYPHILITIC METAPHYSITIS

This is an affection of young infants with congenital syphilis.

Pathology. Several metaphyses are affected. The zone of temporary calcification next to the epiphysial cartilage—normally seen in section as a thin grey line—is widened and yellowish. The adjacent part of the metaphysis is partly replaced by granulation tissue.

Clinical features. The condition affects infants in the first six months of life. There may be severe local pain, in consequence of which the child refuses to use the affected limb (pseudoparalysis): there is no actual loss of muscle power. *On examination* the metaphysial region is thickened and tender.

Radiographic features. Radiographs are characteristic. The part of the metaphysis adjacent to the epiphysial cartilage shows a zone of sclerosis whereas the rest of the metaphysis is rarefied (Fig. 63). Often there is also evidence of periostitis in the form of subperiosteal new bone in the metaphysis and adjacent part of the shaft.

Investigations. The Wassermann reaction is positive.

Diagnosis. The condition may be confused with acute osteomyelitis, but the absence of leucocytosis and the positive Wassermann reaction help to distinguish the two. Metaphysitis may also be confused with scurvy, but the other features of scurvy (haemorrhage from the gums and elsewhere) are absent. Moreover, scurvy occurs in the second six months of life rather than the first.

Treatment. Intensive antisyphilitic measures are rapidly effective.

Figs 63 and 64
Two examples of congenital syphilis of bone. Figure 63—Metaphysitis in an infant. Note white lines at ends of metaphyses, with adjacent zones of rarefaction. Figure 64—Osteo-periostitis in a child. New bone has been laid down in layers under the periosteum.

Fig. 63   Fig. 64

SYPHILITIC OSTEO-PERIOSTITIS

When the diaphysis or body of a bone is infected by syphilis there is usually a combination of osteitis and periostitis, although one or other may predominate. Osteo-periostitis often occurs with metaphysitis in infants; it may occur separately in older children with congenital syphilis (Fig. 64), or in adults with acquired syphilis.

Pathology. Of the long bones, the tibia is most commonly affected. Other bones sometimes involved are the femur, the skull, the clavicle, and the bones of the hand or foot (syphilitic dactylitis). The bone is infiltrated with syphilitic granulation tissue, which may undergo central necrosis. The extent of the lesion varies from case to case. There may be no more than a localised thickening, or there may be diffuse infiltration of the whole of the bone (Fig. 66). The texture of the diseased bone also varies: the bone structure may be partly replaced by granulation tissue, or the formation of much new bone may lead to well marked sclerosis.

Clinical features. Deep boring pain, worse at night, and swelling are the predominant symptoms. *On examination* there is either a localised fusiform swelling over the shaft of the bone or a diffuse thickening of the whole length of the bone.

Radiographic features. Syphilitic bone disease is represented by a variety of radiographic changes ranging from severe osteoporosis to dense sclerosis. The commonest appearances are: 1) widespread subperiosteal new bone (Fig. 64); 2) a localised area of destruction or rarefaction, with dense thickening of the overlying cortex (Fig. 65); and 3) diffuse sclerotic thickening of the whole bone (Fig. 66). Occasionally the predominant change is bone destruction without new bone formation.

Investigations. The Wassermann reaction is positive.

Figs 65 and 66
Acquired syphilis of bone. Two examples of osteo-periostitis seen in diagrammatic section. Figure 65— Zone of destruction surrounded by localised area of thickening. Figure 66—Diffuse sclerotic thickening of the whole shaft.

Fig. 65   **Fig. 66**

Diagnosis. Syphilis of bone or periosteum is easily confused with a malignant bone tumour. Mistakes will be avoided if syphilis is considered as a possibility in every case of localised swelling in a limb. A positive Wassermann reaction lends support to the possibility, and the diagnosis is confirmed if there is rapid improvement under antisyphilitic treatment. This therapeutic test may eliminate the need for biopsy in cases of limb swellings of doubtful nature.

Treatment. The bone lesions usually respond well to intensive antisyphilitic measures.

TUMOURS OF BONE

Bone tumours are subdivided into benign or malignant types, and malignant tumours are further classified as primary or secondary (metastatic). It is necessary here to consider only four types of benign bone tumour and six types of malignant tumour.

BENIGN TUMOURS OF BONE

The following types will be described: 1) osteoma; 2) chondroma; 3) osteochondroma; 4) giant-cell tumour.

OSTEOMA

This forms a smooth rounded prominence upon the surface of a long or a flat bone, or of a skull bone (Fig. 67). It may be composed of hard compact bone (ivory osteoma) or of spongy bone (cancellous osteoma). Apart from visible or palpable swelling there are usually no symptoms.

BENIGN TUMOURS OF BONE

Fig. 67
Osteoma. It may occur on any bone, including the bones of the skull.

Fig. 68
Two types of chondroma: ecchondroma on proximal phalanx; enchondroma in middle phalanx. (See also Figs 31 and 32.)

Fig. 67

Fig. 68

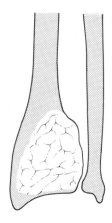

Fig. 69
A small and a large osteochondroma. Originating at the growth cartilage, they have migrated away from it with growth of the bone. Each is capped by cartilage. (See also Fig. 30.)

Fig. 70
Giant-cell tumour (osteoclastoma). Note expansion of cortex and scanty fine trabeculae within the tumour. The tumour extends close up to the articular surface. (See also Fig. 71.)

Treatment. It may either be left alone or excised, according to the circumstances of each case.

CHONDROMA

This is a tumour composed of cartilage.

Pathology. There are two forms of chondroma: in one the tumour grows outwards from a bone (ecchondroma); in the other it grows within a bone and expands it (enchondroma) (Fig. 68). Most *ecchondromata* arise in the hands or feet, or from flat bones such as the scapula or ilium. They often reach a large size. *Enchondromata* are fairly common in the bones of the hands and feet: the affected bone is expanded by the tumour and its cortex is much thinned; so pathological fracture is common.

Chondromata of the major long bones occur mainly in the distinct clinical condition known as dyschondroplasia (multiple chondromatosis or Ollier's disease) (p. 49). In this disorder, which begins in childhood, enchondromata arise in the region of the growing epiphysial cartilages (growth plates) of several bones: they interfere with normal growth at the epiphysial plate and consequently may lead to shortening or deformity (see Fig. 31).

Occasionally a chondroma undergoes malignant change, becoming a chondrosarcoma: when this occurs it is usually in one of the major bones rather than in the small bones of the hands or feet.

Treatment. A chondroma is often best left alone. If it causes trouble or is unsightly it should be removed if removal is practicable.

OSTEOCHONDROMA
(Osteocartilaginous exostosis)

This is the commonest benign tumour of bone.

Pathology. It originates in childhood from the growing epiphysial cartilage plate, but as the bone grows in length the tumours gets 'left behind' and thus appears to migrate along the shaft towards its centre. It grows outwards from the bone like a mushroom (Fig. 69). The stalk and part of the head of the tumour are of bone, but it is capped by cartilage. The tumour continues to enlarge until the cessation of skeletal growth, and even thereafter the cap of cartilage may persist.

The ordinary osteochondroma is single; but in the condition known as diaphysial aclasis (multiple exostoses) (p. 48) the tumours affect several or many bones. Rarely, malignant change to a chondrosarcoma occurs in one of the tumours.

Clinical features. The tumour is noticed as a circumscribed hard swelling near a joint. In severe examples of diaphysial aclasis there is interference with skeletal growth and the patient may be deformed or dwarfed.

Radiographs show the mushroom-like bony tumour but not the cartilaginous cap. The stalk is often narrow.

Treatment. The tumour should be excised if it causes pain or if it enlarges after puberty.

GIANT-CELL TUMOUR
(Osteoclastoma)

This is an important tumour because, though generally classed as benign, it tends to recur after local removal or curettage. In about 10 per cent of cases it behaves as a frankly malignant tumour, metastasising through the blood stream. It occurs most commonly in young adults.

Pathology. The commonest sites are the lower end of the femur, the upper end of the tibia, the lower end of the radius, and the upper end of the humerus—that is, at those ends of the long bones at which most growth occurs. Characteristically it occurs in the end of the bone, occupying the epiphysial region and often extending almost to the joint surface (Figs 70 and 71). It destroys the bone substance, but new bone forms beneath the raised periosteum, so that the bone end becomes expanded. A few bone trabeculae may remain within the tumour, giving a faintly loculated appearance. Pathological fracture is common.

Fig. 71
Giant-cell tumour of bone at a common site. The tumour, faintly loculated, has destroyed most of one femoral condyle. It extends close up to the articular surface.

Histologically the tumour consists of abundant oval or spindle-shaped cells profusely interspersed with giant cells that may contain as many as fifty nuclei (Fig. 72). The giant cells possibly represent fused conglomerations of the oval or spindle-shaped cells. They do not resemble osteoclasts closely, nor do they behave like them: hence the name 'giant-cell tumour' is preferred to 'osteoclastoma'. The actual cell of origin is uncertain.

A giant-cell tumour often recurs after incomplete removal. When it is malignant it metastasises readily, especially to the lungs.

Clinical features. The symptoms are pain at the site of the tumour and a gradually increasing local swelling. Sometimes the patient is made suddenly aware that something is wrong by the occurrence of a pathological fracture. Examination reveals a bony swelling which may be tender on firm palpation.

Imaging. *Radiographs* show destruction of the bone substance, with expansion of the cortex (Fig. 71). The tumour tends to grow eccentrically, and often extends as far as the articular end of the bone. Computerised tomographic scanning or magnetic resonance imaging will help to determine the extent of the tumour.

Radioisotope (technetium) scanning will show increased uptake of the injected isotope in the area of the lesion.

Fig. 72

A typical giant-cell tumour of bone, showing abundant oval and spindle-shaped cells with many multinucleated giant cells scattered among them. (Haematoxylin and eosin × 150.)

Treatment. This depends upon the site of the tumour. If the affected bone is one that can reasonably be dispensed with, such as the clavicle or fibula, excision of part of the bone or even the whole bone is recommended, to ensure complete removal of the tumour. But if the affected bone is one whose removal would cause severe disability, such as the femur, the problem is much more difficult. Curettage followed by packing with bone grafts is often undertaken, but it is attended by a high rate (30–40 per cent) of recurrence, which at the worst may then necessitate amputation. Probably the wisest course, therefore, is to advise wide local excision, even if this entails sacrifice of a major joint such as the knee or shoulder, which may have to be fused by bone grafts or replaced by a metal prosthesis. Radiotherapy is capable sometimes of bringing about permanent cure, but there is a risk that it may itself induce malignant change, perhaps many years later. It should therefore be confined to tumours at sites that are inaccessible to operation, particularly in the spinal column.

MALIGNANT TUMOURS OF BONE

Classification. In the past there has been some confusion in the nomenclature and classification of primary malignant tumours of bone, largely because of difficulties in the interpretation of their histological and radiological features. One difficulty is that tumours of different origin sometimes appear very much alike. For instance, a tumour derived from primitive bone cells (osteosarcoma) may consist predominantly of fibroblasts and may thus resemble a fibrosarcoma; or the predominant tissue may be cartilaginous and thus suggest a chondrosarcoma. Sometimes it is even difficult to distinguish between a primary and a metastatic tumour: a Ewing's sarcoma, for example, may resemble very closely a metastatic neuroblastoma. The fact that the radiological features of many of these tumours are also variable has added to the difficulties of classification. It will be clear from this that the differential diagnosis of a malignant bone tumour may be very difficult. A careful assessment of all the features—clinical, radiological, histological and biochemical—is always required.

It should be noted that primary malignant tumours of bone are uncommon. Secondary (metastatic) tumours are seen much more often than primary tumours.

In this brief review malignant tumours of bone will be classified and described under the following headings (the first five being primary tumours): 1) osteosarcoma (osteogenic sarcoma); 2) chondrosarcoma of bone; 3) fibrosarcoma of bone[1]; 4) Ewing's tumour; 5) multiple myeloma (plasmacytoma); 6) secondary (metastatic) tumours.

OSTEOSARCOMA
(Osteogenic sarcoma)

This is predominantly a tumour of childhood or adolescence. When it occurs in later life it is often a complication of Paget's disease (osteitis deformans).

Pathology. An osteosarcoma arises from primitive bone-forming cells. The commonest sites are the lower end of the femur, the upper end of the tibia, and the upper end of the humerus—that is, in those areas in which, prior to epiphysial fusion, most active growth is occurring. The tumour begins in the metaphysis. It destroys the bone structure and eventually bursts into the surrounding soft tissues, though it seldom crosses the epiphysial cartilage into the epiphysis (Fig. 73). The histological appearance varies widely, because any type of connective tissue may be represented. Thus the tumour may be composed largely of fibrous tissue, of cartilage or of myxomatous tissue; but characteristically there will always be found, in some parts of the tumour, areas of neoplastic new bone or osteoid tissue that indicate the true nature of the lesion, and in some cases newly formed bone is abundant (Fig. 77). The tumour metastasises early by the blood stream, especially to the lungs and sometimes to other bones.

Clinical features. There are local pain and swelling, which gradually increase. Examination reveals a diffuse firm thickening near the end of a bone, close to the joint. The overlying skin is warmer than normal because of the vascularity of the tumour; and the part may be so distended by tumour that the skin appears stretched and shiny.

Imaging. *Plain radiographs* show irregular destruction of the metaphysis. Later the cortex appears to have been 'burst open' at one or more places, but there are always vestiges of the original cortex. There is usually evidence of new bone formation under the corners of the raised periosteum (Codman's triangle) (Fig. 78). Occasionally well marked radiating spicules of new bone are seen within the tumour ('sun-ray' appearance). In a parosteal sarcoma there may be profuse formation of new bone (Fig. 79). A chest radiograph may show pulmonary metastases (Fig. 80).

---

[1]Fibrosarcoma of soft tissue must be considered separately: it is described on page 106.

FOUR MALIGNANT TUMOURS OF BONE

Fig. 73
Osteosarcoma. It arises in the metaphysis. Note the destruction of bone, the raising of the periosteum with new bone formed beneath it, and disruption of the cortex by the tumour. The appearance is variable, and the formation of neoplastic bone by the tumour may be profuse or scanty. (See also Fig. 78.)

Fig. 74
Ewing's tumour. It arises in the diaphysis. Note the central area of destruction and concentric layers of subperiosteal new bone giving an 'onion-peel' appearance.

Fig. 73

Fig. 74

Fig. 75
Multiple myeloma. Small 'punched-out' osteolytic tumours are scattered throughout the skeleton, especially in bone containing abundant red marrow.

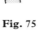

Fig. 76
Metastatic tumours in bone, as found in disseminated carcinoma. Note the circumscribed destruction of bone without any periosteal reaction. Metastatic tumours in bone are very much more common than primary malignant bone tumours.

Fig. 75

Fig. 76

Radioisotope (technetium) scanning shows increased uptake at the site of the tumour and provides additional information on the intramedullary spread by 'skip' lesions. *CT scanning* is more accurate in defining the actual tumour size and the extent of any invasion of soft tissues, though *MRI scanning* is even better for the purpose (Fig. 14, p. 19). CT scanning of the lung fields can also detect small pulmonary metastases before they are apparent in conventional radiographs.

Fig. 77
Section illustrating the varied histological appearance that may be presented by an osteosarcoma. At the extreme left is a darkly-stained remnant of old mature bone. Adjacent to this is an area of fibroblastic tumour tissue. Above this and to the right is atypical immature bone produced by the tumour. (Azan stain × 100.)

Fig. 78
An osteosarcoma at the commonest site. The tumour has destroyed much of the lower end of the femur and has burst through the cortex into the soft tissues. Though profuse new bone formation is a feature of some of these tumours, in this case (as in many others) the tumour is mainly osteolytic and there is evidence of neoplastic bone only in small scattered patches. Another example is shown in Figure 12, page 18.

Diagnosis. In atypical cases an osteosarcoma may be confused with subacute osteomyelitis, with syphilis of bone, or with other bone tumours such as chondrosarcoma, fibrosarcoma, giant-cell tumour, Ewing's tumour, or a metastatic tumour. A representative piece of the tumour should be removed for histological examination (see biopsy p. 35).

Fig. 79

Parosteal sarcoma of femur. At right (above) is a computerised tomographic scan of the normal femur, and (below) a comparable scan of the affected femur at the level of the tumour.

Fig. 80

Pulmonary metastases in a case of osteosarcoma of the tibia. Such metastases are the usual cause of death.

Prognosis. Until recently the mortality—usually from pulmonary metastases—was in the region of 80 per cent even after amputation. Present evidence suggests, however, that the prognosis may be greatly improved—or survival at least extended—by intensive adjuvant treatment by chemotherapy.

Treatment. The introduction of new powerful cytotoxic drugs for adjuvant chemotherapy has revolutionised the treatment of these tumours, because of their ability to prevent or delay the appearance of pulmonary micrometastases. The drugs currently used include high-dose methotrexate, doxorubicin (Adriamycin), cisplatin, and ifosfamide in combinations which are the subject of multi-centre controlled trials. They all have major side effects and should only be used in treatment centres skilled in their use. Chemotherapy is usually commenced before surgical treatment, and is continued intermittently for six months to a year after ablation of the tumour. Commencing chemotherapy before operative treatment allows the pathologist to assess the response of the tumour to the drugs by histological examination of the resected specimen. The ability of chemotherapy to control local recurrence and distant metastatic spread has permitted the increasing use of 'limb salvage surgery' as an alternative to amputation. In selected cases, based on accurate surgical staging from biopsy and modern imaging techniques, it is possible to undertake radical resection and replacement with a metallic prosthesis or a massive bone graft. Recent reports have shown over 70 per cent disease-free survival after five years by this approach in patients with osteosarcoma, with no increase in local recurrence rates when compared with amputation (Goorin and Anderson 1991; Simon 1991).

CHONDROSARCOMA OF BONE

A chondrosarcoma is a malignant tumour derived from cartilage cells, and it tends to maintain its cartilaginous character throughout its evolution.

Pathology. It may develop in the interior of the bone (central chondrosarcoma) or upon its surface (peripheral chondrosarcoma). A *central chondrosarcoma* occurs most commonly in the femur, the tibia or the humerus. It may arise de novo, without there having been a pre-existing lesion, or it may arise from malignant transformation of a previously existing enchondroma (especially in the condition known as dyschondroplasia or multiple chondromatosis (p. 49)).

A *peripheral chondrosarcoma*, on the other hand, tends usually to affect a flat bone such as the innominate bone, the sacrum or the scapula, and it generally arises from malignant transformation of a previously existing osteochondroma (especially in the condition of diaphysial aclasis or multiple exostoses (p. 48)).

Histologically, a chondrosarcoma may be highly cellular. The cartilage cell nuclei tend to be swollen, and double nuclei may be seen. These features, suggestive of malignancy, may be found in only a few microscopic fields, the remainder of the tissue appearing relatively benign.

Clinical features. The patient is often a person of middle age, who complains of pain and local swelling, often in an area where there was known to be a previous lesion, such as diaphysial aclasis or dyschondroplasia. The tumour grows slowly and may attain a large size.

Imaging. *Radiographically,* a central chondrosarcoma is seen to grow at the expense of the bone and may burst through the cortex, whereas a peripheral chondrosarcoma shows as a soft-tissue shadow growing outwards from the surface of the bone. Both types characteristically show blotchy areas of calcification within the tumour mass. *CT* or *MR scanning* helps to define the extent of the tumour.

Prognosis. A chondrosarcoma grows slowly and does not metastasise early; so the prognosis is somewhat more favourable than it is for osteosarcoma.

Fig. 81

Chondrosarcoma of the tibia occurring in a previously existing osteochondroma in a patient with diaphysial aclasis. There is extensive calcification in the posterior extension of the tumour into the soft tissues, seen more clearly in the computerised tomographic scan on the right.

Treatment. When the tumour is favourably placed it may be possible to eradicate it by radical local excision and replacement of the bone by a metal prosthesis or bone graft, thus preserving the limb. Since adjuvant chemotherapy is not effective against chondrosarcoma, amputation must remain the treatment of choice unless adequate surgical margins can be achieved to permit resection.

FIBROSARCOMA OF BONE

Fibrosarcoma of bone is uncommon. It is a fibroblastic connective-tissue tumour which arises within a bone, and is therefore distinct from a fibrosarcoma of soft tissue that has invaded the bone from outside. It occurs mainly in young adults and, as with osteosarcoma, the femur and the tibia are the commonest sites. Pale and fleshy, the tumour grows at the expense of the bone and eventually bursts through the cortex. Histologically, it is composed of rather large fibroblasts which may be well differentiated or poorly differentiated according to the malignancy of the tumour. *Radiographically* the tumour is osteolytic (bone-destroying), and evidence of neoplastic new bone formation is absent. Other imaging techniques are the same as for osteosarcoma.

The prognosis is poor, but in the case of a well differentiated tumour it is more favourable than that of osteosarcoma.

Treatment. Amputation is usually to be advised. Nevertheless if biopsy shows a tumour that appears to be of low malignancy wide local excision may sometimes be considered if it is technically feasible. The tumour responds poorly to irradiation, but more encouraging results have been reported with adjuvant chemotherapy using the combinations of drugs effective in the management of osteosarcoma.

EWING'S TUMOUR
(Endothelial sarcoma of bone)

Ewing's tumour (endothelial sarcoma of bone) is an uncommon but highly malignant sarcoma that arises in bone marrow.

Pathology. The tumour is commonest in the shaft of the femur, tibia, or humerus. Unlike osteosarcoma it arises in the diaphysis rather than the metaphysis of a bone. It probably develops from endothelial elements within the bone marrow, though the precise cell of origin is not known. The tumour tissue is soft and vascular. As it expands it gradually destroys the bone substance. There is a striking reaction beneath the periosteum, where abundant new bone is formed in successive layers (Fig. 74). Histologically the tumour consists of sheets of uniform small round cells. The tumour metastasises early through the blood stream, especially to the lungs, and sometimes to other bones.

Clinical features. Children are the usual victims. Typically, there are local pain and swelling over one of the long bones, usually about the middle of the shaft (contrast osteosarcoma, which arises at the metaphysis). *On examination* the swelling is diffuse or fusiform, and of firm consistency. The overlying skin is warmer than normal owing to the vascularity of the tumour.

Imaging. *Radiographs* show destruction of bone substance and concentric layers of subperiosteal new bone ('onion-peel' appearance) (Fig. 74). *CT or MR scanning* will help to show the extent of the tumour. A chest radiograph or CT scan may show pulmonary metastases. *Radioisotope bone scanning* shows markedly increased uptake of the isotope in the region of the tumour.

Diagnosis. In atypical cases there may be confusion with subacute osteomyelitis, with syphilitic osteo-periostitis, or with other tumours. In particular, it may be confused histologically with a metastasis from a suprarenal neuroblastoma. Biopsy should be undertaken when the tumour is suspected.

Prognosis. The tumour used always to be fatal—usually from pulmonary metastases, with fewer than 15 per cent of patients surviving beyond five years. The advent of adjuvant chemotherapy has changed this gloomy outlook, and now five-year survival rates are recorded in 50–60 per cent of cases.

Treatment. Chemotherapy is slightly different from that used for osteo-sarcoma. A combination of vincristine, cyclophosphamide, actinomycin D and adriamycin is commonly recommended and is commenced as adjuvant therapy prior to any operative treatment. The tumour itself may be treated by radical operative excision with prosthetic replacement, or by amputation. Radiotherapy may be used as an alternative to operation, since the tumour is radiosensitive. Surgical ablation is preferred for lower limb lesions, particularly in young children where leg length discrepancy and joint contractures may follow radiotherapy. Radiotherapy is usually reserved for upper limb tumours and for tumours at inaccessible sites such as the pelvis and spine.

MULTIPLE MYELOMA

(Myelomatosis; plasmacytoma)

This is a uniformly fatal tumour of bone marrow, occurring in adults.

Pathology. It probably arises from the plasma cells of the bone marrow. It is disseminated to many parts of the skeleton through the blood stream, so that by the time the patient seeks advice the tumour foci are usually multiple, affecting chiefly the bones that contain abundant red marrow. Less commonly the tumour may present as a solitary bone lesion, with spread to other skeletal sites only after months or years. The lesions are mostly small and circumscribed (Figs 75 and 82) but occasionally large: the bone is simply replaced by tumour tissue and there is no reaction in the surrounding bone. Pathological fracture is common, especially in the spine (Fig. 82). Histologically the tumour consists of a mass of small round cells of plasma-cell type: the cells may be somewhat larger than normal plasma cells, and less uniform (Fig. 83).

Clinical features. In most cases the tumour affects adults past middle age. There is general ill health, with local pain at one or more of the tumour sites, or sometimes a pathological fracture. *On examination* the patient is pale, from the associated anaemia due to suppression of red marrow function. There is often local tenderness over the affected bones, but there may be no obvious swelling or deformity unless pathological fracture has occurred. The patient is prone to develop infections due to the suppression of normal antibody production.

Imaging. *Radiographs* show multiple small areas of transradiance, especially in bones containing red marrow, such as ribs, vertebral bodies, pelvic bones, skull, and proximal ends of femur and humerus (Figs 75 and 82). Sometimes there is diffuse rarefaction (Table III, p. 64).

Radioisotope bone scanning will show increased uptake of the isotope in the individual lesions.

Investigations. There is microcytic anaemia. The erythrocyte sedi-mentation rate is increased. Bence-Jones·proteose is present in the urine in

Fig. 82

Multiple myeloma. *Left*—Part of pelvis and femur, showing numerous small tumour foci. *Right*—Spine, showing diffuse rarefaction, with partial collapse of the bodies of the second and fourth lumbar vertebrae.

Fig. 83

Multiple myeloma. Sheets of cells resembling plasma cells.
(Haematoxylin and eosin × 400.)

more than half the cases. Serum globulin is increased, often so much that the albumin-globulin ratio (normally 2:1) is reversed. Marrow biopsy usually shows a profusion of plasma cells.

Diagnosis. Iliac or sternal marrow biopsy will often confirm the diagnosis when the clinical and radiographic features are equivocal.

Prognosis. The tumour is uniformly fatal, though its progress can often be checked for several years.

Treatment. The tumour foci respond to radiotherapy for a while, and pain is well relieved. The mainstay of chemotherapy in recent decades has been melphalan, an alkylating agent: this is sometimes used in conjunction with prednisolone. Trials are in progress of combination chemotherapy, melphalan being used in conjunction with doxorubicin, carmustine and cyclophosphamide, or in other combinations. In a favourable case remission for up to four years may be gained. The possible place of bone marrow transplantation is also under investigation.

SECONDARY (METASTATIC) TUMOURS IN BONE

Secondary malignant tumours in bone are much more common than primary tumours; but whereas most primary malignant bone tumours occur in children or young adults, secondary tumours generally occur in later life.

Pathology. The tumours that metastasise most readily to bone are carcinomas of the lung, breast, prostate, thyroid, and kidney (hypernephroma). Metastases occur most commonly in the parts of the skeleton that contain vascular marrow, especially the vertebral bodies, ribs, pelvis, and upper ends of the femur and humerus. The bone structure is simply destroyed and replaced by tumour tissue (Fig. 76). Pathological fracture is common.

Clinical features. Pain is the usual main symptom, but sometimes the disability is insignificant until a pathological fracture occurs. The spine is frequently involved, often with progressive neurological symptoms as well as local pain, from pressure on nerve roots or the spinal cord. In advanced widespread metastatic disease the patient may develop symptoms of hypercalcaemia, with nausea, vomiting, dehydration and even coma. The primary tumour can usually be demonstrated.

Analysis of the different types of clinical presentation has shown that 50 per cent of patients present initially with bone pain, 25 per cent with pathological fracture, 15 per cent with paraplegia or paraparesis, and 10 per cent with local swelling.

Imaging. In *plain radiographs* the bone appears to have been eaten away so that there is a clear circumscribed area of transradiance, without any reaction in the surrounding bone (Fig. 84). Exceptionally, new bone is laid down within the metastasis, causing marked sclerosis—the exact opposite to the usual osteolytic lesion. This type is almost confined to the secondary deposits from prostatic carcinoma. In cases of diffuse infiltration there may be widespread osteoporosis (Table III, p. 64). Chest radiographs should always be obtained because of the possibility that metastases may be present in the lungs.

Technetium isotope scanning is the best technique for detecting occult metastatic deposits in the skeleton as areas of increased uptake. These may be apparent up to eighteen months before they are visible in plain radiographs, making it a very sensitive screening method. Recent studies suggest that *magnetic resonance imaging* may be even more sensitive, particularly for the detection of spinal metastases.

Fig. 84
Typical appearance of a metastatic carcinoma in the humerus. The primary tumour was in the lung. With increasing destruction of bone, pathological fracture is likely to occur.

Investigations. In prostatic metastases the content of acid phosphatase in the plasma is usually increased above the normal range. The increase is specifically in the tartrate labile or 'prostatic' phosphatase. Hypercalcaemia may sometimes occur when there is excessive bone resorption from widespread bone metastases.

Treatment. Radiotherapy is a valuable palliative. Chemotherapy is sometimes appropriate (see p. 89). Radio-active iodine is valuable for metastases from carcinoma of the thyroid. Hormone analogue therapy may be appropriate for metastases from the breast or prostate, and in selected cases adrenalectomy and hypophysectomy have proved worthwhile in slowing the progress of the disease when other measures have failed. In the presence of life-threatening hypercalcaemia, treatment by biphosphonates is valuable in that it inhibits further bone resorption and may also relieve bone pain. Local splintage may be required, but internal fixation is used increasingly for the treatment of impending or established pathological fracture of the long bones as a means of maintaining function. Analgesics and sedatives may be given as required, and selective cordotomy is sometimes justified for severe intractable pain.

BONE CHANGES IN LEUKAEMIA AND LYMPHOMA

This is a convenient place to note that changes may occur in the skeleton in leukaemia and in Hodgkin's disease or related lymphomas. In *leukaemia* the changes are due to infiltration of bone by proliferating white cells, and they are seen most commonly in subacute lymphatic leukaemia in children. Characteristically there are zones of rarefaction with delicate subperiosteal new bone formation in the metaphysial regions of the femur or humerus, or in the spine or pelvis. Leukaemia is also an occasional cause of diffuse widespread rarefaction of the skeleton (Table III, p. 64).

In *Hodgkin's disease* or the related *lymphomas* there may be osteolytic lesions in the proximal limb bones or in the spine or pelvis, denoting destruction and replacement by tumour tissue.

OTHER LOCAL AFFECTIONS OF BONE

There is a miscellaneous group of solitary lesions of bone that do not fall into the category of infection or tumour. The most important members of the group are osteochondritis juvenilis, solitary bone cyst, localised fibrous dysplasia of bone, and osteoid osteoma.

OSTEOCHONDRITIS JUVENILIS
(Osteochondrosis)

The term osteochondritis juvenilis, or simply osteochondritis, is used to describe certain obscure affections of developing bony nuclei in children and adolescents. The term has also been used, wrongly, for some other affections of epiphyses or apophyses that are more likely traumatic in origin. Typically, a bony centre affected by osteochondritis becomes temporarily softened, and while in the softened state it is liable to deformation by pressure. The disease runs a course of variable length (often about three years), but eventually spontaneous rehardening occurs. The precise cause of the disease is unknown, but it is widely believed that temporary interruption of the blood supply to the affected epiphysis is the predominant factor. It should be noted that osteochondritis juvenilis is distinct from osteochondritis dissecans (p. 130).

Sites. Osteochondritis juvenilis is recognised at the following sites (Fig. 85), though the pathology may not be identical at each site: 1) the upper epiphysis of the femur (Perthes' or Legg-Perthes' disease, p. 312); 2) the nucleus of the navicular bone (Köhler's disease, p. 384); 3) Kienböck's disease of the lunate bone (p. 262) presents similar features and may be included in this group despite the fact that it occurs in fully developed adult bone; 4) the disorder of the head of the second or third metatarsal known as Freiberg's disease (p. 399) may possibly fall into the category of osteo-chondritis juvenilis, but there is a tendency now to ascribe it instead to osteochondritis dissecans. A similar radiographic change in the central epiphysis of a vertebral body (Calvé's disease, p. 189) is now generally ascribed to eosinophilic granuloma rather than to osteochondritis. And the affection of the 'ring' epiphyses of the vertebral bodies in the thoracic region known as Scheuermann's disease or adolescent kyphosis (p. 187), again formerly thought to be an example of osteochondritis, is also now believed to be of different pathology. In brief, only the sites shown in Figure 85 are now regarded as those where true osteochondritis commonly occurs.

Fig. 85
Common sites of osteochondritis or related changes. 1. Capital epiphysis of femur (Perthes). 2. Lunate bone (Kienböck). 3. Navicular bone (Köhler). 4. Head of second or third metatarsal (Freiberg).

Radiological appearances that bear some resemblance to the changes of osteochondritis are also seen in cases of pain at the apophysis of the tibial tubercle (Osgood-Schlatter's disease, p. 355) and at the apophysis of the calcaneus (Sever's disease, p. 386). These conditions were formerly thought to be examples of osteochondritis, but it is now recognised that they are traumatic in origin. There is simply a chronic strain of the apophysis from the pull of the tendon that is inserted into it. This type of lesion is now usually termed apophysitis.

Pathology. In a typical example of osteochondritis the histological and radiological evidence suggests that the affected bony centre undergoes partial necrosis, possibly from interference with its blood supply. The necrotic bone is invaded by granulation tissue, broken up, and eventually removed by osteoclasts. During this stage of fragmentation the centre is liable to deformation if subjected to pressure (Fig. 86). The dead tissue is gradually replaced by new living bone trabeculae and eventually the bone texture is restored to normal; but if deformation has been allowed to take place there is permanent alteration of shape.

Fig. 86
The cycle of changes in osteochondritis. 1. Normal epiphysis before onset. 2. The bony nucleus undergoes necrosis, loses its normal texture, and becomes granular. 3. The bony nucleus becomes fragmented during the process of removal of dead bone. 4. If subjected to pressure the softened epiphysis becomes flattened. 5. Re-ossification with restoration of normal bone texture, but deformity may persist. The cycle occupies two to three years.

Clinical features. The age at which the condition arises varies according to the particular bone affected. In general, it occurs during the stage of active development of the bony nucleus. The main symptom is local pain. If the affected epiphysis forms part of a joint, the function of the joint is disturbed and joint movement aggravates the pain. The general health is not impaired.

Imaging. *Radiographic examination.* The cycle of changes can be followed in serial radiographs taken at intervals of a few months. First there is a slight and often patchy increase in density of the bony nucleus. Next the patchy appearance passes to one of fragmentation, representing irregular absorption of dead bone by osteoclasts and the commencing deposition of new bone. At this stage some flattening of the nucleus may be apparent by comparison with the normal side. Later there is a gradual return to normal bone texture, but any flattening that has occurred will remain. *Radioisotope bone scanning* may show absence of uptake of the isotope during the stage at which the epiphysis is avascular.

Prognosis. Osteochondritis in itself is harmless to the general health, but if it leads to distortion of a joint surface it predisposes to osteoarthritis which, in the case of a large joint such as the hip, may cause serious disability in later years.

Treatment. The treatment depends largely upon the site of the affection. When the bony nucleus is relatively unimportant (as for instance that of the navicular bone) treatment may be unnecessary, or it may be sufficient to protect the part in a plaster for six or eight weeks while the pain is severe. But in the case of osteochondritis involving a major joint such as the hip every effort must be made to prevent distortion of the softened epiphysis.

Further details of these disorders will be found in the chapters dealing with individual regions.

SOLITARY BONE CYST
(Simple bone cyst; unicameral bone cyst)

Solitary bone cysts occur mostly in the long bones of children or adolescents, and especially near the proximal end of the humerus. They also occur occasionally in the small bones of the adult carpus, especially in the scaphoid or lunate bone.

Fig. 87
Simple cyst in upper metaphysis of humerus in a child. There has been a pathological fracture, now united with moderate angulation. The cyst has a loculated appearance.

Pathology. The cyst begins as a spherical lesion, but as it enlarges it tends to become oblong with its long diameter in the axis of the bone. In the long bones it tends to lie centrally in the shaft rather than to grow eccentrically, and the remaining cortex may appear expanded equally in all directions. The cyst contains clear fluid. It weakens the bone and often leads to pathological fracture. It is often stated that after a fracture through the wall of a cyst spontaneous filling in of the cyst may occur, but in fact this is unusual.

Histologically, a bone cyst has only a very thin connective-tissue lining. Its wall contains abundant osteoclasts, a fact that has led to confusion with giant-cell tumour.

Clinical features. Single bone cysts often cause no symptoms unless a pathological fracture occurs.

Radiographic features. Plain radiographs show a circumscribed area of transradiance without a surrounding zone of sclerosis (Fig. 87). The cyst may appear faintly loculated and the overlying cortex may be distended or fractured.

Diagnosis. A cyst must be differentiated from other osteolytic lesions. It may be confused with a bone abscess, with a lipoid or eosinophilic granulomatous deposit, with localised fibrous dysplasia, or occasionally with a tumour. It should be remembered also that cyst formation in bones may be a feature of hyperparathyroidism, which must therefore be considered in differential diagnosis. A solitary bone cyst is distinct from an aneurysmal bone cyst (see below).

Treatment. Small uncomplicated cysts do not require treatment, but they should be kept under periodic observation. A large cyst may be curetted and packed with bone chips, but aspiration and corticosteroid injection have now replaced operative treatment as the principal method of management (Scaglietti *et al.* 1982). If fracture occurs each case must be treated on its merits: bone grafting, preferably combined with rigid internal fixation, will sometimes be required.

ANEURYSMAL BONE CYST

Aneurysmal bone cysts also occur in children or young adults, but they are distinct from the solitary bone cysts described above. Their origin is unknown: the term 'aneurysmal' signifies no more than a seeming 'blown-out' distension of one surface of the bone (Jaffe 1958). There is no relationship to arterial aneurysm. The cyst may bulge into the soft tissues, contained only by periosteum and a thin shell of newly formed cortex. The lining consists of connective tissue with numerous vascular spaces and some giant cells; the cyst contains fluid blood.

Radiographic features. Plain radiographs show the cyst to be situated eccentrically in the bone; it presents a characteristic 'blown-out' appearance, as already mentioned. These features distinguish it from the ordinary solitary bone cyst, which is placed centrally in the shaft and expands the bone uniformly.

Treatment. If the bone that is affected can be discarded without consequent disability— for instance the fibula or a rib—the relevant part of the bone may be excised together with the cyst. At other accessible sites the cyst should be curetted out and filled with bone chips.

OSTEOID OSTEOMA

Osteoid osteoma is a benign circumscribed lesion of bone, of uncertain nature. It is generally regarded as a benign tumour, akin to an osteoblastoma.

Pathology. The characteristic feature is the formation of a small nidus of osteoid tissue, seldom more than half a centimetre in diameter, usually in the cortex of a long bone but occasionally in cancellous bone. In the long bones the central nidus of osteoid tissue is surrounded by an extensive zone of dense sclerotic bone which causes localised thickening of the shaft. Sclerosis is slight or absent when the lesion occurs in cancellous bone.

Clinical features. The only symptom is a severe deep 'boring' pain, which is ill localised and worst at night. Characteristically, the pain is eased by aspirin or its derivatives. There may be thickening and local tenderness at the site of the lesion.

Radiographic features. *Plain radiographs* typically show local sclerotic thickening of the shaft (Fig. 88), with a small central area of rarefaction which may however be largely obscured by the sclerotic bone. *Tomography* or *CT scanning* is likely to show the central lesion more clearly. *Radioisotope bone scanning* typically shows a well localised area of markedly increased isotope uptake—a sign that may be helpful in diagnosis.

Diagnosis. This is mainly from low-grade osteomyelitis, and especially from Brodie's chronic bone abscess.

Treatment. The nidus of osteoid tissue should be excised together with a margin of surrounding bone. This operation gives immediate and dramatic relief of pain.

Fig. 88
Osteoid osteoma of femur. Note the extensive thickening of the cortex, with small central nidus.

LOCALISED FIBROUS DYSPLASIA OF BONE
(Monostotic fibrous dysplasia)

In this condition a solitary area of bone is partly replaced by fibrous tissue, in which scanty bone trabeculae may persist. The cause is unknown, as also is its relationship to polyostotic fibrous dysplasia (p. 53). It is not related to the fibrous dysplasia of hyperparathyroidism.

Pathology. One of the limb bones is usually the site affected. The fibrous lesion expands at the expense of the bone, which is much weakened and may fracture.

Clinical features. There may be local pain in the affected bone, but many patients present with a coincidental x-ray finding.

Radiographs show a clear zone of transradiance within the bone. The area has a homogeneous 'ground-glass' appearance.

Treatment. If the lesion is seen to be extending, the affected segment of bone should be excised and replaced by a bone graft. Most lesions, however, are non-progressive and do not require operation.

METAPHYSIAL FIBROUS DEFECT
(Non-ossifying fibroma)

This is a benign defect in the metaphysial region of the cortex of a long bone, found accidentally from time to time in a child or young adult undergoing radiological examination for injury or for some other unconnected reason. The lesion is symptomless. *Radiographs* show a characteristic, well defined notching of the cortex of the affected long bone. Typically it has a scalloped, sclerotic border. *Treatment*, other than observation for a period, is not required, but if the diagnosis is in doubt the lesion should be excised.

References and bibliography, page 403.

6. Affections of soft tissue

INFLAMMATORY LESIONS OF SOFT TISSUE

BURSITIS

Inflammation may occur in a normally situated bursa or in an adventitious bursa. It may arise from mechanical irritation or from bacterial infection.

IRRITATIVE BURSITIS

This is caused by excessive pressure or friction, occasionally by a gouty deposit. There is a mild inflammatory reaction in the wall of the bursa, and there is usually an effusion of clear fluid within the sac. Examples are the common 'bunion' that forms over a prominent metatarsal head in hallux valgus, prepatellar bursitis or 'housemaid's knee', olecranon bursitis (sometimes caused by gout), and subacromial bursitis.

Treatment. In many cases the inflammation subsides with rest if continued pressure or friction is prevented. If the sac is distended the fluid may be aspirated, and the instillation of hydrocortisone through the aspiration needle may help to prevent recurrence. In resistant cases cure can be effected only by operative excision of the bursa.

INFECTIVE BURSITIS

There may be acute inflammation from infection by an organism of the pyogenic group, or chronic inflammation as in tuberculous bursitis. Examples of acute pyogenic bursitis are infected bunion, infected prepatellar bursitis and infected olecranon bursitis. A bursa that is sometimes affected by tuberculosis is the trochanteric bursa.

Treatment. Treatment of acute suppurative bursitis is by surgical drainage and antibacterial drugs. In chronic bursitis excision of the bursa is required.

TENOSYNOVITIS

The term tenosynovitis implies inflammation of the thin synovial lining of a tendon sheath as distinct from its outer fibrous sheath. Like bursitis, tenosynovitis may be caused by mechanical irritation or by bacterial infection.

IRRITATIVE (FRICTIONAL) TENOSYNOVITIS AND PERITENDINITIS

This is caused by excessive friction from over-use. The synovial sheath is mildly inflamed and there is an exudate of watery fluid within it. A similar traumatic inflammation may affect the flimsy paratenon surrounding those tendons that are devoid of synovial sheaths. This is termed paratendinitis (p. 254).

INFECTIVE TENOSYNOVITIS

Bacterial infection of a tendon sheath may be acute or chronic. Acute infective (suppurative) tenosynovitis is caused by an organism of the pyogenic group. There is an acute inflammatory reaction in the wall of the sheath, with a purulent exudate from it. It is an uncommon condition, but it is well recognised in the flexor tendon sheaths in the hand (p. 268).

In chronic bacterial tenosynovitis, also an uncommon lesion in Western countries, the infection is often tuberculous. The synovial wall is much thickened and there is a fibrinous exudate. The flexor sheaths of the forearm and hand are the usual sites (compound palmar ganglion, p. 268).

TENOVAGINITIS

In tenovaginitis there is a mild chronic inflammation or thickening of the fibrous wall of a tendon sheath as distinct from the synovial lining. The cause is unknown: it is not due to bacterial infection. The only common sites are the mouths of the fibrous flexor sheaths in the fingers or thumb ('trigger' finger, p. 279), and the sheaths of the extensor pollicis brevis and abductor pollicis longus tendons at the radial side of the wrist (de Quervain's syndrome, p. 278).

POLYMYALGIA RHEUMATICA

This connective tissue disorder has been recognised with increased frequency in older patients presenting with pain and stiffness in the muscles of the neck and shoulder girdle, or sometimes the low back and buttock regions. Because of these features it may be confused with degenerative disc disease, though characteristically the associated symptoms of malaise, low-grade fever, night sweats and loss of weight should lead to the diagnosis. It tends to be commoner in women than in men, usually affecting patients over the age of 60 years, and in about one-third of cases it is associated with the condition of giant-cell arteritis. This is a more serious disease as it may lead to sudden blindness because of involvement of the cranial arteries.

The clinical features are ill defined muscle pain around the shoulders or low back, with associated stiffness, and the characteristic features of systemic disturbance. When giant-cell arteritis is also present there may be marked tenderness over the temporal arteries. There may be marked elevation of the erythrocyte sedimentation rate, but the rheumatoid factor is negative. When associated giant-cell arteritis is suspected on clinical grounds, urgent administration of prednisolone in high doses is advisable pending confirmation of the diagnosis by biopsy, in order to reduce the risk of blindness. Both conditions show a good response to steroid therapy, usually in a dose of 15 milligrams of prednisolone daily. Once the clinical features have subsided this may be reduced to a maintenance dose of 5 milligrams daily.

FIBROSITIS

Fibrositis is a clinical rather than a pathological entity. Some deny its existence. Certainly its nature is obscure. Nevertheless the term is a useful label for a clinical condition that at present lacks a complete explanation. The main features are pain in certain muscles, with tenderness when they are gripped or squeezed. Small firm nodules may be felt. Joint movements are full and there are no other objective signs. The condition is commonest in the muscles of the back, especially in the trapezius area. Treatment, if required, is by non-steroidal anti-inflammatory medication and active exercises.

TUMOURS OF SOFT TISSUE

The soft-tissue tumours that are met with in orthopaedic practice arise from the connective tissues or blood vessels of the limbs or trunk. They may be benign or malignant. They usually present clinically as painless soft-tissue lumps, and cause symptoms only when quite large.

BENIGN TUMOURS OF SOFT TISSUE

In the soft tissue of the limbs and trunk benign tumours are much more common than malignant tumours. Five types will be described: 1) neurofibroma; 2) fibroma; 3) lipoma; 4) haemangioma; 5) desmoid tumour (fibromatosis).

NEUROFIBROMA

A neurofibroma forms a rather soft, circumscribed, rounded and slightly tender swelling in the skin or deeper tissues. It arises from the interstitial tissue of a peripheral nerve. Histologically it is composed of cellular fibrous tissue arranged in whorls. The tumour may be solitary; but in the condition known as multiple neurofibromatosis (von Recklinghausen's disease) (p. 54) numerous tumours are associated with pigmented areas in the skin. A neurofibroma growing within the spinal canal is an important cause of compression of the spinal cord or cauda equina.

FIBROMA

This is rather uncommon in the extremities and initially is never seen in deep tissues. It is a firm, rounded, painless nodule, usually connected with a fascial or aponeurotic structure such as a digital flexor sheath.

LIPOMA

A lipoma is a common tumour that may arise in almost any part of the body. It usually occurs in the subcutaneous tissues. It forms a soft, often large, lobulated mass enclosed within a thin capsule. It consists of fat, usually with little connective tissue stroma. Less often it contains an abundance of fibrous tissue, which gives it a firm consistency (fibrolipoma).

HAEMANGIOMA

Haemangioma is a benign tumour of blood vessels, usually present at birth. A **capillary haemangioma** forms a dark red, irregular, slightly raised blotch on the skin ('port wine stain'). It is usually congenital. A **cavernous haemangioma** is composed of widely dilated vascular channels with intervening connective tissue. It forms a localised or diffuse tumour within the skin, subcutaneous tissue or muscle. A characteristic feature of diagnostic importance is that the tumour is compressible. It may cause symptoms from its cosmetic appearance, or from the complication of thrombosis, which may be associated with local pain and swelling. When it occurs in a massive form in a limb it may lead to marked increase in growth of the limb as a whole.

Treatment. Superficial capillary haemangiomata fall within the province of the plastic surgeon. A localised deep cavernous haemangioma is usually amenable to excision. Extensive diffuse tumours cannot be eradicated, but improvement may follow transcutaneous arterial embolisation. In the worst cases amputation may be required.

DESMOID TUMOUR
(Musculo-aponeurotic fibromatosis)

This rare tumour occurs mostly in young adults as a slowly growing hard swelling in the musculo-aponeurotic tissues, particularly in the trunk and shoulder regions. It is important because of its histological resemblance to malignant fibrosarcoma. But it has a more benign course and never metastasises, though there is a high risk of local recurrence even after radical excision. This suggests that it may arise from multicentric foci in the same limb.

MALIGNANT TUMOURS OF SOFT TISSUE

Malignant tumours of soft tissue are uncommon, comprising 1 per cent of adult malignant neoplasms. Of mesenchymal origin, they arise from connective tissues such as fascia, aponeurosis, tendon sheath, intermuscular septa, voluntary muscle, and synovial membrane. Such a tumour presents difficulties both in diagnosis and in treatment. It may be indistinguishable from its benign counterpart, presenting as a progressively enlarging but usually painless swelling. It is of firm consistency and may appear to be well localised, though this is usually a false impression. It may spread widely within the soft tissues and the surrounding pseudocapsule forms no barrier. Metastasis occurs through the blood stream, mainly to the lungs.

Investigation of these tumours is aided by computerised tomography (CT scanning) and magnetic resonance imaging (MRI) (see Figs 13 and 14). MRI scans in particular provide good definition of the anatomical extent of the tumour and of its relationship to the neurovascular structures, thereby allowing correct planning of surgical treatment.

Biopsy must be planned in such a way as to minimise the spillage of malignant cells. It may be by needle aspiration or localised incision, but never by local excision of the tumour.

The treatment of most types of soft-tissue sarcoma has been improved by the introduction of potent chemotherapeutic agents used in combination as for bone sarcomas. Radiotherapy may also be of value as an adjunct to operative excision, to reduce the risk of local recurrence. These measures, though, do not remove the need for adequate surgical treatment, which demands excision with wide margins of healthy tissue rather than simple local excision or enucleation, which leads to early recurrence.

The following varieties will be described: 1) malignant fibrous histiocytoma; 2) fibrosarcoma; 3) synovial sarcoma (malignant synovioma); 4) liposarcoma; 5) rhabdomyosarcoma.

MALIGNANT FIBROUS HISTIOCYTOMA

This tumour is composed predominantly of histiocytic-type cells, but may also include cells of fibrous origin. It was formerly included under the diagnosis of fibrosarcoma. It is now regarded as the commonest malignant soft-tissue tumour in older adults. It has a poor prognosis, with local recurrence or metastasis in more than half the patients.

FIBROSARCOMA

Like malignant fibrous histiocytoma this may present as a seemingly localised firm rounded mass arising from the deeper tissues. It has a surrounding false capsule, which does not restrict outward spread of the tumour. Histologically it is composed of spindle cells with elongated nuclei resembling fibroblasts. Infiltration of the surrounding healthy soft tissues is a feature, and early metastasis to the lungs is common.

SYNOVIAL SARCOMA
(Malignant synovioma)

This highly malignant but rare tumour was once thought to arise from the synovial lining of joints or tendon sheaths because of its proximity to these structures. Pathologically it forms a solid, whitish, fleshy mass with a slow but insidious invasion of the soft tissues. It is most common in young and middle-aged adults. It has a poor prognosis, with early pulmonary metastases or spread to local lymph nodes. Histologically the tumour is composed of masses of fusiform cells, but the picture is characterised by the formation of spaces or clefts lined by cuboidal cells which suggest the formation of a synovial cavity—hence the name given to this tumour. Treatment is by wide excision if this is practicable, with pre-operative and post-operative radiotherapy. When the tumour involves a joint amputation offers the best hope of survival.

LIPOSARCOMA

This is one of the commonest of the soft-tissue sarcomas, usually occurring in the deep tissues. It grows as a lobulated mass, usually in the buttock or thigh, and may often attain an enormous size. It has a wide range of behaviour, depending upon its histological appearance and the amount of myxomatous content. Tumours showing predominantly pleomorphic and round cells have a poor prognosis, but the presence of myxoid tissue improves the outlook. Treatment is by radical excision or amputation. Recurrence or metastasis is generally slow.

RHABDOMYOSARCOMA

This rare variety of soft-tissue sarcoma occurs mainly in children or young adults. It affects particularly the trunk or lower limbs. It forms a rapidly growing mass. Histologically it is characterised by cells showing longitudinal and cross striations typical of primitive myoblasts. It metastasises early, mainly to the lungs.

References and bibliography, page 403.

7. Affections of joints

ARTHRITIS

The term arthritis is used here to include both inflammatory and degenerative lesions of a joint.[1] It implies a diffuse lesion affecting the joint as a whole. It does not include localised mechanical disorders such as loose body formation or tears of the menisci of the knee, which are better designated as internal derangements. Nor should it embrace acute injuries of joints.

Clinically, arthritis is generally characterised by pain and restriction of movement at a joint, arising spontaneously; in superficial joints these features are usually accompanied by obvious swelling or thickening. If a joint is not swollen and if it moves freely and painlessly through its normal range it is very unlikely that it is affected by arthritis.

Types of arthritis

It may be said that there are four common types of arthritis, and several less common or rare varieties of which five will be considered here. The incidence of different types varies greatly from country to country and from continent to continent, racial influences or differing standards of general hygiene often being important. Thus tuberculous arthritis is now uncommon in Britain and in most Western countries, whereas it is still common in

---

[1]The term *arthrosis* is sometimes used to denote a degenerative lesion of a joint, *arthritis* being used only for inflammatory lesions. But the use of the word 'arthrosis' to denote degeneration is without valid etymological grounds, and can be justified only on the basis of common usage. Ever since the Greek era *arthritis* has had the connotation 'disease of a joint'. In Greek the word meant simply 'of the joint', νοσος (disease) being understood or sometimes stated. The suffix '-itis' was similarly added to other parts of the body to imply disease of that part. Only more recently has '-itis' been misapplied to denote inflammatory disease. It is therefore still correct to use 'arthritis' as a generic term to cover all types of joint disease, including degenerative disease. The suffix '-osis', also derived from the Greek, had a meaning quite unrelated to disease. It implied a process or activity, as in *hypnosis* or *metamorphosis*. Its use to imply degenerative disease is a comparatively recent extension which cannot be justified etymologically.

Asia and Africa; and osteoarthritis, very common in the white races, is relatively uncommon among Africans and Asians.

The four types of arthritis that are common, taken worldwide, are: 1) pyogenic arthritis; 2) rheumatoid arthritis and juvenile chronic arthritis; 3) tuberculous arthritis; and 4) osteoarthritis. Of these, osteoarthritis and then rheumatoid arthritis are the most common in Britain. Other types of arthritis that will be considered are: 5) gouty arthritis; 6) haemophilic arthritis; 7) neuropathic arthritis (Charcot's osteoarthropathy); 8) the arthritis of rheumatic fever; and 9) ankylosing spondylitis.

PYOGENIC ARTHRITIS
(Infective arthritis; septic arthritis)

In this form of arthritis a joint is infected by bacteria of one of the pyogenic groups. Typically there is acute joint infection of rapid development, but the infection may be subacute or even chronic. When pus is formed within the joint the condition is sometimes termed *suppurative arthritis*.

Cause. The staphylococcus, streptococcus or pneumococcus is usually responsible—occasionally the gonococcus or other organisms.

Pathology. The organisms may reach the joint by three routes: 1) through the blood stream (haematogenous infection); 2) through a penetrating wound; or 3) by extension from an adjacent focus of osteomyelitis— especially when the infected metaphysis is wholly or partly within the joint cavity (as are the upper humeral metaphysis, all the metaphyses at the elbow, and the upper and lower metaphyses of the femur (Fig. 51, p. 71)).

The infection causes an acute or subacute inflammatory reaction in the joint tissues. There is exudation of fluid within the joint: the fluid is turbid or frankly purulent according to the severity of the infection. The outcome varies from complete resolution, with normal function, to total destruction of the joint and fibrous or bony ankylosis (Fig. 89).

Clinical features. The onset is acute or subacute, with pain and swelling of the joint. There is constitutional illness, with pyrexia.

On examination the joint is swollen, partly from fluid effusion and partly from thickening of the synovial membrane. When the affected joint is superficial, the overlying skin is warmer than normal and it is often reddened. All movements are restricted; in severe cases they are almost totally prevented by protective muscle spasm. Attempted or forced movement increases the pain. In cases of haematogenous infection a boil or other primary focus of infection is often to be found elsewhere in the body. In other cases there may be a history of penetrating injury, or of bone infection adjacent to the joint.

Radiographs in the early stages do not show any alteration from the normal (Fig. 90). Later, if the infection persists, there may be diffuse rarefaction of bone adjacent to the joint, loss of cartilage space, and possibly destruction of bone (Fig. 91). Radioisotope bone scanning shows increased uptake of the isotope in the region of the joint.

Investigations. There is a polymorphonuclear leucocytosis. The erythrocyte sedimentation rate is raised. Bacteriological examination of aspirated joint fluid usually identifies the causative organism.

Diagnosis. This is from other forms of arthritis (especially tuberculous arthritis, gouty arthritis, and haemophilic arthritis), and from infections near the joint (especially acute osteomyelitis).

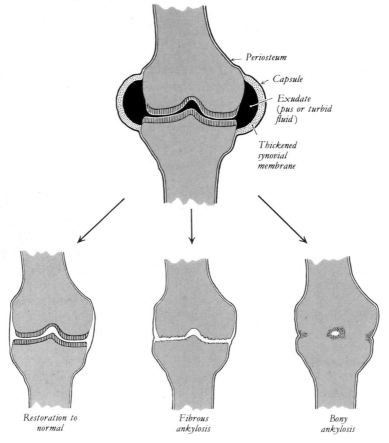

Fig. 89
Pyogenic arthritis, with possible results. In the active phase the joint is distended with pus or turbid fluid; the synovial membrane is inflamed and moderately thickened. The outcome varies with the intensity of the infection and the response to treatment. There may be: 1) restoration to normal; 2) fibrous ankylosis; or 3) bony ankylosis.

Prognosis. This varies widely according to the severity of the infection, the organism responsible, and the promptness with which efficient treatment is begun. Many joints can be saved intact, but many are destroyed more or less completely, with fibrous or bony ankylosis (Fig. 89).

Treatment. Very prompt treatment is essential if there is to be a reasonable prospect of preserving normal joint function.

Constitutional treatment. This is by rest in bed and appropriate antibiotic drugs. Whenever possible the causative organism must be identified by culture of the blood and of joint aspirate and its sensitivity to antibiotics determined, so that the most effective drug may be given. Until that information is available treatment should be begun with flucloxacillin, either alone or in combination with fusidic acid.

Fig. 90   **Fig. 91**

Pyogenic arthritis of the wrist. Figure 90—Initial radiograph, with no apparent abnormality. Figure 91—Four weeks after onset. Note the rarefaction of the bones and the slight but significant narrowing of the cartilage space, indicating destruction of articular cartilage. (See also Fig. 55, p. 73.)

Local treatment. The joint is rested, usually in a plaster splint. In the case of the hip or knee, sustained weight traction is useful in relieving spasm and pain. The fluid exudate, which is often purulent, is removed by aspiration or, if necessary, by incision. At the same time a solution of the appropriate antibiotic drug is injected into the joint. Aspiration and injection of antibiotic solutions are repeated daily so long as the exudate continues to form. Rest is enforced until the infection is overcome, as shown by the subsidence of pyrexia and retrogression of the local signs. Thereafter active movements are encouraged in order to restore the greatest possible function to the joint.

RHEUMATOID ARTHRITIS
(Rheumatoid polyarthritis)

Rheumatoid arthritis is a chronic inflammation of joints, often associated with mild constitutional symptoms. It nearly always affects several joints at the same time (polyarthritis). Joint changes of a similar nature also occur in a number of other conditions such as juvenile chronic arthritis (Still's disease), Reiter's syndrome, psoriasis, lupus erythematosus and other connective tissue or collagen diseases.

Cause. The cause is unknown. At present only two possibilities attract serious consideration: 1) that the disease is due to auto-immunity; and 2) that it is caused by infection. The hypothesis of auto-immunity, possibly to

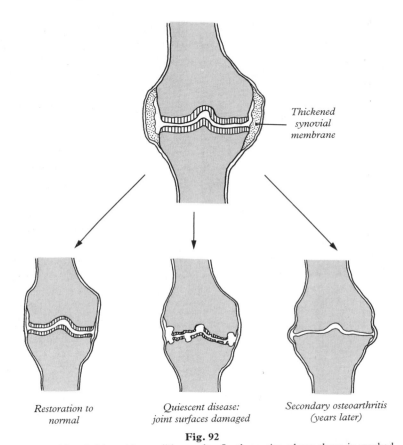

*Thickened
synovial
membrane*

*Restoration to
normal*

*Quiescent disease:
joint surfaces damaged*

*Secondary osteoarthritis
(years later)*

Fig. 92

Rheumatoid arthritis, with possible results. In the active phase there is marked thickening of the synovial membrane. Later, the articular cartilage is often eroded and in severe cases there may be some destruction of bone. The possible results are: 1) restoration to normal (only after mild disease of short duration); 2) continuing mildly active disease with permanently damaged joint surfaces and restricted movement; and 3) secondary osteoarthritis from wear-and-tear degeneration of the damaged joint surfaces.

type II collagen, is based mainly on the observation that the serum of many patients with rheumatoid arthritis contains an antibody known as rheumatoid factor, which reacts with the body protein gamma globulin. When the antibody is present the disease is termed 'sero-positive', as contrasted with sero-negative arthritis when the antibody is absent. The source of the antigen, and many other details of the mechanism by which rheumatoid factor is formed, are unknown.

The hypothesis of infection is likewise without sure foundation. Infection—possibly by a virus or by organisms of the mycoplasma or diphtheroid group—may result in liberation of antigenic type II collagen from the patient's own articular cartilage.

Pathology. The synovial membrane is thickened by chronic inflammatory changes: characteristically it is infiltrated with macrophage-like cells and T-cell lymphocytes (Fig. 92). Later the articular cartilage is gradually softened and eroded, and the subchondral bone may also be eroded, characteristically at the joint margins—probably from the action of lytic enzymes and inflammatory mediators produced in the thickened synovial membrane. The eroded surfaces become covered by a soft membrane of inflammatory tissue known as 'pannus'.

The pathological changes are not confined to joints. The synovial lining of tendon sheaths may be similarly inflamed and thickened, both in the hands and in the feet. The contained tendons may become softened and may rupture, aggravating any existing deformity. Inflammatory nodules may form in the soft tissues.

After months or years of activity the disease process tends to become less active, usually leaving a number of joints that are permanently damaged, with consequent deformity, instability, or ankylosis.

Clinical features. The patient is usually a young or middle-aged adult, and is more likely to be a woman than a man. Any joint may be affected, but the incidence is higher in the more peripheral joints such as the hand joints, wrists, feet, knees, and elbows than in the lumbar or thoracic spine, shoulders, or hips. The onset is gradual, with increasing pain and swelling of a joint. Soon a number of other joints are similarly affected. Pain and stiffness are often worst when activity is resumed after resting. Often there is constitutional disturbance, with tiredness and anaemia, and occasionally fever.

On examination the affected joints are swollen from synovial thickening. The overlying skin is warmer than normal. The range of joint movements is restricted, and movement causes pain, especially at the extremes. These clinical features are often more severe in sero-positive disease than when rheumatoid factor is absent from the serum.

It is important always to study the condition of the cervical spine, which is commonly affected. Despite relatively minor symptoms, destruction of ligaments and bone may sometimes lead to subluxation of such degree that the spinal cord is in jeopardy, and it is important always to be wary of this possibility.

Extra-articular features may include enlargement of lymph nodes, muscle wasting, subcutaneous rheumatoid nodules, and anaemia.

Imaging. *Radiographic features:* At first there is no alteration from the normal. Later, there is diffuse rarefaction in the area of the joint. Eventually destruction of joint cartilage may lead to narrowing of the cartilage space and, in severe cases, to localised erosion of the bone ends (Fig. 94). *Radioisotope bone scanning* shows increased uptake of the isotope in the region of affected joints.

Investigations. Both the erythrocyte sedimentation rate and C-reactive proteins are raised during the active phase. The latex fixation test and if necessary the Rose-Waaler sheep cell agglutination test are used to determine whether or not rheumatoid factor is present in the serum.

Fig. 93

Joint damage in rheumatoid arthritis. *Left*—Long-established rheumatoid arthritis of the knee. Note the rarefaction and loss of cartilage space. *Right*—Destruction of the elbow joint in a case of severe rheumatoid arthritis of long duration.

Diagnosis. The clue to the diagnosis is the simultaneous involvement of several joints, with raised sedimentation rate. The presence of rheumatoid factor in the blood is highly suggestive, though the tests are not specific for rheumatoid arthritis; and rheumatoid factor may be absent in about 20 per cent of patients even in well established rheumatoid arthritis.

A search should always be made for evidence of one of the distinct medical entities that may be associated with joint changes of a rheumatoid type. The most important of such conditions are: 1) psoriasis; 2) Reiter's syndrome (urethritis, arthritis, conjunctivitis, and hyperkeratotic eruptions on the skin); 3) lupus erythematosus (scaly erythema of face or other parts); and 4) scleroderma. These conditions are all sero-negative, and they may be associated with ankylosing spondylitis.

Course. There is a tendency for rheumatoid arthritis to become quiescent after remaining active for months or years. In most cases there is permanent impairment of joint function. In certain joints—especially in the knees—degenerative changes are often superimposed upon the previous rheumatoid condition, and lead to increasingly severe disability even though the original rheumatoid affection is no longer active.

Treatment. The treatment of rheumatoid arthritis is unsatisfactory. No specific cure has been found. Innumerable drugs have been tried and many are in use; yet it is by no means certain—opinions differ on this point—that any of them has an influence on the duration of the disease or on its eventual outcome in a particular case. Undoubtedly some drugs can mitigate the symptoms—if only by an analgesic effect—but this may well be the sole extent of their benefit.

Methods of treatment may be classified into the following categories: 1) rest and constitutional treatment; 2) drugs, which include mainly the various non-steroidal anti-inflammatory agents; the 'second-line' drugs such as gold salts, sulphasalazine and penicillamine; and (rarely) the 'third-line' corticosteroids; 3) intra-articular injections of hydrocortisone; 4) physiotherapy; 5) occupational therapy; and 6) operation.

Rest and constitutional treatment. Rest is thought to be beneficial, especially in the early stages of the disease and during an exacerbation. At many centres patients are admitted to hospital at the outset for a period of rest lasting one or two months, and sometimes this temporary removal from the home environment, with skilled nursing, regular food and proper sleep, has a remarkably good effect on the general health, which is often impaired in these cases. Rest for individual joints is also helpful during the initial active stage of inflammation, provided it is not enforced for too long. Convenient light splints for this purpose may be made from expanded polystyrene, or plaster of Paris may be used. Splintage is seldom required for more than two months, and should be followed by graduated exercises under the supervision of a physiotherapist.

Drugs. Drugs used in rheumatoid arthritis fall mainly into the categories of non-steroidal anti-inflammatory drugs, and the potent anti-inflammatory agents grouped under the heading corticosteroids. A logical plan is to use aspirin or a related salicylate as the first-line drug and to follow with other drugs if the response is unsatisfactory. Aspirin has both analgesic and mild anti-inflammatory properties but to be effective it may have to be given in fairly large doses. Alternative first-line drugs, after aspirin, should probably be chosen from the group of non-steroidal anti-inflammatory drugs which includes indomethacin, ibuprofen, naproxen, flufenamic acid and piroxican. Due regard must be paid to the risk of side effects: gastric pain is a common complaint with most of these drugs, and more serious complications, such as gastric bleeding, are seen occasionally.

A different class of anti-rheumatic agents, to be regarded as second-line drugs, includes the potentially toxic group of compounds containing gold salts, usually given by intramuscular injection. These must be used with care, but they are thought to be sometimes beneficial and therefore justified in severely afflicted patients who have failed to respond to the first-line drugs. Sulphasalazine, a derivative of sulphapyridine, is now also used increasingly as a second-line drug. Its mode of action is uncertain, but it has the advantage over gold salts of oral administration and fewer side effects. Another drug in this second-line category is penicillamine, the effect of which is comparable to that of gold. This also is potentially toxic for the kidneys and must be used with caution. Also included in this category are certain immuno-suppressive agents, such as azathioprine and methotrexate.

The place of corticosteroids in rheumatoid arthritis is still controversial. There is wide agreement that because of their serious side effects they should be avoided altogether in the great majority of patients; otherwise there is a real risk that the ill effects of treatment may be actually worse than those of the disease itself. There is, however, a small proportion of severely afflicted patients in whom the advantages outweigh the hazards.

Intra-articular injections. Injections of corticosteroids (usually hydrocortisone) into an affected joint can produce worth-while relief, but their disadvantages have precluded their widespread use. The main disadvantages are: 1) risk of infection, especially with repeated injections; 2) risk of accelerating a degenerative reaction, the mechanism of which is not yet clear; 3) the short duration of the relief obtained; and 4) repeated injections at several sites may become so irksome to the patient as to be unacceptable. In general, it is wise to avoid repeated injections.

Physiotherapy. Physiotherapy is widely used and generally beneficial, even though some of the benefit may result from suggestion or 'placebo effect' rather than from a direct effect on the disease process. Heat in the form of infra-red radiation or short-wave diathermy is commonly used, but probably the most useful contribution of physiotherapy is active exercises, designed both to keep joints as mobile as possible and to maintain useful function in the muscles that control them.

Occupational therapy. Occupational therapy is useful mainly in helping seriously disabled patients to find ways in which they can more easily carry out the various activities of everyday life—bathing, toilet, cooking, feeding, boarding public transport, and many others. Many useful aids for the disabled are available, and those that are appropriate should be brought to the patient's notice.

Operation. Operation has an important place in treatment, but each operation must be considered as a component in the overall plan of management and not as a substitute for other measures. Operation may be applicable to the early stages of the disease, or it may be used in the later stages to salvage a joint that has been permanently damaged and remains a source of persistent pain.

In the early stages the operation most commonly used is synovectomy—excision of thickened and inflamed synovial membrane from joint or tendon sheath. As well as relieving pain, this may possibly slow down the inflammatory process and so help to preserve articular cartilage in an affected joint. It is undertaken mainly in the knee and wrist, and in the small joints and tendon sheaths of the hand.

Operation may also be required in the hand for repair or replacement of ruptured tendons, or for correction of finger deformities. In the painful elbow there is often a place for excision of the diseased radial head, and at the wrist excision of the lower end of the ulna may bring worth-while relief in selected cases.

Operations used in the later stages are osteotomy, arthroplasty, and arthrodesis. *Osteotomy* is useful mainly for the correction of deformity, particularly at the knee. *Arthroplasty* is applicable particularly to the hip and knee, and sometimes to the shoulder or elbow, and to the joints of the fingers and toes. *Arthrodesis* is usually the operation of choice for the joints of the spine, the wrist and the ankle, and sometimes for the shoulder, the elbow and the knee.

Further details are given in the sections on individual joints.

JUVENILE CHRONIC ARTHRITIS
(Juvenile rheumatoid arthritis; Still's disease)

Juvenile chronic arthritis is uncommon. In the past the general term 'Still's disease' was often used broadly to cover all its manifestations, but almost certainly the disease is not a single entity. Rather it comprises a number of conditions that are more or less distinct, though features common to all are pain, swelling and stiffness of joints. Recognised types include: 1) seropositive polyarthritis (adult type); 2) classical Still's disease (a) with systemic manifestations, (b) with polyarthritis, and (c) with pauciarticular arthritis; 3) sero-negative polyarthritis with sacro-iliitis; 4) arthritis asso-ciated with psoriasis, ulcerative colitis or Crohn's disease. These subgroups vary in age of onset, sex incidence, course, complications and prognosis.

Sero-positive juvenile rheumatoid arthritis is similar in all respects to the same disease in adults. It tends to begin rather late in childhood and affects girls more often than boys.

Classical Still's disease begins in early childhood. In the systemic type there is swinging pyrexia with enlargement of lymph glands and of the spleen, with joint involvement simul-taneously or later. The eventual outlook is favourable, as it is with the sero-negative polyarticular and pauciarticular variants—though the pauciarticular disease is complicated rather frequently by iridocyclitis necessitating local or systemic steroid therapy.

The sero-negative disease with sacro-iliitis is commoner in boys than in girls and tends not to begin until late in childhood: it may lead on to ankylosing spondylitis in early adult life. Most of such patients show a positive test for HLA-B27 antigen and there is often clinical overlap between these patients and relatives with ankylosing spondylitis, Reiter's disease, ulcerative colitis or Crohn's disease. It is thus probable that there is a hereditary factor in the causation.

Treatment. This is similar to that for rheumatoid arthritis in adults, with reliance on aspirin in the first instance and resort later if necessary to non-steroidal anti-inflammatory agents and possibly—in florid sero-positive disease—to gold therapy or penicillamine. Corticosteroid therapy should usually be avoided except for patients with iritis or iridocyclitis. General management includes adequate rest, temporary splinting of inflamed joints, graduated exercises with the physiotherapist, and occasionally operation—for instance, correction of fixed deformity or arthroplasty of the hip.

TUBERCULOUS ARTHRITIS

In Britain the incidence of tuberculous arthritis, formerly common, de-creased markedly in the years following the Second World War, probably because of the general improvement in living standards and the intro-duction of streptomycin and other antituberculous drugs. Pasteurisation of milk and elimination of infected cattle have virtually abolished bovine infection. In some Asiatic and African countries tuberculous infection is still common, and cases are now seen regularly among immigrants to Britain.

Whereas formerly a joint affected by tuberculosis was nearly always destroyed, with modern treatment good recovery of function may now be expected in most patients treated early.

Cause. Tuberculous arthritis is caused by infection of a joint with tubercle bacilli, human or (rarely) bovine. The infection is commonly contracted from another patient with open pulmonary tuberculosis.

Pathology. No joint is immune, but the joints most often affected are the intervertebral joints of the thoracic or lumbar spine, and next in frequency the hip and knee. The organisms reach the joint through the blood stream from a focus elsewhere. The synovial membrane is much thickened (Fig. 94) by the tuberculous inflammatory reaction, which is of charac-teristic type, with round-cell infiltration and giant-cell systems. Unless the disease is arrested the articular cartilage is soon destroyed and the under-lying bone is eroded. Sometimes the infection begins in bone adjacent to a joint rather than in the joint itself; thence it extends into the joint by direct continuity. The slow formation of an abscess—a 'cold' or chronic abscess in contradistinction to the florid abscess that may accompany an acute pyogenic infection—is a common feature. The abscess often makes its way towards the skin surface and may eventually rupture, giving rise to a chronic tuberculous sinus. This may provide a route for the entry of secondary infecting organisms.

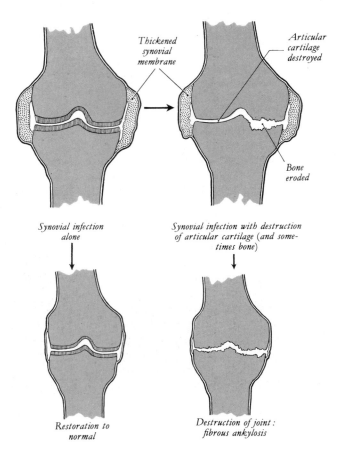

Fig. 94

Tuberculous arthritis, with possible results. When infection is purely synovial there is marked thickening of the synovial membrane but the articular cartilage is intact (note similarity to early rheumatoid arthritis). With efficient treatment begun at this stage restoration to normal is possible; but if neglected the disease progresses to involve the articular cartilage and bone: the joint is destroyed, and fibrous ankylosis is the natural outcome.

If healing occurs before the articular cartilage and bone have been damaged the function of the joint is restored virtually to normal; but if cartilage or bone has been damaged before healing is secured permanent impairment—often complete loss of function— is inevitable (Fig. 95).

Clinical features. Children and young adults are most commonly affected. There is often a history of contact with a patient with active pulmonary tuberculosis. In general, the predominant symptoms are pain, swelling, and impairment of function of the affected joint. There is usually some impairment of the general health. *On examination* the characteristic features are increased warmth of the overlying skin, swelling from synovial thickening, and restriction of movement in all directions. Forced movement causes sharp pain and induces protective muscle spasm. The muscles controlling the joint are usually wasted. An abscess or sinus is often apparent. A tuberculous lesion may be found elsewhere in the body.

Imaging. *Radiographic features.* The earliest change in tuberculous arthritis is diffuse rarefaction throughout a fairly wide area of bone adjacent

Fig. 95
Tuberculous arthritis of right hip. Note the rarefaction, loss of joint cartilage, and early erosion of bone surfaces. The normal side is shown for comparison.

to the joint. If the disease is arrested early there may be no further change; but if the infection progresses the cartilage space is narrowed and the underlying bone is eroded (Fig. 96). As the disease heals the bones harden up again—that is, the rarefaction becomes gradually less apparent until the bone density is restored to normal.

Radioisotope bone scanning shows increased uptake of the isotope in the region of the joint.

Investigations. The erythrocyte sedimentation rate is raised in the active stage. Its gradual decrease is an indication of healing. The Mantoux test is positive. Aspiration of the joint may yield a little turbid fluid, in which organisms can seldom be demonstrated, but culture may prove its tuberculous nature. Examination of pus withdrawn from an abscess often reveals tubercle bacilli. Biopsy of thickened synovial membrane shows the typical histological features of tuberculosis.

Complications. These are: 1) sinus formation; 2) secondary infection through a sinus track; 3) spread of disease to another part of the body. Other complications are peculiar to special regions—for example, compression of the spinal cord by an abscess in tuberculosis of the spinal column.

Course. This depends largely upon the conditions in which the patient lives, and upon the promptness with which treatment is begun and its efficiency. Under favourable conditions early treatment usually promotes gradual healing, with preservation of a useful or even a normal joint; but where conditions tend to be poor and the disease florid, as in many countries of the East, the joint may be largely or totally destroyed.

Treatment. The principles of treatment are the same no matter which joint is affected, with antibacterial drugs as the mainstay of treatment; variations in detail will be discussed in the sections on individual joints.

Antibacterial drugs. There is now a choice of several antituberculous drugs, including rifampicin, isoniazid, pyrazinamide, streptomycin and ethambutol. Regimens vary: a common combination of drugs is rifampicin, isoniazid and pyrazinamide, with the addition if appropriate (depending upon the resistance of the organisms) of streptomycin or ethambutol. The course of drug treatment should continue for six to nine months, with streptomycin or ethambutol (if used) discontinued after two months.

Careful watch must be kept for undesirable side effects, especially with ethambutol, which may cause optic atrophy; and with streptomycin, which may cause auditory impairment. Liver function must be monitored during treatment because rifampicin, isoniazid and pyrazinamide may be harmful to liver cells. Streptomycin carries the additional disadvantage that it has to be administered by intramuscular injection.

Local treatment varies according to the particular joint that is affected. Tuberculosis of a large joint such as the hip or knee may demand a period of rest in bed, at any rate in the early stages; whereas a patient with disease of a smaller joint—particularly in the upper limb—may be up and about throughout the period of treatment. Immobilisation of the affected joint in a plaster or splint is usually advisable in the early stages, both to relieve pain and to provide favourable conditions for healing. Splintage should generally be continued for two to four months, depending on the severity of the disease. Meanwhile abscesses should be aspirated or drained surgically.

Subsequent management depends on progress. If cartilage and bone are preserved intact and the local signs of inflammation subside, with improvement in the sedimentation rate, the outlook is good and activity may be progressively increased. If however the disease progresses to the point of eroding articular cartilage and underlying bone, a further period of immobilisation may be required, and fusion of the joint—usually by operation—may become the ultimate objective.

OSTEOARTHRITIS
(Degenerative arthritis; arthrosis; osteoarthrosis; hypertrophic arthritis; post-traumatic arthritis)

Osteoarthritis is a degenerative wear-and-tear process occurring in joints that are impaired by congenital defect, vascular insufficiency, or previous disease or injury. It is by far the commonest variety of arthritis.

Cause. It is caused by wear and tear. If a joint were never put under stress it would never become osteoarthritic. Hence the relatively lightly stressed joints of the upper limb are, in general, less prone to osteoarthritis than the heavily stressed joints of the lower limb. Nearly always, however, there is a predisposing cause that accelerates the wear-and-tear process. Almost any abnormality of a joint may be responsible, indirectly, for the development of osteoarthritis—often many years later. The main predisposing factors are: 1) congenital ill-development; 2) irregularity of joint surfaces from previous fracture; 3) internal derangements, such as a loose body or a torn meniscus; 4) previous disease, leaving a damaged articular cartilage (for example, rheumatoid arthritis or haemophilia); 5) mal-alignment of a joint from any cause (for example, bow leg); 6) obesity and overweight. Age alone is not a cause of osteoarthritis, though it may be associated with an impaired capacity for tissue repair after injury, and this may be an indirect causative factor.

Fig. 96
Osteoarthritis. The main changes are in the articular cartilage and underlying bone. The cartilage is gradually worn away, disappearing first at the points of greatest pressure. The subchondral bone becomes sclerotic, and at the joint margins it hypertrophies to form osteophytes.

Pathology. Any joint may be affected, the lower limb joints more often than the upper. The articular cartilage is slowly worn away until eventually the underlying bone is exposed (Fig. 96). This subchondral bone becomes hard and glossy ('eburnation'). Meanwhile the bone at the margins of the joint hypertrophies to form a rim of projecting spurs known as osteophytes. There is no primary change in the capsule or synovial membrane, but the recurrent strains to which an osteoarthritic joint is subject often lead to slight thickening and fibrosis.

Clinical features. Most patients with osteoarthritis are past middle age. When it occurs in younger patients there is usually a clear predisposing cause such as previous injury or disease of the joint. The onset is very gradual, with pain that increases almost imperceptibly over months and years. Movements slowly become more and more restricted. In some joints (notably the hip) deformity is a common feature in the later stages. This means that the joint cannot be placed in the neutral (anatomical) position.

On examination slight thickening is often found on palpation; it is mainly a bony thickening caused by the marginal osteophytes. There is no increased warmth. Movements are impaired slightly or markedly according to the degree of arthritis; in most joints movement is accompanied by palpable or audible crepitation of a rather coarse type. Fixed deformity (that is, inability of the joint to assume the neutral anatomical position) is often found in the hip, and sometimes in other joints.

Fig. 97
Osteoarthritis of the right hip, with the sound hip shown for comparison. Note the narrowing of the cartilage space, the subchondral sclerosis, and the marginal osteophytes. Note also the adduction deformity: this is a common feature.

Radiographic features. The characteristic features of osteoarthritis are: 1) diminution of cartilage space; 2) subchondral sclerosis; and 3) spurring or 'lipping' of the joint margins from the formation of osteophytes (Fig. 97).

Diagnosis. This is usually made clear by the history, clinical findings, and radiographic features. Osteoarthritis is not easily confused with inflammatory forms of arthritis, because there is no synovial thickening, no increased local warmth, and no muscle spasm; radiographs show sclerosis rather than rarefaction, and the erythrocyte sedimentation rate is not increased.

Course. Osteoarthritis usually increases slowly year by year. In many cases the disability never reaches the stage at which treatment is required. In others increasing pain, stiffness, or deformity drives the patient to demand measures for its relief.

Treatment. The management of osteoarthritis exemplifies well the three categories of treatment that should be considered in every orthopaedic problem—namely: 1) no treatment, but advice and reassurance only; 2) conservative treatment; and 3) operative treatment (p. 22).

In many cases treatment is not required. The patient may have sought advice only because of anxiety lest some grave disease be present. Reassurance, with advice to restrict the wear and tear on the affected joint, is all that is required.

When more active treatment is called for, conservative measures should usually be tried first. The methods available include physiotherapy (often by local heat and muscle-strengthening exercises), analgesic drugs, local injections of hydrocortisone, and supportive bandages or appliances. In addition, the stress that is put upon the affected joint should be reduced—for instance, in the case of the joints of the lower limb by restricting the amount of walking or by the use of a stick.

When severe disability is unrelieved by conservative treatment operation may be justified. Chief among the operations available are osteotomy to realign a joint; arthroplasty (the construction of a new joint) (p. 30); and arthrodesis (elimination of the joint by fusion (p. 29). Osteotomy is useful mainly at the knee, to correct varus or valgus deformity, and at the hip. Arthroplasty is applicable particularly to the hip, knee, shoulder, elbow, certain joints of the hand, and the metatarso-phalangeal joints. For a few joints arthrodesis may be the operation of choice. Further details of treatment will be given in the sections on individual joints.

GOUTY ARTHRITIS
(Podagra; urate crystal synovitis)

Gout is the clinical manifestation of a disturbed purine metabolism. It is characterised by deposition of uric-acid salts—especially sodium biurate—in connective tissues such as cartilage (of joints, or of the ear), the walls of bursae, and ligaments.

Cause. The precise cause of the disturbance of metabolism is unknown. There is an inherited predisposition to the disease. In susceptible persons an attack may be induced by excessive consumption of purine-rich foods such as liver, kidneys, sweetbreads, shellfish, beer or heavy wines, or by recent injury or operation.

Pathology. The primary fault is an impaired excretion of uric acid by the kidneys. In consequence the level of urate in the plasma is increased, sometimes to 0.5 mmol per litre or more (normal = 0.1–0.4 mmol per litre (2.0–7.0 mg per 100 ml)). In the blood the uric acid is in solution in a loose combination with proteins; it comes readily out of solution as a sodium salt (sodium biurate) to be deposited in the form of crystals in certain connective tissues, especially those that have been injured or those that have a sluggish blood supply, such as the articular cartilage of the joints of the foot. The deposited crystals set up an inflammatory reaction. In acute gout the deposit is microscopic in amount and is soon reabsorbed, with restoration of the tissue to normal. In chronic gout, however, widespread deposits of sodium biurate in joint cartilages, ligaments and the articular ends of bones lead to considerable disorganisation of affected joints. Gouty deposits, known as tophi, are also common at other sites, notably in the olecranon bursa and in the cartilage of the ear, where they may form rounded nodules.

Clinical features. The patient is nearly always over 40, and is more likely to be a man than a woman, in the ratio of 10:1. The chief clinical manifestations are arthritis and bursitis.

Arthritis. Gout affects principally the peripheral joints such as the joints of the toes, tarsus, and ankle, and the small joints of the hands. It occurs in recurrent attacks. The first attack is usually in the great toe; later attacks may affect other joints. In an acute attack the onset is sudden—often during the night. The affected joint is swollen, red and glossy. Pain is very severe. Movements are greatly restricted because of the pain. The attack subsides after a few days and the joint is normal between attacks.

In chronic gout several joints are affected together. They are thickened and nodular, and painful on movement.

Bursitis. The bursa most commonly affected by gout is the olecranon bursa. It becomes distended with fluid, and there may be palpable deposits of uric acid salts.

Other manifestations. Deposits of uric acid salts (tophi) are common in the ear cartilages, where they form palpable nodules. They may also occur at other sites.

Radiographic features. In acute attacks of articular gout the joints do not show any radiographic change. In chronic gout the deposits of uric acid salts in the bone ends show as clear-cut erosions adjacent to the articular surfaces, for the deposits are transradiant.

Investigations. There is sometimes a mild leucocytosis and the erythrocyte sedimentation rate may be increased. The plasma uric acid content is raised. Aspiration of swollen joints may yield a small quantity of turbid fluid, but never organisms. Polarised light microscopy of synovial fluid usually reveals needle-shaped crystals showing negative birefringence.

Diagnosis. Acute gout has to be distinguished from other forms of arthritis of acute onset, especially from acute pyogenic arthritis, acute 'pseudogout' (see below), haemophilic arthritis, and rheumatic fever. Features suggestive of gout are: a history of previous attacks, with symptom-free intervals; a raised plasma urate content; the presence of tophi in the ears or elsewhere; detection of crystals in synovial fluid; and a favourable response to treatment.

Chronic gout involving several joints may simulate rheumatoid arthritis.

Course. Gout usually occurs in recurrent attacks. Early attacks subside in a few days, leaving the joint clinically normal. In chronic gout the affected joints are gradually disorganised, and permanent disability is inevitable.

Treatment. For acute attacks reliance is usually placed upon a non-steroidal anti-inflammatory drug such as indomethacin or naproxen. Colchicine is also effective. The affected joint should be rested until the attack has subsided. A large effusion in a major joint such as the knee should be aspirated and replaced by an instillation of hydrocortisone.

For patients with frequent attacks or with chronic gout, especially if the plasma urate level is persistently raised, long-term drug therapy to reduce the plasma urate level may be required. The two types of drug available are represented by: 1) probenemid, which paralyses renal tubular reabsorption of urates and thus increases their excretion in the urine; and 2) allopurinol, which reduces the formation of uric acid by inhibiting the enzyme xanthine oxydase. Provided its long-term use is not associated with toxic reactions, allopurinol is probably to be preferred because it does not increase the load of urate in the urine, with its hazard of stone formation.

PYROPHOSPHATE ARTHROPATHY
(Pseudogout)

With the general acceptance of the idea that joint manifestations in gout are caused by the presence of urate crystals, it has more recently come to be appreciated that similar manifestations may be induced by the crystals of other salts. In most such cases the crystals are composed of calcium pyrophosphate showing positive birefringence, and characteristically calcification of articular cartilage or of menisci is demonstrable radiologically

Fig. 98
Pyrophosphate arthropathy of the knee. Note the faint but characteristic calcification of the medial and lateral menisci and of articular cartilage.

(Fig. 98). Arthritis of this type, due to crystals other than urate crystals, has been termed 'pseudogout'. It usually presents as a chronic arthritis with characteristic calcification of cartilage, but it may occur in an acute form, from the shedding of crystals into the synovial fluid. Treatment should be by rest, aspiration of joint fluid, and a non-steroidal anti-inflammatory agent.

HAEMOPHILIC ARTHRITIS

Joint manifestations are common in haemophilia, but examples are seen only infrequently because haemophilia is itself an uncommon disease.

Pathology. The term 'haemophilia' is used loosely to embrace a group of different defects in the process of coagulation of the blood. Classical haemophilia, the commonest of the group, occurs in males but is transmitted by females. There is an inherited deficiency of a specific clotting factor known as antihaemophilic factor (factor VIII). In consequence the clotting time of the blood is prolonged and there is a tendency to undue bleeding when even quite small vessels are cut or torn. Joint manifestations are caused by haemorrhage into a joint, occurring after a minor strain or even without any known injury. The joints most commonly affected are those most vulnerable to strain—especially the knee, elbow, and ankle. The joint cavity is distended with blood (haemarthrosis), which is later slowly reabsorbed if the joint is rested. Recurrent haemarthroses lead eventually to degenerative changes in the articular cartilage and to fibrosis of the synovial membrane.

Clinical features. The boy is often a known sufferer from haemophilia or can recall previous episodes of bleeding. He suddenly finds that a joint has become painful and swollen. *On examination* the findings vary according to the phase and duration of the arthritis. In the absence of specific treatment the joint remains swollen for several weeks after the acute onset—partly from effused blood and partly from the synovial thickening that results from interstitial extravasation. The overlying skin is abnormally warm. Joint movements are restricted and very painful.

In the quiescent phase between attacks of haemarthrosis there is moderate thickening of the joint from synovial fibrosis, movements are slightly impaired, and often there is some degree of fixed deformity—for instance, inability to straighten the knee fully.

Diagnosis. Because of the synovial thickening, increased warmth of the skin, and restriction of joint movements, haemophilic arthritis is easily mistaken for acute or chronic inflammatory arthritis. The history of previous episodes of bleeding, the sudden onset, and the recurrent nature of the attacks are important diagnostic features; and the prolonged clotting time of the blood is confirmatory evidence.

Treatment. When the necessary facilities are available, the correct treatment for a recent acute incident is to promote coagulability of the blood by the administration of antihaemophilic factor in the form of factor VIII concentrate or of cryoprecipitate, and then to treat the joint as for ordinary traumatic haemarthrosis by aspiration and temporary support in a plaster splint. Early treatment on these lines should reduce the incidence of irreversible fibrosis of the synovial membrane, hitherto a cause of serious permanent disability.

Failing adequate supplies of antihaemophilic factor, resort must be had to prolonged splintage.

In the chronic degenerative phase that follows repeated haemarthroses it is often necessary to give permanent support to the joint by means of a moulded plastic splint or other appliance. Operation must be avoided whenever possible, though it may if necessary be undertaken safely as long as adequate cover by antihaemophilic factor can be provided.

The future outlook for haemophilic patients is much improved by the new-found ability to manufacture factor VIII in commercial quantities by genetic engineering technology. If such a product can be developed to the point of being effective when taken by mouth the advantage will clearly be even greater.

NEUROPATHIC ARTHRITIS

(Charcot's osteoarthropathy)

In neuropathic arthritis a joint is disorganised by repeated minor injuries because it is insensitive to pain.

Cause. The underlying cause is a neurological disorder interfering with deep pain sensibility. In patients with involvement of joints of the lower limb the commonest cause in the past was tabes dorsalis, a manifestation of syphilis; but tabes is now uncommon, and there has been a corresponding decline in the incidence of neuropathic arthritis in the lower limb. Other causes are diabetic neuropathy, cauda equina lesion, and in some countries leprosy. In those with upper limb involvement the usual cause, apart from leprosy, is syringomyelia.

Pathology. Any of the large joints may be affected, including the joints of the spine. The knee, ankle and subtalar joint are most commonly affected in the lower limb, and the elbow in the upper limb. In a normal joint harmful strains are prevented by a protective reflex whereby muscle contraction is evoked by incipient pain. When joint sensibility is destroyed the protective function of pain is lost. Strains are unrecognised and, cumulatively, they lead to severe degeneration of the joint. The changes may be regarded as a much exaggerated form of osteoarthritis. The articular cartilage and subchondral bone are worn away, but at the same time there is sometimes massive hypertrophy of bone at the joint margins. The ligaments become lax and the joint is unstable. Indeed it is often subluxated or even dislocated.

Clinical and radiographic features. The patient is usually in adult life. The main symptoms are swelling and instability of the affected joint. Since the joint is insensitive pain is slight or, sometimes, absent. *On examination* the joint is thickened, mostly from irregular hypertrophy of the bone ends. The range of movement is moderately restricted, and there is marked lateral laxity leading to instability. In extreme cases the joint may be dislocated. Further examination will reveal evidence of the underlying neurological disorder. *Radiographs* show severe disorganisation of the joint. The changes are basically those of osteoarthritis, but enormously exaggerated. There are loss of cartilage space and some absorption of the bone ends, often with considerable hypertrophy of bone at the joint margins (Fig. 199, p. 238, and Fig. 312, p. 342).

Treatment. In most instances the best treatment is simply to provide support for the joint by a suitable appliance. Sometimes operation may be undertaken to fuse the joint, but fusion may be difficult to achieve. The primary neurological disorder will usually demand appropriate treatment.

ARTHRITIS OF RHEUMATIC FEVER

In adolescent children and young adults arthritic manifestations are a prominent feature of rheumatic fever. This has now become an uncommon disease in Western countries; so joint manifestations from this cause are hardly ever seen except in under-developed parts of the world.

Cause. Rheumatic fever is ascribed to a sensitivity reaction associated with infection by a haemolytic streptococcus. There may be an inherited predisposition to the disease.

Pathology. Any joint may be affected. The synovial membrane is acutely inflamed, but there is no suppuration. Clear fluid is effused into the joint.

Clinical features. The patient is usually a child over 10, or a young adult. There is constitutional illness, with malaise and pyrexia. A joint becomes painful and swollen, and soon afterwards other joints are likewise affected. *On examination* an affected joint is swollen, partly from contained fluid and partly from synovial thickening. The overlying skin is warmer than normal. Movements are markedly restricted, and painful if forced. Other features of rheumatic fever, such as carditis and chorea, should be looked for. *Radiographs* of affected joints do not show any alteration from the normal. *Investigations*: There is a mild leucocytosis. The erythrocyte sedimentation rate is increased.

Diagnosis. Arthritis of rheumatic fever has to be distinguished from other forms of arthritis—especially from acute pyogenic arthritis, rheumatoid arthritis, gout and haemophilic arthritis—and from acute osteomyelitis. Features suggestive of rheumatic fever are: onset in adolescence; affection of several joints together or in succession; severe pain with signs of acute inflammation, but without suppuration; a mild rather than a marked leucocytosis; a concomitant cardiac lesion; and a rapid favourable response to salicylates.

Treatment. For joint involvement alone salicylates are adequate, but prednisone or a related steroid may be required if the heart is affected. A therapeutic course of penicillin should also be given to eliminate streptococci, and thereafter twice-daily oral penicillin should be continued well into adult life to reduce the risk of recurrent attacks.

ANKYLOSING SPONDYLITIS
(Spondylitis ankylopoietica; Marie-Strümpell arthritis)

As the name implies, ankylosing spondylitis is primarily a disease of the spine, though in a few cases the arthritic changes involve also the proximal joints of the limbs, especially the hips. Briefly, it is a chronic inflammatory affection of the joints and ligaments of the spine, beginning in the sacro-iliac joints. It progresses slowly, the changes gradually creeping up the spinal column from below. The natural outcome is bony ankylosis of the affected joints, but the disease may be arrested at any stage short of this.

Typically, ankylosing spondylitis affects men in early adult life, with a strong hereditary link to the HLA-B27 gene. After remaining active for several years it tends eventually to become quiescent, always leaving some degree of permanent stiffness of the spine. A fuller description is given in Chapter 10 (p. 184).

DISLOCATION AND SUBLUXATION OF JOINTS

A joint is dislocated or luxated when its articular surfaces are wholly displaced one from the other, so that all apposition between them is lost (Fig. 101). A joint is subluxated when its surfaces are partly displaced but retain some contact one with the other (Fig. 100).

Dislocation or subluxation may be congenital, spontaneous, traumatic, or recurrent.

| Fig. 99 | Fig. 100 | Fig. 101 |

To show the difference between subluxation and dislocation of a joint Figure 99—The normal state: joint surfaces congruous. Figure 100—Subluxation: incomplete loss of contact between the joint surfaces. Figure 101—Dislocation: total loss of contact between the joint surfaces.

CONGENITAL DISLOCATION OR SUBLUXATION

The most important representative of this group is congenital dislocation of the hip (p. 292). Congenital club foot (talipes equino-varus) (p. 372) may be regarded as congenital subluxation of the talo-navicular joint. Congenital displacement of other joints is rare.

TRAUMATIC DISLOCATION OR SUBLUXATION

Injury is by far the commonest cause of dislocations. Traumatic dislocations are described in textbooks of fractures and joint injuries, and they will not be considered further here.

SPONTANEOUS (PATHOLOGICAL) DISLOCATION OR SUBLUXATION

Displacement may occur spontaneously at any joint in consequence of a structural defect or of destructive disease. It is encountered frequently in the spine, where the stability of the intervertebral joints may be impaired by structural defects, by previous injury, or by destructive arthritis (pyogenic, rheumatoid, or tuberculous). It is common for a phalanx to become dislocated dorsally at the metatarso-phalangeal joint in cases of severe clawing of the toes; and in the hands interphalangeal subluxation may occur in rheumatoid arthritis. Another example is the dislocation of the hip that sometimes complicates severe tuberculous arthritis or pyogenic arthritis. Spontaneous subluxation or dislocation is also a common feature of neuropathic arthritis (p. 126).

RECURRENT DISLOCATION OR SUBLUXATION

Certain joints are liable to repeated dislocation or subluxation. Usually, but not always, there has been an initial violent dislocation which causes permanent damage to the ligaments or articular surfaces. The joints most often affected are the shoulder (p. 217), the patello-femoral joint (p. 350), and the ankle (p. 371).

INTERNAL DERANGEMENTS OF JOINTS

The term internal derangement implies a localised mechanical fault which interferes with the smooth action of a joint. An internal derangement is distinct from arthritis, which is nearly always a diffuse lesion involving the joint as a whole.

Internal derangements will be considered in three groups: 1) interposition of soft tissue; 2) loose body formation; and 3) osteochondritis dissecans.

INTERPOSITION OF SOFT TISSUE IN JOINTS

The smooth action of a joint may be obstructed by a displaced mass of soft tissue within it. The soft tissue most often responsible is an intra-articular fibrocartilage, expecially a meniscus in the knee (p. 343). As a rule a fibrocartilage can be displaced only when it is torn. Other soft tissues that are occasionally interposed are synovial fringes and ligamentous tags.

Clinical features. Disorders of this type are common only in the knee. The characteristic features are recurrent sudden 'locking' or giving way of the joint, with later an effusion of clear fluid within it.

LOOSE BODIES IN JOINTS

Intra-articular loose bodies may be derived from bone, cartilage, or synovial membrane. They may be entirely free within the joint or they may retain a pedicle of soft tissue.

Causes. The commonest causes of loose bodies are: 1) osteochondritis dissecans (one to three loose bodies); 2) osteoarthritis (one to ten loose bodies); 3) chip fracture of the articular end of a bone (one to three loose bodies); and 4) synovial chondromatosis (fifty to five hundred loose bodies).

Pathology. *Osteochondritis dissecans* (see below). The loose body is derived from a part of the articular surface that undergoes necrosis and separates.

Osteoarthritis. The bodies may be derived from marginal osteophytes, in which case they often retain firm soft-tissue attachments and may cause little trouble. Free bodies may be derived from shed flakes of articular cartilage: nourished by synovial fluid, these gradually enlarge.

Fracture of articular margin (osteochondral fracture). Fractures only occasionally cause intra-articular loose bodies. A well recognised example is a fracture-separation of the medial epicondyle, which may be sucked into the elbow joint while still retaining its muscle attachments.

Synovial chondromatosis (osteochondromatosis). This is a rare disease of synovial membrane. A large number of villous folds become pedunculated and their bulbous extremities undergo metaplasia to cartilage. Eventually they separate from their pedicles to become free mobile bodies, and many of them become calcified. The disease may affect any joint—or even the synovial lining of a bursa.

Clinical features. Loose bodies do not necessarily cause symptoms unless they become caught between the joint surfaces. In that event the characteristic feature is sudden painful but usually momentary locking of the joint, succeeded after some hours by an effusion of clear fluid within it.

Treatment. When a loose body causes trouble it should be removed. In synovial chondromatosis this may be combined with subtotal synovectomy.

OSTEOCHONDRITIS DISSECANS

Osteochondritis dissecans is a localised disorder of convex joint surfaces in which a segment of subchondral bone becomes avascular and, with the articular cartilage that covers it, may slowly separate from the surrounding bone to form a loose body.

Common sites. The only joints commonly affected are the knee and the elbow. In the knee the site of the lesion is nearly always the medial femoral condyle, and in the elbow, the capitulum of the humerus. Occasionally the hip joint (femoral head) and the ankle joint (talus) are affected. The disorder of a metatarsal head known as Freiberg's disease (p. 399) is thought by some to be an example of osteochondritis dissecans and by others to represent osteochondritis juvenilis. It shows some features common to both conditions.

Cause. The precise cause is unknown. Impairment of blood supply to the affected segment of bone and cartilage—possibly by thrombosis of an end artery—has been suggested. The significance of injury is uncertain. There is probably an inborn susceptibility to the disease, for it may occur in several joints of the same patient, or in several members of a family.

Pathology. A segment of the articular surface of a bone becomes avascular (Fig. 102), and a line of demarcation slowly forms between the avascular segment and the surrounding normal bone (Fig. 103). The

Fig. 102   **Fig. 103**   **Fig. 104**

Evolution of osteochondritis dissecans. Figure 102—Segment of articular surface of medial femoral condyle deprived of blood supply. Figure 103— A line of demarcation has formed and the avascular fragment is separating from the surrounding healthy bone. Figure 104—Fragment loose in joint. A cavity remains in the articular surface.

affected segment varies in size: in the knee it often measures about one to three centimetres in diameter and half a centimetre in depth. It is always on the convex joint surface. If the segment is small it is sometimes re-attached spontaneously, especially in adolescents; but in most cases it finally separates to form a loose body in the joint, still covered by its articular cartilage (Fig. 104). The resulting cavity in the articular surface of the bone fills with fibrous tissue, but there is inevitably some irregularity of the joint surface which predisposes to the later development of osteoarthritis.

Clinical features. The patient is an adolescent or a young adult. The early symptoms and signs are those of a mild mechanical irritation of the joint—namely a tendency to aching after use, with recurrent effusion of clear fluid. After separation of a fragment from the articular surface the clinical features are those of an intra-articular loose body—recurrent sudden locking of the joint accompanied by sharp pain and followed by effusion.

Radiographs show a clearly defined shallow excavation in the articular surface of the bone, with a discrete bone fragment lying either within the cavity or elsewhere in the joint.

Treatment. Until a loose body has separated or appears 'ripe' for separation treatment should be expectant. In the case of a small lesion in early adolescence rest in plaster for two months may help to allow spontaneous re-attachment of the fragment. When a fragment has separated it should usually be removed, though in the case of a large fragment it may be practicable to fix it back in position with a pin. Further details will be found in the appropriate sections on the knee (p. 347), the elbow (p. 239), and the foot (p. 399).

References and bibliography, page 403.

8. Neurological disorders

POLIOMYELITIS
(Anterior poliomyelitis; infantile paralysis)

Poliomyelitis is a virus infection of nerve cells in the anterior grey matter of the spinal cord, leading in many cases to temporary or permanent paralysis of the muscles that they activate. In many countries the incidence of the disease increased so much in the years succeeding the Second World War that its management—or rather the management of the paralytic disabilities that it produces—became one of the foremost problems of orthopaedic surgery. However, in the 1950s the incidence decreased very markedly in Western countries, in consequence of nationwide programmes of prophylactic vaccination; so much so that the disease has now been virtually eliminated. Nevertheless it still occurs frequently in certain countries of Asia and Africa.

Cause. It is caused by infection with a virus, of which at least three types have been identified.

Pathology. After gaining access to the body through the nasopharynx or the gastro-intestinal tract, the virus finds its way to anterior horn cells of the spinal cord (Fig. 105) and sometimes to nerve cells in the brain stem. According to the virulence of the infection the cells may escape serious harm, or they may be damaged or killed. If cells are damaged there is paralysis of the corresponding muscles but recovery is possible; if the cells are killed paralysis is permanent. The extent and distribution of the lesions vary widely from case to case.

Clinical features. Although it is still commonest in children, poliomyelitis often attacks young adults. For descriptive purposes the disease is conveniently divided into five stages.

Stage of incubation. This is the interval between infection and onset of symptoms. It is thought to be about two weeks. There are no symptoms.

Stage of onset. This lasts about two days. The symptoms are like those of influenza: headache, pains in the back and limbs, and general malaise. Examination may show mild pyrexia, often with neck rigidity if flexion is attempted, and tenderness of muscles. Lumbar puncture may show an increase of round cells in the cerebrospinal fluid.

133

In many cases the disease does not progress beyond this stage, the patient making a rapid and complete recovery.

Stage of greatest paralysis. This stage, when it occurs, lasts about two months. Paralysis develops rapidly and is usually at its greatest within a few hours, thereafter remaining unchanged throughout this stage. The extent and distribution of the paralysis vary enormously. There may be no paralysis at all, or it may be total. In this stage muscle pain continues, and unparalysed muscles are often painful if stretched. If the respiratory muscles are paralysed preservation of life will be dependent upon the use of a mechanical respirator.

Stage of recovery. When any recovery of power occurs it may continue for about two years.[1] The degree of recovery varies within the widest limits. There may be complete recovery or there may be none.

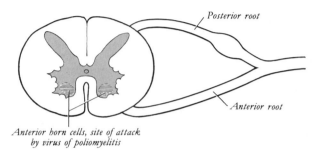

Posterior root

Anterior root

Anterior horn cells, site of attack by virus of poliomyelitis

Fig. 105

Section of spinal cord. The virus of poliomyelitis attacks the anterior horn cells. If the cells are killed there is permanent paralysis of the corresponding muscle fibres. If the cells are damaged but not killed the paralysis is recoverable.

Stage of residual paralysis. Paralysis or weakness persisting after two years is permanent. Its degree and extent vary from insignificant local weakness to almost total paralysis of the trunk and all four limbs. Weakness or paralysis is accompanied by obvious wasting of the affected muscles. This in turn is associated with defective growth of the bones and consequent shortening if the disease occurs in childhood.

Prognosis. In round figures, it may be stated that half of all patients clinically infected with poliomyelitis have no paralysis at any time. Of those with paralysis, 10 per cent die (usually from respiratory paralysis); 30 per cent recover fully; 30 per cent have moderate permanent paralysis; and 30 per cent have severe permanent paralysis.

Prophylaxis. In Britain prophylactic vaccination is by an attenuated living virus, taken by mouth.

Treatment. No specific treatment is available. In few diseases is the doctor so powerless to influence recovery: the patient either will or will not recover his muscle power, depending upon the severity of the neurological damage; and there is very little that the doctor can do about it. The main duties of the orthopaedic surgeon are to prevent deformity, to assist returning muscle power by graduated exercises, and to reduce residual disability in the final stage by the provision of appropriate appliances or by operations on joints or muscles. The treatment appropriate to each stage of the disease is best considered separately.

Stage of onset. The patient should rest in bed and may be given sedatives as required.

Stage of greatest paralysis. In this stage artificial respiration by a mechanical respirator may be necessary to preserve life if the respiratory muscles are paralysed. Paralysed limbs may have to be supported by splints in a neutral position to prevent the development of contractures with consequent deformity. Fixed equinus deformity of the ankle and foot is

---

[1]It will be observed that the figure 2 appears in the stated duration of each of the first four stages—2 weeks, 2 days, 2 months, 2 years. These are only very approximate figures, but they are easily memorised.

particularly liable to develop in cases of paralysis of the anterior leg muscles unless the foot is maintained at a right angle to the leg. Joints should be put through a full range of movement daily, so far as pain allows. Muscle pain may be eased by warmth, as from hot packs. Whether or not the patient must remain in bed in this stage will depend upon the degree and distribution of the paralysis.

Stage of recovery. The patient should be under the close supervision of a skilled physiotherapist. Any muscle that is seen to be regaining power must be exercised, gently and patiently at first, but later very strenuously, to encourage the greatest possible redevelopment. It should be remembered that power may improve partly as a result of recovery of the damaged nerve cells, but partly also from hypertrophy of muscle fibres that have escaped paralysis. When possible, walking should be resumed at this stage, if necessary with the aid of appliances, crutches or sticks.

Stage of residual paralysis. The disability in this stage can often be reduced either by the provision of suitable external appliances (orthoses), or by operation.

Fig. 106   **Fig. 107**   **Fig. 108**

Orthoses for residual paralysis after poliomyelitis. Figure 106—Caliper with lockable knee flexion hinge, used in a case of quadriceps paralysis. Figure 107—Below-knee brace with T-strap for stabilising a weak ankle and foot. Figure 108—A simple drop-foot appliance used to prevent dropping of the foot in paralysis of the anterior leg muscles. This is only one of many types that are available: in some a spring is concealed within the shoe.

Appliances. The purpose of external appliances or orthoses is to support joints that have lost their normal muscle control. They are required more often for the lower limbs and spine than for the upper limbs. The following are commonly prescribed: 1) spinal brace, to support a weakened spine; 2) abdominal support, to check abdominal protrusion when the abdominal muscles are weak; 3) knee caliper (Fig. 106), to hold the knee extended in cases of severe quadriceps paralysis; 4) below-knee brace (Fig. 107), to stabilise a flail ankle or foot; 5) single below-knee steel (lateral or medial) with ankle strap, to control varus or valgus deformity of the foot; 6) drop-foot spring (Fig. 108), to hold the foot up when the dorsiflexor muscles are paralysed.

Operative treatment. Two main groups of operations are available: 1) arthrodesis of joints; and 2) muscle or tendon transfers. *Arthrodesis* is a valuable method of stabilising joints that have lost their controlling muscles. It is particularly applicable to the shoulder, elbow, wrist, spine, ankle, and foot. In *muscle* or *tendon transfer* operations the object is to use a healthy muscle to replace the function of one that is paralysed. The method finds its chief application in the upper limb. Examples are the transfer of part of the pectoralis major muscle to replace the function of paralysed elbow flexors, transfer of wrist flexors to serve as extensors of the fingers, and transfer of a flexor digitorum superficialis tendon to replace a paralysed opponens muscle.

CEREBRAL PALSY
(Spastic paralysis; spastic paresis; Little's disease)

The term *cerebral palsy* embraces a number of clinical disorders, mostly arising in childhood, the feature common to all of which is that the primary lesion is in the brain. The incidence of these disorders is such that cerebral palsy constitutes a major social and educational problem.

Cause. There is no single cause. Any event that results in damage to the brain may be responsible. Thus the causes may be classified into three groups: pre-natal, natal, and post-natal. *Pre-natal* causes include congenital defective development of the nervous system, and erythroblastosis leading to icterus gravis in the child, with consequent damage to the basal nuclei (kernicterus). *Natal* causes include damage to the brain from birth injury, and anoxaemia with consequent cerebral anoxia. Prematurity is believed to be an important factor. *Post-natal* causes include infections such as pertussis, encephalitis and meningitis, head injuries, and, in later life, cerebro-vascular accidents. In children it is not always easy to ascribe the fault in a given case, but probably the commonest causes are damage to the brain during difficult labour and cerebral anoxia during birth.

Types. A number of clinical types may be recognised, of which the most important are: 1) spastic paresis; and 2) athetosis. Mixed types also occur.

SPASTIC PARESIS

Pathology. Part of the motor cortex of the brain is replaced by areas of gliosis. There is degeneration of the pyramidal tracts.

Clinical features. Usually within the first year it is noticed that the child has difficulty in controlling the movements of the affected limbs, and there is delay in sitting up, standing and walking. Commonly the upper and lower limbs of one side are affected (hemiplegia). Less often there is involvement of a single limb (monoplegia), of both lower limbs (paraplegia), or of all four limbs (tetraplegia[1]). The trunk and face muscles may also be affected. *On examination* the features that are found constantly are weakness, spasticity, and imperfect voluntary control of movement. Usually there is also deformity, and in some cases there may be mental deficiency, impaired vision, or deafness. These various features are best considered separately.

Weakness. There is no true paralysis, but there may be fairly marked weakness of muscles. The weakness seldom affects all the muscles of a limb

[1]Also termed (though less correctly because Latin is mixed with Greek) diplegia or quadriplegia.

equally; often there is marked muscle imbalance which may lead to deformity.

Spasticity. The muscles are 'stiff': they resist passive movement of the joints, but when steady pressure is applied for some time they slowly relax, allowing the joint to be moved. When the pressure is released the spasm immediately returns. The tendon reflexes are exaggerated and muscle clonus may be elicited.

Lack of voluntary control. This is a striking feature, especially in severe cases. When the patient attempts to move a single group of muscles, other groups contract at the same time.

Deformity. When spasm and muscle imbalance are pronounced they lead eventually to the development of fixed deformity. The stronger muscles hold the limb constantly in an unnatural position, and secondary adaptive changes take place in the muscles and periarticular tissues. The commonest deformities in the upper limb are flexion contracture of the elbow, pronation deformity of the forearm, flexion of the wrist, and adduction of the thumb. In the lower limb the common deformities are adduction of the hip, flexion of the knee, and equinus of the ankle.

Mental deficiency. Impairment of mental capacity is sometimes present, but usually intelligence is normal. Lack of control of the facial and speech muscles may suggest mental impairment when in fact none exists. It is important that the medical advisers be not misled in this respect. *Defective vision* and *deafness* may also retard the child's progress.

The severity of the disability varies widely from case to case. In the mildest examples the child is able to lead a normal active life with very little handicap, whereas in the worst cases the patient is almost helpless.

Prognosis. Since an essential part of the brain is destroyed and cannot be replaced complete cure is impossible. All that can be hoped for is improvement. To achieve even this requires endless patience on the part of the patient and the attendants. Yet perseverance is nearly always well rewarded, and there are few cases in which worth-while improvement cannot be gained. Thus a patient formerly dependent upon others in many daily activities may often gain independence, and many who were previously unable to work become capable of earning their own living.

Treatment. Up to the age of about 5 years treatment may be carried out at non-residential centres, but after the age of 5 a child who is considerably disabled should be admitted to a special residential school where adequate facilities and trained staff are available.

The methods of treatment available are muscle training, corrective splinting, speech therapy, and operations on tendons, bones, or nerves.

Muscle training. This is an important part of the management of all except the mildest cases, and it is best carried out by a physiotherapist with experience of this very demanding work. The principles of muscle training are to teach the child to relax spastic muscles, to develop the use of individual muscle groups, and to improve coordination. Repetitive rhythmic movements are valuable. Stage by stage the child is instructed in dressing, toilet, feeding, and walking.

Corrective splinting. Splints or plasters are especially useful in overcoming the deformities induced by spastic muscles. Deformity is first corrected by gradual stretching of the contracted muscles, if necessary under anaesthesia. The limb is held by plaster in the over-corrected position for six to eight weeks. Thereafter removable braces or splints (orthoses) may be used indefinitely to prevent recurrence of the deformity.

Speech therapy. Many spastic children have a speech defect which, with constant grimacing and salivation, may lead one to suppose that there is mental deficiency when in fact this is not so. In these cases the speech therapist is sometimes able to achieve a marked improvement.

Operative treatment. Operations for spastic paralysis should be approached with caution: striking benefit may be achieved in appropriate cases, but injudicious operation in unsuitable cases has often led to disappointing results. Operation may be upon tendon, joint, or nerve.

TENDON DIVISION OR ELONGATION. Division or lengthening of the tendon of a spastic muscle reduces its mechanical advantage and improves muscle balance. Examples are lengthening of the calcaneal tendon in a case of spastic equinus deformity, and tenotomy of the adductors of the hip for adduction deformity.

TENDON TRANSFER. At certain sites transfer of the insertion of a muscle that is aggravating deformity may so modify the muscle's action that it acts beneficially instead of as a deforming force. An example is the transfer of the insertion of the hamstring tendons from the tibia to the back of the femoral condyles in a case of flexion deformity of the knee: this eliminates the undesirable action of the spastic hamstrings in flexing the knee, while enhancing their desirable action as hip extensors.

ARTHRODESIS. When skeletal growth is complete it is sometimes of benefit to fuse a joint in the position of function, to overcome persistent deformity from the pull of spastic muscles. Thus a wrist that lies constantly flexed may be fused in a neutral or slightly extended position, with consequent improvement in function.

NEURECTOMY. The principle is to divide part or the whole of a nerve that supplies an overacting spastic muscle. An example is division of the anterior branch of the obturator nerve to overcome spastic adduction at the hip.

ATHETOSIS

Pathology. The main damage is in the basal nuclei.

Clinical features. The principal feature is the occurrence of generalised overlaid involuntary movements which have no pattern and which interfere with the performance of normal movements. Any part or the whole of the muscular system may be affected.

In mild cases the child is able to lead a fairly normal life, but in the worst examples the patient may be unable to sit up, walk, feed himself, or express himself in words, even though the mental state may be good.

Treatment. In all except the mildest cases residential treatment is desirable, as for spastic paresis. The first essential in treatment is to teach the child general relaxation. Once this has been achieved, purposeful voluntary movements can be taught. Splints and appliances may be required, but in pure athetosis there is no place for operations on the limbs. In some cases of severe athetosis improvement has been reported after surgical ablation of the globus pallidus.

SPINA BIFIDA

The term *spina bifida* implies a failure of the enfolding of the nerve elements within the spinal canal during early development of the embryo. The defect varies in degree and in its site (Fig. 109). In the mildest cases there is no more than a failure of fusion of one or more of the vertebral arches posteriorly, in the lumbo-sacral region. This is often of no clinical significance. Less often, the posterior bony deficiency is marked on the surface by an abnormality of the overlying skin, in the form of a dimple, a tuft of hair, a lipomatous mass or a dermal sinus. In these cases there may be an underlying abnormality involving nerves of the cauda equina. These relatively minor varieties of spina bifida, in which the defect is not obvious at the skin surface, are termed *spina bifida occulta*. This contrasts with *spina bifida aperta*, in which there is a major defect of enfolding of the nerve elements, involving not only the bony vertebral arches but also the overlying soft tissues and skin, and often the meningeal membranes enclosing the

Fig. 109
Spina bifida. Diagrams showing four grades of severity of the posterior defect of the spinal canal. *From left to right:* Spina bifida occulta, meningocele, myelomeningocele, rachischisis.

spinal canal, so that the neutral tube itself is exposed and open (Fig. 109). This major variant of spina bifida may occur anywhere in the spine but is commonest in the thoraco-lumbar region, and it is attended by grave impairment of nerve function.

SPINA BIFIDA OCCULTA
(Occult spinal dysraphism)

As noted above, the bony defect is simply a failure of fusion of the vertebral arches posteriorly. When there is neurological involvement the overlying skin nearly always shows an abnormality, as already described.

Impairment of nerve function may be caused in some such cases by tethering of the dura, and through this the spinal cord, to the skin surface by a fibrous membrane. Traction on the cord becomes gradually worse as the spinal column elongates disproportionately to the spinal cord, so that the neurological deficit may be progressive. A rather similar effect is caused by tethering of the distal end of the spinal cord by the filum terminale. Rarely, too, a bifid cord is transfixed by a delicate bar of bone crossing the spinal canal in the antero-posterior plane (diastematomyelia) with consequent tethering and progressive neurological impairment. In yet other cases the neurological fault may be a consequence of myelodysplasia, a congenital defect of development of nerve tissue.

In cases of occult spinal dysraphism there is no close correlation between the severity of the bony defect and the degree of neurological impairment. Often there is no neurological involvement; but on the other hand it may be severe. Clinically, the common manifestation of nerve involvement is muscle imbalance in the lower limbs, often with selective muscle wasting and deformity of the foot which often takes the form either of equino-varus or of cavus.

Investigation and treatment. The patient may be brought for advice because of an abnormality of the skin over the lumbo-sacral region, because of abnormality of the feet or perhaps just a limp, or because of urinary incontinence. A plain radiograph will show the extent of the bony deficiency.

If evidence of neurological impairment is lacking, treatment is not required. If neurological impairment or incontinence is present—and especially if there has been progressive deterioration—further investigations, including CT or MR scanning and radiculography, are required. These may point to the presence of one of the structural lesions mentioned above, and in such a case neurosurgical intervention may be required: its object is to prevent further deterioration rather than to promote complete recovery (James and Lassman 1962; Till 1969).

SPINA BIFIDA APERTA

(Overt spinal dysraphism; variations include rachischisis, myelomeningocele and meningocele)

The neurological deficit that complicates the more severe forms of spina bifida leads to varying degrees of motor, sensory and visceral paralysis, and the consequent orthopaedic disability in the lower limbs may be complex. The number of children demanding orthopaedic care for such disabilities has increased in recent years because a far higher proportion of children born with myelomeningocele survived when the associated hydrocephalus was controlled by a ventriculo-cardiac or ventriculo-peritoneal shunt. Nevertheless the incidence is likely to fall dramatically since the advent of antenatal screening for alpha-fetoprotein, high-resolution ultrasound, and amniocentesis, with the option of termination of pregnancy in positive cases.

The cause is unknown: genetic factors may play a part but environmental factors are also probably involved. In particular, the influence of certain drugs—notably anti-epileptic drugs such as sodium valproate—has been recognised.

Pathology. The basic structural defect—failure of total closure of the embryonal neural tube or of mesodermal tissue to invest it—varies in degree (Fig. 109). In the most serious defect, *rachischisis*, the neural tube is open and exposed on the surface. Cerebrospinal fluid leaks from the exposed upper end of the central spinal canal. In *myelomeningocele* the neural tube is closed by a membrane but the skin covering is deficient. The spinal cord and the nerve roots are displaced posteriorly into the sac and are outside the line of the vertebral canal (Fig. 109). In *meningocele* the bulging sac consists of meninges and fluid only, the nerve elements being normally situated. The skin may or may not be intact.

The distinction between closed lesions, with intact skin, and open lesions in which skin is deficient and nerve tissue is exposed on the surface of the body, is fundamental because open lesions may demand operation within a few hours of birth to close the defect, if indeed active intervention is deemed advisable.

The neurological lesion. Neurological deficit may be primary or secondary. Primary paralysis is present at birth and implies failure of development of part of the spinal cord—myelodysplasia. This varies widely in degree. In a fairly common example there may be normal innervation down to the level of the fourth lumbar segment and failure of development below that level. But the lesion may be either less extensive or more extensive than this.

Secondary paralysis develops after birth, either from drying or infection of exposed nerve tissue when closure of an open lesion has been delayed; from stretching of tethered nerve fibres as growth occurs; or from compression of nerve tissue within the abnormal spinal canal.

Clinical assessment. It is difficult in small infants to assess accurately the extent of motor and of sensory paralysis, and particularly to determine the state of bladder function. Nevertheless the important objective at the outset is to determine the level at which normal function of the spinal cord ceases. This is done by observing what movements the child makes, and correlating these with the root level. Sensibility can be determined by stimulating the skin lightly with a pin moved upwards from the limbs to the trunk until the child is awakened.

Motor paralysis. Motor paralysis affects mainly the lower limbs and to some extent the trunk. The extent of limb paralysis corresponds to the degree of dysplasia or of secondary damage in the spinal cord. It varies from the very mild, in which there may be no more than minor weakness of a single muscle group, to the very severe, in which there is total paralysis of the limbs. In the instance quoted above of normal cord function down to the fourth lumbar segment with loss of function below that, motor power is present only in the flexors and adductors of the hips, the quadriceps and the tibialis anterior: the remaining muscles are paralysed. This is a fairly common distribution but only one of an almost infinite variety. This uneven paralysis, with consequent muscle imbalance, leads commonly to secondary contractures with fixed deformity of hips, knees or feet. It may also lead to dislocation of the hip, a common sequel to gluteal and abductor paralysis in the presence of strong flexors and adductors.

Sensory paralysis. Motor paralysis is nearly always accompanied by sensory paralysis of approximately the same distribution. This makes treatment more difficult because the use of corrective splints is hampered by the risk of pressure sores on the insensitive skin.

Visceral paralysis. Incontinence of bladder and bowel is present in a high proportion of patients.

Hydrocephalus. Associated hydrocephalus, usually due to the Arnold-Chiari malformation of the hind-brain, is common and was formerly largely responsible for the poor rate of survival among children with severe spina bifida.

Treatment. Every child with major neurological or visceral dysfunction from spina bifida should be admitted immediately to a special centre where a team of experienced specialists—including paediatrician, paediatric surgeon, neurosurgeon and orthopaedic surgeon—may cooperate in deciding upon a programme that is best suited to the child. The team must first decide whether or not any surgical treatment, including closure of the defect, is to be advised. This selective approach arose from review of large series where closure was universal: in the worst cases, with gross neurological deficit or hydrocephalus, the results were disastrous. In these it is probably better to adopt an expectant attitude, accepting the situation and relying simply on careful nursing and feeding. It has to be taken as inevitable that many of these badly affected infants will fail to survive.

The problems that are to be tackled when more active treatment is undertaken are often very complex. No firm rules can be laid down because there is so much variation between individual cases. It is sufficient here to indicate the main principles of orthopaedic treatment. These are: 1) to correct deformity; 2) to maintain correction; and 3) to promote the best possible function in the affected limbs (Sharrard and Grosfield 1968; Sharrard 1969). In general, orthopaedic treatment should be deferred until the age of one to three years, to ensure that the child is thriving well and that the problems of hydrocephalus and renal function are satisfactorily controlled. This may have required a ventriculo-cardiac or ventriculo-peritoneal shunt to drain the excess cerebrospinal fluid, and urinary diversion to an artificial bladder for reasons of hygiene.

Correction of deformity. Deformity, whether of the hip, knee or foot, should be corrected in the simplest way possible with the object of providing a limb that is straight, mobile, and with a plantigrade foot—that is, a limb that is best suited for weight bearing. This may be achieved by a combination of splintage and surgical treatment, depending on the level of paralysis and the joints affected. Splints and plasters are useful for controlling flail joints and for maintaining correction after operative procedures, but they must be fitted and used with care because of the risk of pressure sores involving the insensitive skin. When fixed deformity is present as a result of unbalanced or spastic muscle action operation is needed to divide or elongate tight structures—tendon, muscle, ligament or joint capsule—in order to achieve a neutral anatomical position. Paralytic dislocation of the hip is common and may necessitate posterior transfer of the iliopsoas muscle to the greater trochanter (to act as a hip abductor), sometimes combined with femoral or pelvic osteotomy, to maintain stability. In the more severe lesions, where wheelchair locomotion is inevitable, it may be better to leave the dislocation unreduced while preserving mobile hips. Spinal deformity, often a combination of kyphosis and scoliosis, may require surgical correction and fusion, but the complications of pseudarthrosis and pressure sores are common (Drummond *et al.* 1980).

Development of limb function. Even when lower limb paralysis is severe it is often possible to get the child walking with crutches once deformities have been overcome. In many cases external bracing in the form of limb calipers or swivel walkers is also required, and prolonged training by a skilled physiotherapist is essential if maximal function is to be achieved (Rose *et al.* 1983).

PERIPHERAL NERVE LESIONS

Disorders of the peripheral nerves come largely within the sphere of the neurologist, but the orthopaedic surgeon is concerned with lesions that have a mechanical basis and with those that lend themselves to reconstructive surgery.

Pathology. Nerves may be damaged by laceration, contusion, traction, compression, friction, burns or ischaemia. According to its severity, a nerve lesion may be classified as neurapraxia, axonotmesis, or neurotmesis (Seddon 1942). In *neurapraxia* the damage is slight and it causes only a transient physiological block. Recovery occurs spontaneously within days or weeks. In *axonotmesis* the internal architecture of the nerve is preserved, but the axons are so badly damaged that peripheral degeneration occurs. Recovery can occur spontaneously, but it depends upon regeneration of the axons and may take many months (about 2.5 centimetres a month is the usual speed of regeneration). In *neurotmesis* the structure of the nerve is destroyed by actual division or by severe scarring. Recovery is possible only after excision of the damaged section and end-to-end suture of the stumps, or after nerve grafting.

Clinical features. The effects of complete loss of conductivity of a nerve are motor, sensory, and autonomic. They are localised to the distribution of the nerve affected. *Motor changes:* The muscles are paralysed and wasted. Changes occur in the electrical reactions, but they take between two and three weeks to develop. These changes were described on page 20. *Sensory changes:* There is loss of cutaneous, deep, and postural sensibility. *Autonomic changes:* These include loss of sweating, loss of pilomotor response to cold ('goose-skin'), and temporary vasodilation with increased warmth, which, however, is followed later by vasoconstriction and coldness.

Complications. Injury to a peripheral nerve trunk is occasionally followed by severe burning pain in the distribution of the nerve. This is termed *causalgia.* It is a complication of incomplete rather than of complete lesions, and with few exceptions it is confined in the upper limb to the brachial plexus or the median nerve, and in the lower limb to the sciatic nerve or the tibial nerve. It may be a very disabling complication, the only effective treatment of which is by sympathetic denervation of the limb.

Treatment. *Open injuries.* If a nerve is believed to have been divided—for example, by a penetrating injury—the wound should be explored and the nerve identified. If the nerve is severed the ends should be examined carefully to determine the extent to which they have been damaged by laceration or bruising. Only in the case of a clean-cut division with minimal damage to the severed ends should primary suture be carried out. If these criteria are not satisfied it is better simply to tack the ends together with one or two sutures and to delay definitive repair—preferably with a magnification technique—until two or three weeks after the injury. At that time the extent of the scarring, and consequently the length of nerve to be resected, can be determined accurately, and thickening of the nerve sheath makes suture technically easier.

Closed injuries. In closed injuries complicated by nerve paralysis it is usually assumed that the nerve is in continuity, and expectant treatment is adopted at first. If signs of recovery are not observed within the expected time (calculated from the site of injury and length to be regenerated) exploration is advised. Evidence of muscle re-innervation may be derived from electromyography at an earlier stage than from clinical examination. Such exploration should seldom be delayed for more than three or four months, because long delay prejudices successful repair if the nerve has been divided.

When a nerve lesion has been caused by stretching, compression or ischaemia the essential principle of treatment is to ensure that the harmful conditions are relieved, if necessary by operation to free the nerve or to remove a compressing agent.

Nerve grafting. When the gap to be bridged between healthy neurones proximally and distally is large, nerve grafting is preferable to attempted direct suture under tension. A thick nerve may be bridged by multiple grafts from a thinner nerve—for example the sural nerve. By microsurgical techniques it is also now possible to transfer a nerve complete with its blood supply, to bridge a major defect. Freeze-thawed muscle grafts have been used experimentally as an alternative to nerve grafts. They may provide a chemotactic stimulus for nerve regeneration as well as providing a micro-skeleton to guide axonal fibres across the gap, which should not exceed three centimetres.

BRACHIAL PLEXUS INJURIES

Injuries of the brachial plexus are a major cause of partial or complete loss of function of the upper limb. Most of them are caused by forcible distraction of the upper extremity away from the neck by violent depression of the shoulder. The main injury is sustained by the upper roots of the plexus, which may be stretched, torn, or even avulsed from the spinal cord. There is consequent paralysis of the muscles supplied through the upper roots—chiefly the abductor and lateral rotator muscles of the shoulder and the flexors of the elbow (Erb type of paralysis). A less common type of brachial plexus injury is caused by forcible elevation of the arm and shoulder. This tends to drag on the lower roots of the plexus, with consequent motor and sensory paralysis mainly in the forearm and hand (Klumpke type of paralysis). In the most severe injuries the whole plexus is torn or avulsed and there is total paralysis of the upper limb.

Brachial plexus lesions in infants. In infants, brachial plexus injuries are usually caused during delivery (obstetrical palsy), and the risk is greatest in difficult breech deliveries. The upper arm type (Erb's palsy) is the more common. Soon after birth it is noticed that the child does not move the arm as he normally should. Unopposed action of the unparalysed muscles tends to bring the arm into a position of adduction and medial rotation, and secondary contracture of the soft tissues may lead to fixed deformity in that position.

Prognosis depends upon the severity of the stretching injury. If this was mild full recovery may occur, though it may take many months; but in a severe case there may be permanent loss of power and sensibility. The prognosis is less favourable in the rare lower arm type of lesion (Klumpke type) than in the commoner upper arm type.

Treatment. In a mild case the mother should be taught to move the limb frequently through the full range, to prevent fixed contracture. In a severe case seen early it may be possible, if the requisite expertise is available, to restore continuity of the damaged nerves by operation. In late cases with permanent paralysis and deformity there is a place for late reconstructive operations such as corrective (rotation) osteotomy of the humerus, arthrodesis of the shoulder or tendon transfer operations.

Brachial plexus lesions in adults. In adults brachial plexus injuries are usually caused by forcible depression of the shoulder. By far the commonest cause is a motorcycling accident.

It is important to distinguish between preganglionic lesions, in which the nerve roots are avulsed from the spinal cord, and postganglionic lesions, in which the nerves are torn more distally. Preganglionic lesions are irrecoverable, whereas there is potential for some recovery in postganglionic lesions. Clinical and electrical tests may indicate the approximate site of the lesion, but special investigations are needed for more accurate assessment. Initially, spinal root imaging by radiculography may show dural pouches at the sites of nerve avulsion. CT scanning with contrast gives the best information on the extent of the damage and is superior to MRI scanning. In the last resort surgical exploration may be needed to localise the lesion definitively, especially in the first few days after injury when the prospect of successful repair is most favourable. The measurement of intra-operative nerve action potentials is valuable: when these are present distal to the lesion a substantial number of large fibres have survived the injury, so excision and grafting are unnecessary.

Treatment. For irrecoverable (preganglionic) lesions all that can be done is to make the best use of any function that remains. Tendon or muscle transfers, to replace the action of paralysed muscles, may be appropriate in selected cases, and arthrodesis of the shoulder may sometimes be indicated if strong scapular muscles and useful hand function are preserved.

If however it is confirmed at operation that the roots have been torn across rather than avulsed, repair by nerve grafting—a vascularised nerve graft may be inserted by microsurgical techniques—may be attempted with some hope of success. Nerve transfers that have been used include: accessory nerve to suprascapular nerve, to improve shoulder function; and third or fourth intercostal nerve to musculocutaneous nerve, to restore elbow flexion. Even limited recovery is well worthwhile, and may reduce the level of severe causalgic pain; nevertheless the outlook for good recovery of motor and sensory function is always very doubtful, especially in the forearm and hand, and severe permanent disability is usually to be expected.

References and bibliography, page 403.

PART THREE

REGIONAL ORTHOPAEDICS

In this part the features of the common disorders of the trunk and limbs will be outlined against the background of the systematic descriptions covered in Part 2.

9. Neck and cervical spine

The commonest orthopaedic cause of neck disorders is degeneration of a cervical intervertebral disc. This may lead to protrusion of part of the disc contents (prolapsed cervical disc) or, more often, it may give rise to secondary osteoarthritic changes in the intervertebral joints (cervical spondylosis). These conditions together make up a large proportion of the disabilities of the neck encountered in an orthopaedic out-patient department.

A disorder of the cervical spine often interferes with the roots of the brachial plexus, causing radiating pain, muscle weakness, or sensory impairment in the corresponding upper limb. Indeed, the clinical importance of a cervical disorder often lies in its neurological effects rather than in the local lesion itself.

SPECIAL POINTS IN THE INVESTIGATION OF NECK COMPLAINTS

History. It is important to ascertain the relationship of the present symptoms to any previous neck disorder. Has there been any previous injury to the neck? Or a sudden jerk of the head that might have jarred the cervical spine? Is there a history of 'stiff neck'—a common feature in the early stages of prolapsed cervical disc?

If pain in the upper limb is a prominent symptom, it is important to determine its exact distribution and its nature. Pain caused by pressure upon a nerve in the cervical region follows a clearly defined course which depends upon the particular nerve involved, and it is usually severe. It commonly extends throughout the upper arm into the forearm and hand, radiating to one or more of the digits. It is often accompanied by paraesthesiae, described as 'pins and needles' or 'numbness'. In contrast, pain referred down the limb from a lesion of the shoulder or humerus is more diffuse and ill defined, and it seldom extends below the elbow.

Exposure. The patient must be stripped to the waist. Preferably he should stand, or he may sit upon a stool.

Steps in clinical examination. A suggested routine for clinical examination of the neck is summarised in Table IV.

Deformity. The cervical spine normally has a slight anterior curvature (lordosis). Straightening of this curve, or an angulation in the reverse direction (kyphosis) is sometimes significant and may suggest an underlying abnormality. Any lateral or rotational deformity must also be noted.

Movements. The movements to be examined are flexion, extension, lateral flexion to right and left, and rotation to right and left. Flexion-extension movements occur mainly at the occipito-atlantoid joint but to some extent throughout the cervical spine. Lateral flexion takes place throughout the cervical spine. Rotation occurs largely at the atlanto-axial joint, with a small range of movement at the other joints. It is important to find out whether movement causes pain and, if so, whether the pain is felt locally in the neck or whether it is referred down the upper limbs. It should be noted also whether movement is accompanied by audible or palpable crepitation.

Table IV
Routine clinical examination in suspected disorders of the neck

1. LOCAL EXAMINATION OF NECK, WITH NEUROLOGICAL AND VASCULAR SURVEY OF UPPER LIMBS

Inspection
    Bone contours: ?deformity
    Soft-tissue contours
    Colour and texture of skin
    Scars or sinuses

Movements
    Flexion-extension
    Lateral flexion
    Rotation
    ? Pain on movement
    ? Crepitation on movement

Palpation
    Skin temperature
    Bone contours
    Soft-tissue contours
    Local tenderness

Neurological state of upper limb
    Muscular system
    Sensory system
    Sweating
    Reflexes

Vascular state of upper limb
    Colour
    Temperature
    Pulses

2. EXAMINATION OF POTENTIAL EXTRINSIC SOURCES OF NECK SYMPTOMS

Symptoms suggestive of a neck disorder may arise from the ears or throat. Symptoms in the upper limb suggesting a neck disorder with involvement of the brachial plexus may arise from shoulder, elbow, or nerve trunks in their peripheral course.

3. GENERAL EXAMINATION

General survey of other parts of the body. Neck symptoms may be only one manifestation of a more widespread disease.

Neurological examination of upper limbs. This is an essential step in the investigation of the neck because cervical lesions so often interfere with the brachial plexus.

Muscular system. The muscles of the shoulder girdle, arm, forearm, and hand must be examined for wasting or fasciculation, a comparison being made on the two sides. The tone and power of each muscle group are then tested in turn and a comparison is made with the opposite limb.

Sensory system. Examine the patient's sensibility to touch and pin prick. In appropriate cases test also the sensibility to deep stimuli, joint position, vibration, and heat and cold. In the assessment of sensory loss it should be remembered that the middle or long finger, representing the central axis of the limb, is innervated mainly from the seventh cervical nerve. The radial half of the hand is innervated by the proximal roots of the brachial plexus (C.5, C.6) whereas the ulnar half is innervated from the more distal roots (C.8, T.1).

Sweating. Feel whether the digits are moist or dry. Sweating is dependent upon intact sudomotor nerve fibres.

Reflexes. Compare on the two sides the biceps jerk (mainly C.6), the triceps jerk (mainly C.7), and the brachioradialis jerk (mainly C.6).

From the findings elicited it should be possible to determine whether there is a neurological disturbance and, if so, whether it is of upper or lower motor neurone type, and the identity of the roots, trunks, or branches involved.

Vascular examination of the upper limb. The subclavian artery is sometimes interfered with by a lesion of the neck. The efficiency of the circulatory system in each upper limb must therefore be determined. Judge and compare on the two sides the colour and warmth of the forearm, hand and fingers. Test and compare the radial pulses, first with the limb at rest, then with the shoulder depressed and the head rotated towards the side examined.

Extrinsic causes of neck symptoms
Occasionally neck symptoms have their origin outside the neck itself. Thus pain may be referred to the neck from the ears or throat. These sites should be examined routinely for evidence of disease.

Symptoms in the upper limb that might suggest the possibility of a neck disorder involving the brachial plexus may in fact have their origin in the shoulder or elbow, or at any point along the peripheral distribution of the nerve trunks.

Diagnostic imaging
Radiographic examination. Routine radiographs of the cervical spine include an antero-posterior and a lateral projection. Additional projections are often required when it is desired to show a particular structure more clearly. For a study of the dens (odontoid process) of the axis a special antero-posterior projection is made through the open mouth. Oblique projections are essential for a proper investigation of the intervertebral foramina and the facet joints, and an oblique view of the lower cervical region is valuable in revealing the size and shape of a cervical rib. In cases of special difficulty tomography, comparative lateral views in flexion and in extension, cineradiography, or stereoscopic radiography may be helpful.

Other techniques of imaging. Radioisotope scanning, computerised tomography (CT scanning) and magnetic resonance imaging (MRI) must be considered in appropriate circumstances.

CLASSIFICATION OF DISORDERS OF THE NECK AND CERVICAL SPINE

Deformities
Infantile torticollis
Congenital short neck
Congenital high scapula

Arthritis of the spinal joints
Rheumatoid arthritis
Ankylosing spondylitis
Osteoarthritis of the cervical spine
(cervical spondylosis)

Infections of bone
Tuberculosis of the cervical spine
Pyogenic infection of the cervical spine

Mechanical derangements
Prolapsed intervertebral disc
Cervical rib
Cervical spondylolisthesis

Tumours
Benign and malignant tumours
in relation to the cervical
spine and nerve roots

INFANTILE TORTICOLLIS

('Congenital' torticollis; muscular torticollis)

In infantile torticollis (wry neck) the head is tilted and rotated by contracture of the sternomastoid muscle of one side. Strictly this is not a true congenital deformity because it arises after birth. With improvements in obstetrical practice it is now seen much less often than it was in the past.

Cause. This is uncertain. Probably there is interference with the blood supply of the sternomastoid muscle, caused by injury during birth.

Pathology. In the established condition, part of the affected muscle is replaced by contracted fibrous tissue. In some cases contracture is known to have been preceded, in early infancy, by a tumour-like thickening of the muscle ('sternomastoid tumour'), the histology being that of muscle infarction and replacement by fibrous tissue.

Clinical features. The child, often between 6 months and 3 years old when brought for consultation, is noticed to hold the head on one side. *On examination*, the contracted muscle is felt as a tight cord. The ear on the affected side is approximated to the corresponding shoulder. In long-established cases there is retarded development of the face on the affected side, with consequent asymmetry (Fig. 110).

Fig. 110
Infantile torticollis. Note the tense cord-like left sternomastoid muscle and the facial asymmetry.

Diagnosis. The condition has to be distinguished from other forms of wry neck, including structural deformities of the cervical spine, ocular torticollis, muscle spasm from a local inflammatory lesion such as infected glands, and psychogenic (hysterical) torticollis. The important diagnostic features are the history, the cord-like contracted sternomastoid, and the facial asymmetry.

Treatment. If the condition is seen at the stage of 'sternomastoid tumour', repeated stretching of the muscle under the supervision of a physiotherapist is effective. In established cases the contracted muscle should be divided at its lower attachment. After operation corrective exercises should be encouraged.

CONGENITAL SHORT NECK

(Klippel-Feil syndrome)

This is an uncommon non-familial congenital malformation of the cervical spine characterised clinically by short neck and limitation of head movements. The cause is unknown.

The degree of abnormality varies widely. The bony deformity consists in fusion of two or more of the cervical vertebrae. Clinically, the neck appears short or absent, and the hair-line is low. The neck may also be webbed to the shoulder. Movements of the head are restricted. *Radiographs* show the underlying bony abnormality.

Treatment. Operation is seldom indicated, but upper thoracoplasty has sometimes been undertaken simply for cosmetic improvement.

CONGENITAL HIGH SCAPULA

(Sprengel's shoulder)

Congenital high scapula is an uncommon congenital deformity characterised by an abnormally high position and relative fixity of the scapula. The cause is unknown. The anomaly represents a failure of the scapula—originally a cervical appendage—to descend during development to its normal thoracic position. The scapular muscles are ill developed and may be represented only by tough fibrous bands.

Clinically, the scapula on one or both sides is abnormally high. Its attachments seem almost rigid and it does not rotate freely during abduction of the arm. The range of shoulder abduction is consequently impaired, but the functional disability is slight.

Treatment. The condition is often best left alone, but some cases are suitable for operation. The upper part of the scapula (above its spine) is excised after division of the contracted levator scapulae muscle and of tight fascial hands. The blade of the scapula is then divided vertically throughout its length near the vertebral border. This allows the main (lateral) part of the scapula to be displaced downwards relative to the medial strip, and the two parts are re-united with sutures through drill holes (Wilkinson and Campbell 1980).

TUBERCULOSIS OF THE CERVICAL SPINE

(Tuberculous cervical spondylitis)

Tuberculosis is far less common in the cervical spine than in the thoracic and lumbar regions. It is now seldom seen in Britain. The general features of tuberculosis of bone were described in Chapter 5 (p. 76).

Pathology. The organisms reach the cervical spine through the blood stream from a pre-existing focus—latent or overt—elsewhere in the body. The infection begins in the front of a vertebral body, or in an intervertebral disc (Fig. 111). Destruction of bone and intervertebral disc leads to anterior collapse with consequent cervical kyphosis (Fig. 112). The degree of destruction varies widely, depending upon the virulence of the organism and the resistance of the patient. Formation of pus leads either to a retropharyngeal abscess (behind the prevertebral fascia), which may eventually point at the posterior margin of the sternomastoid muscle, or, if the pus tracks posteriorly, to a suboccipital abscess. The spinal cord may be damaged by direct pressure of an abscess, or by secondary thrombosis of the vessels of the cord.

Clinical features. The disease occurs mainly in children and young adults. There is pain in the neck and occiput, aggravated by movement. In addition, one or more of the following symptoms may be present: difficulty in swallowing; abscess or sinus at the side or back of the neck; neurological symptoms from spinal cord dysfunction, the upper limbs being affected before the lower. *On examination* the head is held rigidly, often supported by the hands. The cervical muscles stand out in spasm. One or more of the spinous processes may appear prominent, due to cervical kyphosis. There is local tenderness on firm palpation over the spinous processes. All movements of the head and neck are restricted, and cause pain if forced. An abscess may be present in the suboccipital region, behind the sternomastoid muscle, or behind the pharynx (see below). Associated tuberculous lesions elsewhere are common.

Radiographic features. Radiographs always show diminution of disc space, usually some destruction of bone (Fig. 112), and sometimes an abscess shadow.

Investigations. The erythrocyte sedimentation rate is raised in the active stage. The Mantoux test is positive. Pus obtained by aspiration of an abscess may yield tubercle bacilli.

Complications. *Retropharyngeal abscess.* This causes difficulty in swallowing (dysphagia), and the posterior wall of the pharynx is seen to bulge forwards in the midline. Eventually the abscess may point behind the sternomastoid muscle. If neglected, it may rupture into the pharynx.

Spinal cord dysfunction. If the spinal cord is affected there will be neurological signs (sensory, motor, and visceral) at and below the level of the lesion, which may progress to complete paralysis.

Fig. 111	**Fig. 112**

Tuberculosis of the cervical spine. Figure 111—The infection begins at the front margin of a vertebral body close to the intervertebral disc, or possibly in the disc itself, as indicated by the shaded area. Figure 112—The opposing surfaces of the bodies of C.4 and C.5 have been eroded and the intervening disc is destroyed. Pus has collected behind the prevertebral fascia, forming a bulging retropharyngeal abscess.

Diagnosis. Important diagnostic features are the history (contact with tuberculosis, or tuberculous lesions elsewhere), spasm of the neck muscles with restriction of all movements, abscess formation and the radiographic findings.

Treatment. The principles of treatment are the same as for other forms of skeletal tuberculosis. *Antibacterial therapy:* Combinations of antituberculous drugs were described on page 120. *Local treatment* is by support for the cervical spine by plaster of Paris or by a plastic collar until the disease is quiescent—often a matter of several months.

Operation is sometimes required and the following are the main indications: 1) to drain a retropharyngeal abscess that threatens to rupture or to cause asphyxia; 2) in a florid case, to remove necrotic bone and debris and then to embed a bone graft in the cavity; 3) to decompress a spinal cord damaged by pressure of abscess or granulation tissue; 4) in the quiescent stage, to fuse the affected region of the spine if it is judged to be unstable.

PYOGENIC INFECTION OF THE CERVICAL SPINE
(Pyogenic cervical spondylitis)

Infection of the cervical vertebrae or intervertebral discs with pyogenic organisms is uncommon. It is usually caused by the staphylococcus, streptococcus or pneumococcus, and occasionally by other bacteria, including salmonella organisms or brucella abortus.

Pathology. The organisms reach the spinal column by the general blood stream (from a septic focus elsewhere), by lymphatic channels (from a local infection, for instance in the pharynx), or possibly by the spinal venous plexus (from a focus in the pelvis) (Batson 1940). As in tuberculous spondylitis, there is destruction of bone and intervertebral disc, with or without abscess formation. The spinal cord may be damaged by direct pressure or by thrombosis.

Clinical features. The onset is usually acute or subacute, with pyrexia. The clinical features resemble those of tuberculous spondylitis (p. 150), but the course is more rapid. A suppurative process elsewhere in the body (for instance, in the pharynx or pelvis) is usually present. *Radiographs* show local osteoporosis or erosion of bone, diminution of disc space, and sometimes subligamentous new bone formation.

Investigations. The erythrocyte sedimentation rate is raised and polymorphonuclear leucocytosis is to be expected. Appropriate agglutination tests may be positive.

Diagnosis. The condition must be distinguished from tuberculous spondylitis. A history of pre-existing septic focus, the relatively rapid onset and course, with pyrexia and leucocytosis, and identification of the causal organism in pus, are the main diagnostic criteria.

Treatment. Appropriate antibiotic drugs (see p. 111) should be given systemically. The cervical spine must be immobilised in a plaster collar or brace; sometimes sustained head traction is required for relief of spasm. When there is an abscess it should be drained, especially if the spinal cord is threatened. Spontaneous fusion of the affected vertebrae usually makes operative fusion unnecessary.

RHEUMATOID ARTHRITIS
(General description of rheumatoid arthritis, p. 111)

The cervical spine is often affected in rheumatoid polyarthritis, especially in sero-positive disease. It is important that it be recognised, because there is a risk that destruction of the intervertebral joints may allow gradual forward subluxation of a cervical vertebra upon the one next below it, with danger to the integrity of the spinal cord. There is a particular risk of subluxation at the atlanto-axial joint due to softening of the transverse ligament of the atlas (see Fig. 126), and it is important to remember that these destructive changes may occur insidiously without significant symptoms; thus they may be overlooked until the onset of paralysis. If erosion of intervertebral joints and subluxation are shown radiologically to be occurring, the neck must be supported either by a suitable plastic collar or, in selected cases, by local intervertebral fusion.

ANKYLOSING SPONDYLITIS

Ankylosing spondylitis creeps up the spine from below. In a high proportion of cases—though by no means in all—it extends to involve the cervical region, with aching pain and permanent stiffness—sometimes total rigid ankylosis—of the intervertebral joints. The disease as a whole will be described in the chapter on the spine (p. 184).

CERVICAL SPONDYLOSIS
(Cervical spondylarthritis; cervical spondylarthrosis; cervical osteoarthritis; cervical osteoarthrosis)

Degenerative changes are common in the cervical spine. Indeed, they are found almost universally in some degree in persons over 50 years of age. Beginning in the intervertebral discs, they affect the posterior intervertebral (facet) joints secondarily, causing pain and stiffness of the neck, sometimes with referred symptoms in an upper limb.

Cause. The primary degenerative changes are often initiated by injury. In other cases the condition is simply a manifestation of normal wear and tear.

Pathology. Degenerative arthritis occurs most commonly in the lowest three cervical joints. The changes affect first the central intervertebral joints (between the vertebral bodies) and later the posterior intervertebral (facet) joints. In the central joints there is degenerative narrowing of the intervertebral disc, and bone reaction at the joint margins leads to the formation of osteophytes (Fig. 113). In the posterior intervertebral joints the changes are those of osteoarthritis in any diarthrodial joint—namely, wearing away of the articular cartilage and the formation of osteophytes (spurs) at the joint margins (Fig. 114).

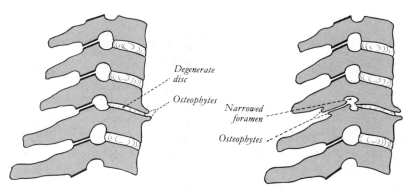

| **Fig. 113** | **Fig. 114** |

Osteoarthritis of the cervical spine. At first there is simply degeneration and narrowing of the intervertebral disc, with the formation of osteophytes anteriorly (Fig. 113). Later, the posterior or facet joints are affected: the articular cartilage is worn away and marginal osteophytes may encroach upon the intervertebral foramen (Fig. 114).

Secondary effects. Osteophytes commonly encroach upon the intervertebral foramina, reducing the space for transmission of the cervical nerves (Fig. 114). If the restricted space in a foramen is reduced still further by traumatic oedema of the contained soft tissues, manifestations of nerve pressure are likely to occur. Exceptionally, the spinal cord itself may suffer damage from encroachment of osteophytes within the spinal canal.

Clinical features. The symptoms are in the neck or in the upper limb, or both.

Neck symptoms consist chiefly of aching pain in the back of the neck or in the trapezius area, a feeling of stiffness, and 'grating' on movement. Usually slight, they are liable to periodic exacerbations, probably from unremembered strains or repetitive movements. Occipital headache may be a feature if the upper half of the cervical spine is affected.

In the *upper limb* there may be a vague, ill defined and ill localised 'referred' pain spreading over the shoulder region, or there may be more serious symptoms from interference with one or more of the cervical nerves in their foramina. The main feature of nerve root irritation is radiating pain along the course of the affected nerve or nerves, often reaching the digits. There may also be paraesthesiae in the hand, in the form of tingling or 'pins and needles'. Noticeable muscle weakness is uncommon.

Fig. 116

Fig. 115

Figs 115–116
Cervical spondylosis. Note in the lateral view (Fig. 115) the narrowed intervertebral space, with marginal osteophyte formation, at C.5–C.6 and at C.6–C.7. The oblique view (Fig. 116) shows severe encroachment of osteophytes upon an intervertebral foramen (compare with the normal foramen below).

On examination, the neck may be slightly kyphotic. The posterior cervical muscles may be somewhat tender but they are not in spasm. Movements are not markedly diminished except during acute exacerbations or when the degenerative changes are very advanced. Audible crepitation on movement is common. In the upper limb objective findings are usually slight or absent, for nerve pressure is seldom great enough to produce well defined objective neurological signs (compare prolapsed intervertebral disc). Thus demonstrable motor weakness or sensory impairment is exceptional. Depression of one or more of the tendon reflexes is, however, fairly common.

Radiographic features. There is narrowing of the intervertebral disc space, with formation of osteophytes at the vertebral margins, especially anteriorly (Fig. 115). Encroachment of osteophytes upon an intervertebral foramen is demonstrated best in oblique projections (Fig. 116).

Diagnosis. Distinction has to be made: 1) from other causes of neck pain; and 2) from other causes of upper limb pain (Fig. 117).

Other causes of neck pain. These include prolapsed cervical disc, tuberculous or pyogenic infection, tumours involving the vertebral column, and fibrositis.

Other causes of upper limb pain. These are as follows: *Central lesions*—Tumours involving the spinal cord or its roots; cervical spondylolisthesis. *Plexus lesions*—Tumours at the thoracic inlet (Pancoast); cervical rib; prolapsed intervertebral disc. *Shoulder lesions* with radiating pain in the upper arm. *Skeletal lesions* such as a tumour, infection, or Paget's disease of a bone of the upper extremity. *Elbow lesions,* such as tennis elbow or arthritis. *Distal nerve lesions* such as friction neuritis of the ulnar nerve at the elbow or compression of the median nerve in the carpal tunnel.

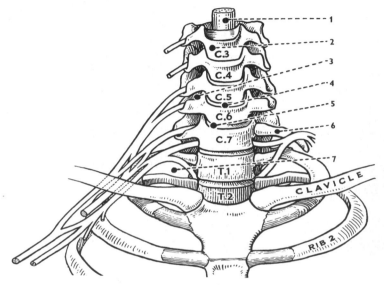

Fig. 117
Seven causes of interference with the brachial plexus or its roots. 1. Tumour of cord. 2. Tumour of spinal column. 3. Tumour of nerve root. 4. Prolapsed cervical disc. 5. Cervical spondylosis (osteoarthritis). 6. Cervical rib. 7. Tumour at thoracic inlet.

Osteoarthritis of the cervical spine is common in patients beyond middle life, and it is often symptomless: consequently, if osteoarthritic changes are found radiographically during the investigation of neck or upper limb pain it does not necessarily follow that the symptoms are caused by the arthritis. The diagnosis is at best presumptive, never unequivocal; before it is justified, other causes of similar symptoms must be excluded by full and careful investigation (Fig. 117).

Complications. If the spinal canal is markedly narrowed by osteophytes the spinal cord may be damaged, with progressive upper motor neurone disturbance affecting all four limbs and possibly the bladder. This complication is serious but uncommon.

Treatment. There is a strong tendency for the symptoms of cervical spondylosis to subside spontaneously, though they may persist for many months and the structural changes are clearly permanent. Treatment is thus aimed towards assisting natural resolution of temporarily inflamed or oedematous soft tissues. In mild cases such measures include analgesic drugs and various forms of physiotherapy (ultrasound, short-wave diathermy, massage, traction, or exercises). Manipulation is sometimes recommended, but in the presence of extensive osteophytes it is hazardous because it may damage the spinal cord; it should therefore be employed with extreme caution, and only by those familiar with a gentle technique. In the more severe cases it is wise to provide rest and support for the neck by a closely-fitting collar of plaster or plastic (see Fig. 121), which should be worn for one to three months according to progress.

In the exceptional cases in which the spinal cord is constricted, decompression either from in front or by laminectomy may be required, and thereafter it may be advisable to fuse the affected segments of the spinal column by a bone-grafting operation.

PROLAPSED CERVICAL DISC

Displacement of intervertebral disc material in the cervical spine is much less common than it is in the lumbar region. It is characterised by pain and stiffness in the neck, often with neurological manifestations in the upper limb and occasionally with signs of spinal cord compression.

Cause. Jarring injury is a predisposing factor, though a history of injury cannot be obtained in every case. Probably an intrinsic change in the substance of the disc makes it prone to rupture and displacement.

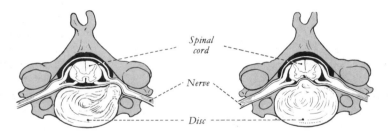

Fig. 118   **Fig. 119**

Prolapsed cervical disc. Figure 118 shows a postero-lateral prolapse, with compression of the issuing nerve. Figure 119 shows the much less common central prolapse, with impingement upon the spinal cord.

Pathology. The disc between C.5–C.6 and that between C.6–C.7 are those most frequently affected. Part of the gelatinous nucleus pulposus protrudes through a rent in the annulus fibrosus at its weakest part, which is postero-lateral; or part of the annulus itself may be displaced. If slight, the protrusion bulges against the pain-sensitive posterior longitudinal ligament, causing local pain in the neck. If large, the protrusion herniates through the ligament and may impinge upon the nerve leaving the spinal canal at that level (postero-lateral prolapse) (Fig. 118), or occasionally upon the spinal cord itself (central prolapse) (Fig. 119). Healing is probably by shrinkage and fibrosis of the extruded material rather than by its reposition within the disc. *Secondary effects*: Prolapse of a disc accelerates its degeneration and predisposes to the development of osteoarthritis in later years.

Clinical features. *Central protrusions.* These lead to manifestations of spinal cord compression and may be confused with spinal cord tumours or other central neurological disorders. They fall within the province of the neurosurgeon rather than the orthopaedic surgeon.

Postero-lateral protrusions. A typical clinical picture is as follows. The patient sustains an injury to the neck—often a jarring or twisting strain— which may seem slight at the time and may cause no immediate effects. Hours or days later there is a rapid development of acute 'stiff neck' with severe pain made worse by coughing or similar strains. Hours or days later still, the pain begins to radiate over the shoulder and throughout the length of the upper limb; it is felt strictly in the course of a cervical nerve, and characteristically it is severe. Paraesthesiae are felt in the digits. *On examination,* there is limitation of certain neck movements by pain, but movement in at least one direction (often lateral flexion) is free. In the upper limb there is a full range of joint movements. There are slight muscle wasting and slight sensory impairment in the distribution of a cervical nerve. The corresponding tendon reflex (biceps jerk in C.5–C.6 lesions; triceps jerk in C.6–C.7 lesions) is depressed or absent.

Variations. The characteristic features described are not always present. Variations are common. Thus a history of injury is not always obtainable. The symptoms may be confined to the neck, the upper limb being spared; or they may be confined entirely to the upper limb. Motor changes (wasting and weakness) may be marked, sometimes amounting to almost complete paralysis of a muscle or a group of muscles; or on the other hand they may be absent. Similarly, wide variations in the degree of sensory impairment are noted.

Imaging. *Radiographs* characteristically show a normal appearance in the first attack, but narrowing of one of the disc spaces (usually C.5–C.6 or C.6–C.7), denoting long-standing disc degeneration, is often demonstrable. *Magnetic resonance imaging* may show the displaced disc material; and myelography may show a filling defect.

Diagnosis.[1] Prolapsed cervical disc has to be differentiated: 1) from other causes of neck pain; and 2) from other causes of upper limb pain (Fig. 117). The main conditions that may be confused with it are the same as those listed in the differential diagnosis of cervical spondylosis (p. 155). A confident diagnosis is justified only when a suggestive history is associated with the signs of a lesion of a single cervical nerve, and provided always that other possible causes have been excluded by careful investigation. Diagnostic myelography is seldom justified unless a spinal tumour is seriously suspected, or unless there are signs of compression of the spinal cord. It has largely been superseded by magnetic resonance imaging (MRI).

---

[1]Postero-lateral protrusions only are considered here. Central protrusions with spinal cord compression fall within the province of the neurosurgeon.

Relationship between prolapsed disc and cervical spondylosis.
The clinical features of the two conditions are similar. Distinction is difficult
if the radiographs show arthritic changes, because the arthritis may be only
incidental and itself symptomless. Nerve pressure is probably greater in

Fig. 120   **Fig. 121**

Figure 120—Light resilient collar made from expanded polystyrene. It
provides some support but restricts movements only to a moderate extent.
Figure 121—Moulded polythene collar, used when much firmer support is
needed.

prolapsed disc than in osteoarthritis: consequently the symptoms tend to be
more clearly defined and pain very severe; and the objective signs are more
marked. Fortunately differentiation is not important in practice because the
treatment of both conditions is usually similar.

Course. There is a strong tendency to spontaneous recovery, but symptoms often persist with decreasing severity for as long as six months or more.

Treatment.[1] This depends upon the nature and severity of the
individual case. When the symptoms are slight no treatment other than
perhaps a mild analgesic drug is required. In the more severe cases
treatment is advisable, especially in the early acute stage. If the neck is 'stiff'
and if movements aggravate the neck and limb pain, rest for six weeks in a
supportive collar made from plaster of Paris or from plastic (Figs 120 and
121) is the most satisfactory method.

Pain is usually severe, necessitating fairly intensive analgesic therapy. As
the acute symptoms gradually subside, physiotherapy in the form of short-
wave diathermy or ultrasound, massage and graduated neck exercises to
restore full mobility is often helpful.

Operative removal of postero-lateral disc protrusions is potentially
dangerous and is seldom justified.

---

[1]Postero-lateral protrusions only are considered here. Central protrusions with spinal cord
compression fall within the province of the neurosurgeon.

CERVICAL RIB

A cervical rib is a congenital over-development, bony or fibrous, of the costal process of the seventh cervical vertebra. It often exists without causing symptoms, especially in the young, but in adult life the tendency to gradual dropping of the shoulder girdle may lead to its causing neurological or vascular disturbance in the upper limb.

Pathology. The over-developed costal process may be unilateral or bilateral. It may be of any size from a small bony protrusion, often with a fibrous extension, to a complete supernumerary rib. The subclavian artery and the lowest trunk of the brachial plexus arch over the rib. In a proportion of cases the nerve trunk suffers damage at the site of pressure against the rib; this accounts for the neurological manifestations. The vascular changes are probably similarly accounted for by local damage to the subclavian artery, from which thrombotic emboli may be repeatedly discharged into the peripheral vessels of the upper limb.

Fig. 122
Cervical rib. Typical appearance of a small supernumerary rib. This one caused severe neurological symptoms and signs. A cervical rib is shown best in an oblique radiograph such as this.

Clinical features. Cervical rib is often symptomless. When symptoms occur, they usually begin during early adult life. They may be neurological, vascular, or combined.

Neurological manifestations. The sensory symptoms are pain and paraesthesiae in the forearm and hand, most marked towards the medial (ulnar) side, and often relieved temporarily by changing the position of the arm. The motor symptoms include increasing weakness of the hand, with difficulty in carrying out the finer movements.

On examination, there is usually an area of sensory impairment—sometimes complete anaesthesia—in the forearm or hand. The affected area does not correspond in distribution to any of the peripheral nerves, but may be related to the lowest trunk of the brachial plexus. There may be wasting of the muscles of the thenar eminence or of the interosseous and hypothenar muscles.

Vascular manifestations. The changes that have been observed range from dusky cyanosis of the forearm and hand to gangrene of the fingers. The radial pulse may be weak or absent.

Radiographic features. Radiographs show the abnormal rib: if small, it is seen best in oblique projections (Fig. 122). In cases of suspected vascular obstruction arteriography is required.

Diagnosis. Radiographic demonstration of a cervical rib does not prove that it is the cause of symptoms. The condition has to be distinguished: 1) from other causes of pain and paraesthesiae in the forearm and hand; 2) from other causes of muscle wasting in the hand; and 3) from other causes of peripheral vascular changes in the upper limb.

Other causes of pain in the forearm and hand (Fig. 117). The important alternative causes are as follows: *Central lesions*—Tumours involving the spinal cord or its roots; cervical spondylolisthesis. *Plexus lesions*—Tumours at the thoracic inlet (Pancoast); prolapsed cervical disc; cervical spondylosis. *Distal nerve lesions*—Friction neuritis of the ulnar nerve at the elbow; pressure upon the median nerve in the carpal tunnel.

Other causes of muscle wasting in the hand. These include: *Central lesions*— Syringomyelia; tumour of spinal cord; poliomyelitis; motor neurone disease; cervical spondylolisthesis. *Plexus lesions*—Tumours at the thoracic inlet (Pancoast); prolapsed cervical disc (especially at C.7–T.1). *Distal nerve lesions*—Friction neuritis of the ulnar nerve at the elbow; pressure upon the median nerve in the carpal tunnel; toxic neuritis. *Muscle lesions*—Muscular dystrophy.

Other causes of upper limb peripheral vascular lesions. These include peripheral arterial disease and Raynaud's disease.

The diagnosis of symptomatic cervical rib depends upon the detection of the characteristic neurological signs or vascular disturbance in association with a demonstrable supernumerary rib. Prolapsed intervertebral disc at C.7–T.1 gives a similar clinical picture neurologically, and indeed it may often be the true cause of symptoms ascribed to a cervical rib; but in prolapsed disc there is a strong tendency to natural recovery, which is not the case with cervical rib. Arteriography may be conclusive by revealing obstruction of the subclavian artery.

Treatment. This depends upon the severity of the subjective and objective manifestations. In mild cases physiotherapy in the form of 'shrugging' exercises, to improve the tone of the elevator muscles of the shoulder girdle, is adequate. But if the neurological or vascular signs are well marked, and especially if they are increasing, operation is advisable. First the scalenus anterior muscle is divided. If this does not demonstrably release the lowest nerve trunk from constricting pressure the scalenus medius should be divided and the abnormal rib removed.

Occlusion of the subclavian artery may be amenable to reconstruction by vein grafting if the diagnosis is made before irreversible changes in the limb have occurred.

SCALENUS SYNDROME

(First rib syndrome; thoracic outlet syndrome)

Occasionally the neurological manifestations characteristic of cervical rib occur in the absence of a demonstrable skeletal abnormality. They have been ascribed to trapping of nerves between the first rib and the clavicle (costo-clavicular compression), or between the first rib and the scalenus anterior muscle; and to stretching of the lowest trunk of the brachial plexus over the normal first rib. More often, they are caused by a tough fibrous band in the scalenus medius muscle, which may lead to kinking of the lowest trunk of the brachial plexus, demonstrable at operation (Bonney 1977). The symptoms are easily confused with those from a prolapsed intervertebral disc between C.7 and T.1. Treatment should be conservative at first, as for prolapsed disc. Gradual improvement would support that diagnosis. But if the symptoms persist with undiminished intensity for a long time a true scalenus syndrome is probably the cause. In that event it may be justifiable to explore the plexus, to divide the scalenus anterior and the scalenus medius, and if necessary to excise the first rib.

CERVICAL SUBLUXATION AND DISLOCATION

(Spontaneous subluxation of the cervical spine; cervical spondylolisthesis)

In some conditions the cervical spine undergoes spontaneous displacement, usually forwards, of a cervical vertebra upon the one next below it.

Causes and pathology. There are three types, caused by: 1) congenital failure of fusion of the dens (odontoid process) with the axis; 2) inflammatory softening of the transverse ligament of the atlas; and 3) instability from previous injury or from rheumatoid arthritis.

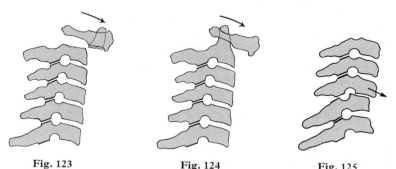

| Fig. 123 | Fig. 124 | Fig. 125 |

Three types of cervical spondylolisthesis or spontaneous subluxation. Figure 123—Displacement of atlas with the dens permitted by congenital or post-traumatic non-fusion of the dens with the axis. Figure 124—Displacement of atlas on axis, from softening of the transverse ligament of the atlas. Figure 125—Subluxation of the fifth on the sixth cervical vertebra due to instability of the intervertebral joint after previous injury. Instability may also be caused by rheumatoid arthritis.

Congenital or acquired non-fusion of dens. Occasionally the dens fails to fuse with the body of the axis by bone, being attached only by fibrous tissue. Under the constant stress of superimposed weight the fibrous bond slowly stretches, allowing the dens, and with it the atlas and skull, to slide gradually forwards upon the axis (Fig. 123). A similar condition may exist after fracture of the dens.

Inflammatory softening of the transverse ligament of the atlas. In this type the underlying cause is an inflammatory lesion in the upper part of the neck, such as rheumatoid arthritis or an infection of the throat or glands. There is rarefaction of the atlas, with softening of the transverse ligament. In consequence the atlas is able to slide forwards upon the axis (Fig. 124).

Instability from previous injury or from arthritis. A traumatic fracture-dislocation or subluxation at any level in the cervical spine may cause permanent instability, with a liability to slow redisplacement months or years after the initial injury (Fig. 125). Instability at any level may also arise from severe rheumatoid arthritis of long duration.

In all types the upper segment is displaced forwards in relation to the lower. The spinal canal becomes progressively more flexed and narrowed, and there is always a grave risk of compression of the spinal cord.

Clinical features. In the inflammatory type the patient is often a child with an acute infective lesion in the ear, throat, or neck, or an adult with rheumatoid arthritis. There is complaint of 'stiff neck'. The head is held rigidly, the cervical muscles being in spasm. In subluxation from congenital or post-traumatic instability there are discomfort and stiffness in the neck, and flexion deformity is apparent. *Radiographs* will show the displacement, and its type (Fig. 126).

Complications. In all types the complication to be feared is compression of the spinal cord. The first symptoms appear in the upper limbs and consist of root pain, paraesthesiae, motor weakness, or sensory impairment. Eventually, increasing cord compression may lead to spastic paralysis below the level of the lesion, and to bladder and bowel dysfunction.

Treatment. This depends upon the underlying cause and upon whether or not neurological disturbance is present.

Inflammatory type. The displacement is reduced by head traction, which is continued for two weeks. Thereafter the neck is immobilised in extension in a plaster jacket for two months. Atlanto-axial fusion may be required.

Fig. 126
Rheumatoid affection of the cervical spine. The atlas is displaced forwards upon the axis, and the axis vertebra is displaced slightly forwards upon the third cervical vertebra.

Congenital or post-traumatic instability. If subluxation is not complicated by neurological disturbance, treatment may be expectant (observation only), by a plastic collar to give support (Fig. 121), or by local fusion of the spine, according to the severity of the displacement and of the local symptoms. If neurological disturbance is present, treatment is by preliminary skull traction to reduce the displacement, followed by operative fusion of the affected segments of the spine.

TUMOURS IN RELATION TO THE CERVICAL SPINE
AND EMERGING NERVES

Tumours involving the cervical spine or the related nerves may arise: 1) in the spinal column itself; 2) in the meninges or, rarely, the spinal cord; 3) in the fibrous components of a peripheral nerve (neurofibroma); or 4) in adjacent soft tissues.

Tumours of the spinal column are more often malignant than benign, and predominantly metastatic rather than primary. A meningeal tumour (meningioma) is an uncommon cause of compression of the spinal cord. A tumour arising in nerve (neurofibroma) occurs occasionally within an intervertebral foramen, where it may grow inwards to compress the spinal cord and outwards towards the surface ('dumb-bell' tumour). A tumour at the apex of the lung (Pancoast's tumour) is a well recognised cause of severe pain from invasion of the brachial plexus.

Clinical features. The effects of these tumours vary according to their site and nature. Broadly, there may be: 1) local destruction and collapse of cervical vertebrae; 2) spinal cord compression; or 3) interference with the brachial plexus.

Destruction and collapse of cervical vertebrae. The commonest cause is a metastatic carcinoma (Fig. 127). The clinical features are local pain and, usually, flexion deformity. The spinal cord or the issuing cervical nerves may be involved, with corresponding signs of spinal cord compression or peripheral nerve defect.

Fig. 127
Partial destruction of the body of the third cervical vertebra by a metastasis from a renal carcinoma.

Spinal cord compression. Interference with the function of the spinal cord may be caused by tumours of the cord itself or of its meninges, by tumours of nerves (neurofibroma), or by tumours of the bony spinal column. The clinical manifestations depend upon the location of the tumour. Typically, root pains at the level of the lesion are followed by lower motor neurone changes at the same level and by progressive upper motor neurone paralysis and visceral dysfunction below the lesion.

Fig. 128
Tumour at the thoracic inlet (apical lung carcinoma or Pancoast tumour) causing well marked opacity at the apex of the right lung. This tumour should always be borne in mind in the differential diagnosis of pain in the upper limb.

Interference with the brachial plexus. Nerves forming the plexus may be involved by tumours of the nerves themselves (neurofibroma), by bone tumours, or by tumours at the thoracic inlet (Fig. 128). The predominant features are severe pain along the course of the nerve or nerves affected (neck or upper limb) and increasing motor and sensory impairment in the distribution of the nerves.

Imaging. Plain radiographs will usually help in discovering a tumour arising in the bones of the spinal column or eroding the bones from outside (Fig. 127). They may also reveal a tumour at the thoracic inlet (Fig. 128). Computerised tomography or magnetic resonance imaging may give more precise information. Radiculography is helpful in the diagnosis of intraspinal tumours, but it has been largely superseded by magnetic resonance imaging. Radiographs of the chest may reveal an apical lung tumour or pulmonary metastases.

References and bibliography, page 403.

10. Trunk and spine

Pain in the back is the commonest symptom encountered in orthopaedic practice. Indeed, if accident cases are excluded, it probably accounts for nearly a third of all orthopaedic out-patient attendances.

When this huge mass of material is sifted and categorised it is found that the cases fall into two broad groups. In the first group clear-cut physical signs, with or without distinctive radiographic changes or other abnormal findings, allow a precise determination of the nature of the lesion and of its site. The diagnosis is positive, and rational treatment can be applied. In the second group, almost as large as the first, there are few or no abnormal findings on clinical and radiographic examination; so the pathology is unclear. Diagnosis is largely a matter of conjecture, and treatment is empirical. For want of more accurate knowledge these rather vague and unsatisfactory cases are generally classed as 'chronic ligamentous strain' or 'postural back pain'.

Lumbar back pain is often accompanied by radiating pain in the buttock, thigh or leg, usually on one side but occasionally on both sides. This pain is generally referred to as sciatica, though the term should strictly be reserved for pain in the distribution of the sciatic nerve. It should be noted that sciatica is often a much more disturbing and persistent symptom of back disorders than the back pain itself, which indeed may be slight or transient.

SPECIAL POINTS IN THE INVESTIGATION OF BACK AND SCIATIC SYMPTOMS

History
Special attention should be paid to the mode of onset of the symptoms, whether they are periodic or constant, whether they are getting worse or better, and what relieves them or aggravates them. The precise location of the back pain and its character should be determined. The patient should be asked to what he attributes his symptoms: a history of a jarring strain, a fall, or an unaccustomed lifting job may be pertinent. Exacerbation of the pain on coughing or sneezing is indicative of an organic lesion.

Significance of sciatica. If pain radiates into the lower limb its character and exact distribution must be ascertained. Two distinct types of sciatica can be recognised. If the pain is severe and radiates in a well defined course that can be outlined on the skin surface, and especially if it is accompanied by motor, sensory, or reflex impairment, it suggests mechanical interference with nerve fibres of the lumbar or sacral plexus. On the other hand, if it takes the form of a vague diffuse ache, ill defined in its distribution, it is more likely to be a 'referred' pain originating in a disordered joint or ligament.

Exposure

The patient should be stripped completely, except for undergarments and, in women, a brassiére.

Steps in routine examination

A suggested plan for the routine clinical examination of the back is summarised in Table V.

Assessment of deformity

Any visible or palpable alteration of shape or posture of the spinal column should be noted. Deformity may occur in the sagittal plane, in the form of kyphosis (excessive forward curve or stoop) or lordosis (hollow back); or it may occur in the coronal plane as a lateral curvature (scoliosis). Combined curves and rotational deformity may also occur.

Table V
Routine clinical examination in suspected disorders of the back

---

1. LOCAL EXAMINATION OF THE BACK, WITH NEUROLOGICAL SURVEY OF THE LOWER LIMBS

(Patient standing)

Inspection
  Bone contours and alignment:
    (?visible deformity)
  Soft-tissue contours
  Colour and texture of skin
  Scars or sinuses

Palpation
  Skin temperature
  Bone contours
  Soft-tissue contours
  Local tenderness

Movements
  Spinal joints
    Flexion
    Extension
    Lateral flexion
    Rotation
    ? Pain on movement
    ? Muscle spasm

Costo-vertebral joints
  Range indicated by chest
  expansion

Sacro-iliac joints
  (Impracticable to assess range)
  ? Pain on movement imparted
    by lateral compression of
    pelvis

(Patient recumbent)

Palpation of iliac fossae
  Examine specifically for abscess
  or mass

Neurological state of lower limbs
  Straight leg raising test
  Muscular system
  Sensory system
  Reflexes

---

2. EXAMINATION OF POTENTIAL EXTRINSIC SOURCES OF BACK PAIN AND SCIATICA

This is important if a satisfactory explanation for the symptoms is not found on local examination. The investigation should include: 1) the abdomen; 2) the pelvis, including rectal examination; 3) the lower limbs; and 4) the peripheral vascular system.

---

3. GENERAL EXAMINATION

General survey of other parts of the body. The local symptoms may be only one manifestation of a widespread disease.

Movements of the spinal column and related joints

The spinal column. The joints of the spinal column must necessarily be considered as a group, for it is impracticable to study the movement of each joint independently. The movements to be examined are flexion, extension, lateral flexion to right and left, and rotation to right and left. It should be noted particularly whether the spinal muscles go into protective spasm when movement is attempted. *Flexion:* Instruct the patient to stretch his fingers towards the toes, keeping the knees straight. It is important to judge what proportion of the movement occurs at the spine and how much is contributed by hip flexion (Figs 129 and 130). Some patients can almost reach their toes, despite a stiff back, simply by flexing unusually far at the hips. (Normally the hamstrings limit hip flexion to about 90 degrees when the knees are straight.) The range may be expressed roughly as a percentage of the normal, or as the distance by which the fingers fail to reach the floor; or more accurately as the linear widening of the interspinous spaces as indicated by a tape measure laid along the line of the spinous processes. *Extension:* Instruct the patient to arch the spine backwards, looking up at the ceiling. Judge the range and express approximately as a percentage of the normal. *Lateral flexion:* Instruct the patient to slide each hand in turn down the lateral side of the corresponding thigh. Observe the range. *Rotation:* With the feet fixed, the patient rotates the shoulders towards each side in turn. Hold the pelvis steady, and note the range of spinal rotation as distinct from that which occurs at the knees and hips.

Fig. 129	**Fig. 130**

Figure 129—Normal flexion of lumbar spine. A tape measure laid along the line of the spinous processes will show widening of the interspinous spaces as the column flexes. Figure 130—Apparent or false flexion due entirely to movement at the hips, the hamstrings being unusually lax. A tape measure laid along the line of the spinous processes shows little excursion of their tips. In assessing trunk flexion it is important to judge in this way how much of the movement occurs at the spinal joints and how much at the hips.

Related joints. *The costo-vertebral joints:* The mobility of the costo-vertebral joints is judged from the range of chest expansion. The normal difference in chest girth between full inspiration and full expiration is about 7 or 8 centimetres. A marked reduction of chest expansion is of particular significance when ankylosing spondylitis is suspected. *The sacro-iliac joints:* It is not practicable to measure the range of sacro-iliac movement. But the joints should be moved passively to determine whether pain is produced, as it will be in arthritic conditions of the joints. A simple method is to grip each iliac crest and compress the pelvis strongly from side to side.

Palpation of iliac fossae and groins

Palpation of the iliac fossae and groins is an essential step in the examination of the back. Its specific purpose is to determine whether or not there is a soft-tissue thickening or abscess. It should be remembered that a 'psoas' abscess originating from a tuberculous lesion of the lumbar spine first becomes palpable deep in the iliac fossa. Such an abscess is felt most easily by pressing the flat palmar surface of the hand and fingers against the flat inner aspect of the iliac bone. To do this the surgeon must stand at the side of the couch corresponding to the side being examined—that is, he must stand on the right of the patient to examine the right iliac fossa and on the left to examine the left iliac fossa (Fig. 131).

Fig. 131
Palpating the iliac fossae for abscess. This is an essential step in the routine examination of the spine.

Fig. 132
The straight leg raising test, an important part of the neurological examination of the lower limbs.

Neurological examination of the lower limbs
Disorders of the back are so frequently accompanied by radiating pain, paraesthesiae, or other manifestations in the lower limb that a neurological survey should be carried out as a routine.

Straight leg raising test. Holding the knee straight, lift each lower limb in turn to determine the range of pain-free movement (normal = 90 degrees; often more in women) (Fig. 132). When associated with clearly defined sciatica (and in the absence of gross disease of the hip), marked impairment of straight leg raising by pain suggests mechanical interference with one or more of the roots of the sciatic nerve. The pain is easily explained. Even a normal sciatic nerve is tautened by straight leg raising, though not to the point of causing pain by dragging on the meningeal sheath that encloses the nerve root. If a nerve is already stretched or anchored, as by a protruded piece of an intervertebral disc or a tumour, the further tautening entailed in lifting the limb is sufficient to cause pain.

When a nerve is tensely stretched, raising the straight leg on the unaffected side may cause pain on the affected side. This sign, termed the crossed sciatic reflex, is a well recognised feature of prolapsed lumbar intervertebral disc with nerve pressure.

Fig. 133   **Fig. 134**
Figure 133—Girth measurement at the widest part is a reliable method of comparing the bulk of the calf muscles on the two sides. Figure 134—Measurement is less reliable in comparing the bulk of the thigh muscles because of the conical shape of the thigh and the difficulty of taking the measurement at an exactly comparable level on each side.

Muscular system. Examine the muscles for wasting, hypertrophy, and fasciculation. Note the tone and test the power of each muscle group, comparing it with its counterpart in the opposite limb. Circumferential measurement is a reliable method of comparing the bulk of the calf muscles, the girth being measured at the widest part or 'equator' (Fig. 133). Circumferential measurement of the thighs, on the other hand, tends to be inaccurate, and may be misleading, on account of the conical shape of the thigh (Fig. 134). Often a more accurate assessment of the relative volume of the two thighs is obtained from inspection and palpation. If the thighs are measured the girth should be taken on each side at an equal distance above the knee—12 or 15 centimetres above the upper margin of the patella is usually a convenient level.

Power of the muscles is estimated in comparison with the opposite side. Not only the major muscle groups should be tested: significant information may emerge from assessing the power of the toe muscles, and in particular of the extensor hallucis longus, which characteristically is weakened by lesions (such as prolapsed intervertebral disc) involving the fifth lumbar nerve.

Sensory system. Examine the patient's sensibility to touch and pin prick. When indicated, test also the sensibility to deep stimuli, joint position, vibration, and heat and cold.

Reflexes. Compare on the two sides the knee jerk (dependent mainly on the L.4 nerve) and the ankle jerk (mainly S.1). It is important to note not only the presence or absence of the response, but also any difference of intensity (Figs 135 and 136). Test the plantar reflex.

Fig. 135   **Fig. 136**

Figure 135—The patellar reflex is dependent mainly on L.4 nerve. Figure 136—In testing the calcaneal reflex (mainly S.1 nerve), slight inequalities between the two sides can best be detected if the patient lies prone, with the knee flexed 45 degrees and the ankle at 90 degrees.

Electromyography. Electromyographic examination of selected muscles in the lower leg may have an occasional place in helping to establish whether or not there is degeneration in the innervating lumbar or sacral nerve, as indicated by abnormal potentials in the resting muscle. For instance, abnormal potentials in the lateral half of the gastrocnemius muscle or in the extensor digitorum brevis suggest degeneration of the fifth lumbar nerve, whereas abnormal potentials in the medial half of the gastrocnemius or in the soleus indict the first sacral nerve.

Imaging

Radiographic examination. If the complaint is clearly localised to the thoracic spine, antero-posterior and lateral radiographs of that area alone will usually suffice. If the lumbar spine is the part complained of, radiographs should include not only antero-posterior and lateral views of the lumbar spine but also at least one view of the sacro-iliac joints, pelvis, and hip joints. In cases of doubt additional projections may be required. Oblique projections—from half right and half left—are essential for the proper study of the sacro-iliac joints and the posterior intervertebral (facet) joints of the lumbar region. For doubtful lesions of the vertebral bodies tomographs are often helpful. If a spinal tumour is suspected, myelography or radiculography is required.

Other methods of imaging. *Radioisotope bone scanning* (p. 16) is of particular value in examination of the spinal column, especially in the early detection of metastatic deposits.

Computerised tomography (CT scanning) (p. 17) is valuable in selected cases. It gives cross-sectional images of the trunk that reveal bony abnormalities very clearly, and in favourable circumstances the soft-tissue contents of the spinal canal may also be demonstrated. The technique is also valuable in the elucidation of certain lesions of, or within, the pelvis.

Magnetic resonance imaging (MRI), though not yet available everywhere, is even more informative than CT scanning, for it can show the intervertebral disc substance and the nerve roots.

Discography (radiography after injection of radio-opaque fluid into the nucleus pulposus) indicates the integrity or otherwise of the disc, but the technique has been largely superseded by magnetic resonance imaging.

Ascending spinal venography may be a useful supplementary method of outlining the spinal theca.

Extrinsic sources of back pain and sciatica

The back offers many pitfalls in diagnosis. Sometimes there are no local symptoms to indicate that the spine is the seat of the disorder, pain being referred entirely to the buttock or to the lower limb. Thus patients often complain only of pain 'in the hip' or 'in the leg' when the true source of the trouble is the lumbar spine. Conversely, the symptoms may suggest a spinal lesion when in fact they arise from an affection of the abdomen, pelvis, or lower limb, or from occlusion of a major artery or a leaking aortic aneurysm. Finally, it should always be remembered that back symptoms may be no more than a local manifestation of a generalised skeletal disease.

Thus the investigation of back or sciatic symptoms must extend further than a study of the spine itself; it must include an examination of the abdomen, pelvis, lower limbs and vascular system, and a general survey of the rest of the body.

CLASSIFICATION OF DISORDERS OF THE TRUNK AND SPINE

Congenital abnormalities
Lumbar and sacral variations
Hemivertebra
Spina bifida

Deformities
Scoliosis
Kyphosis
Lordosis

Infections of bone
Tuberculosis of the thoracic or lumbar spine
Pyogenic infection of the thoracic or lumbar spine

Arthritis of the spinal joints
Rheumatoid arthritis
Osteoarthritis
Ankylosing spondylitis

Other local affections of bone
Scheuermann's kyphosis
Calvé's vertebral compression

Mechanical derangements
Prolapsed lumbar disc
Acute lumbago
Spondylolysis
Spondylolisthesis
Spinal stenosis

Tumours
Tumours in relation to the spinal column, spinal cord, or nerve roots
Other tumours of the trunk

Chronic strains
Chronic lower lumbar ligamentous strain
Coccydynia

Miscellaneous
Senile osteoporosis

Disorders of the sacro-iliac joints
Tuberculosis of a sacro-iliac joint
Ankylosing spondylitis
Other forms of arthritis
Sacro-iliac ligamentous strain

LUMBAR AND SACRAL VARIATIONS

Minor variations of the bony anatomy are common, especially in the lumbar and sacral regions. Most are of little practical importance. They include: deficient or rudimentary lowest ribs; incomplete or complete incorporation of the fifth lumbar vertebral body in the sacrum (sacralisation of the fifth

Fig. 137   Fig. 138

Fig. 139

Three congenital anomalies of the spine. Figure 137—Hypertrophied transverse process forming false joint with ilium. Figure 138—Hemivertebra, an occasional cause of scoliosis. Figure 139—Four examples of spina bifida. In all, the neural arch of the vertebra is deficient posteriorly. In the first diagram, representing spina bifida occulta, there is no other deficiency; the skin and soft tissues are intact. In the second diagram overlying soft tissues are also deficient and the spinal theca bulges backwards to form a meningocele. In the third diagram nerve elements are also displaced backwards within the bulging sac (myelomeningocele). In the final diagram skin is deficient as well, and nerve elements are exposed on the surface (rachischisis).

lumbar vertebra); persistence of the first sacral segment as a separate vertebra (lumbarisation of the first sacral vertebra); and over-development of the fifth lumbar transverse process on one or both sides with, in marked cases, a false joint between the hypertrophied process and the ilium (Fig. 137). In the last-mentioned condition the false joint is sometimes a source of pain.

HEMIVERTEBRA

In this anomaly a vertebra is formed in one lateral half only. The defect may occur at any level. The body of the half-vertebra is wedge-shaped, and the spine is angled laterally at the site of the defect (Fig. 138). This anomaly is a rare cause of scoliosis.

SPINA BIFIDA

(Spinal dysraphism)

The basic fault in spina bifida is a failure of the embryonic neural plate to fold over to form a closed neural tube, or of mesodermal tissue fully to invest the neural tube as it does in the normal embryo to form the vertebral arch with its spinous process and the surrounding muscles and ligaments. Different grades of the anomaly are shown in Figure 139.

In most cases spina bifida is of minor degree and not a cause of disability. Indeed it is often found incidentally during radiography for some other reason. The importance of spina bifida lies in the fact that in the more severe forms there is a co-existing lesion of the nerve elements. The subject of spina bifida with neurological involvement was discussed in Chapter 8 (p. 138).

SCOLIOSIS

The term *scoliosis* denotes lateral curvature of the spine. The deformity may be 'structural', implying a permanent change in the bones or soft tissues, or it may be no more than a temporary disturbance produced by reflex or postural activity of the spinal muscles. Five types can be recognised: 1) infantile scoliosis, a type seen in very young children which may either resolve or progress; 2) primary or idiopathic structural scoliosis, a well defined group of unknown cause arising in children; 3) secondary structural scoliosis, a miscellaneous group in which the curvature is secondary to a demonstrable underlying disorder; 4) compensatory scoliosis; and 5) sciatic scoliosis, a temporary deformity.

INFANTILE SCOLIOSIS

Infantile scoliosis begins in the first year of life as a simple curve, usually convex to the left, without known cause. There are two subgroups—resolving and progressive—and it is usually possible to distinguish them by the radiographic appearance (Mehta 1972).

IDIOPATHIC STRUCTURAL SCOLIOSIS

Idiopathic scoliosis is the commonest and the most important type of structural scoliosis. It begins in childhood or adolescence and tends to increase progressively until the cessation of skeletal growth. It sometimes leads to severe and ugly deformity, especially when the thoracic region is the part affected. The exact cause of the growth disturbance is unknown: the children are otherwise healthy. The condition is much commoner in girls than in boys, which, with its frequent onset at puberty, suggests a possible link with the hormonal control of bone growth.

Pathology. Any part of the thoraco-lumbar spine may be affected. There is a primary structural curve, with secondary compensatory curves above and below. The pattern of curve and its natural evolution are fairly constant for each site, and the following types are recognised: lumbar scoliosis, thoraco-lumbar scoliosis and thoracic scoliosis (Fig. 140). The lateral curvature is constantly accompanied by rotation of the vertebrae on a vertical axis, the body of the vertebra rotating towards the convexity of the curve and the spinous process away from the convexity. By thrusting the ribs backwards on the convex side this rotation increases the ugliness of the deformity (Figs 140 and 141).

Fig. 140

Fig. 141
With rotation of the vertebrae the ribs are thrust backwards on the convex side, increasing the ugliness of the deformity. This rotation is a constant feature of structural scoliosis.

Fig. 140
Idiopathic scoliosis in an adolescent girl. The main curve is in the thoracic region. There is marked rotation of the vertebrae, causing posterior prominence of the ribs on the side of the convexity. In lumbar scoliosis the deformity is much less noticeable.

Clinical features. The onset is usually in middle childhood—often between the ages of 10 and 12 years, at the time of the adolescent growth spurt.

In children deformity is usually the only symptom. Pain is occasionally a feature in adults with long-standing deformity, particularly with structural curves in the lumbar region of the spine.

Course and prognosis. The outlook depends upon the age at onset and upon the site of the primary curve. The ultimate visible deformity tends to be worst in thoracic scoliosis and least in lumbar scoliosis. The curvature tends to increase until the end of the period of spinal growth, but not significantly thereafter. In general, therefore, the earlier the onset the worse the prognosis.

Treatment. The first essential is to assess the prognosis for progression of the deformity from a consideration of the age of onset and the site of the curve. When the prognosis is good (for instance, in most cases of lumbar scoliosis) expectant treatment, with regular reviews every six months, may be all that is required. But when the prognosis is poor (as in thoracic scoliosis with early onset) active treatment is advised. This usually necessitates operation, and much surgical endeavour has been spent in the quest for an effective and safe method of correcting the deformity and maintaining the correction. Surgical treatment is usually deferred until early adolescence to minimise the loss of height which may result from fusion of a significant length of the growing spine. To prevent further deterioration in the curvature during this waiting period, conservative management with various types of orthotic bracing may be required.

Fig. 142
Left—Milwaukee distraction brace, formerly widely used to control scoliosis in young children awaiting correction and spinal fusion. *Right*—The Boston brace, designed to control lateral curvature by flattening excessive lumbar lordosis. It is more acceptable to patients than the Milwaukee brace.

For many years the brace most commonly employed was the Milwaukee brace (Fig. 142). This uses the principle of three-point correction by distracting the spine between a pelvic band and an occipito-cervical support with additional lateral pressure from a pad applied to the chest wall at the apex of the curvature. It has adjustable anterior and posterior uprights to allow for growth in height. To be effective it must be worn almost continuously day and night, with one hour off for exercise and toilet purposes. Recently doubt has been cast on the effectiveness of this type of bracing, which has never been subjected to proper prospective controlled trials and may merely mask the natural history of variable rates of progression of the curves. Because of this uncertainty, and because of frequent problems of acceptance by the patient, an alternative under-arm thoraco-lumbar jacket, or Boston brace (Fig. 142), has been used increasingly for the conservative management of the deformity. This provides only two-point correction and it acts by flattening the lumbar lordosis; thus it is most suitable for lower curvatures with an apex below the ninth thoracic vertebra.

The principle of surgical treatment is to fuse the joints of all the vertebrae within the primary curve, after having first achieved the greatest possible correction of the curvature. When surgical treatment was first introduced correction was obtained by pre-operative traction or corrective plaster casts. It is now routinely gained at the time of operation by the use of a Harrington distraction rod or other internal corrective implant. This is inserted posteriorly in the concavity of the curve between two hooks placed under the laminae of the top and bottom vertebrae and then forcibly elongated to produce straightening. After operation the correction must be protected while fusion is occurring by immobilisation in a plaster jacket. The results from this technique are encouraging, with up to 50 per cent correction of the lateral curvature, though this is not necessarily reflected in impressive improvement of the cosmetic deformity, which largely results from vertebral rotation. Some improvement in the rotational deformity has been reported from the addition of segmental sublaminar wiring, wires being passed beneath the laminae and round the Harrington rod at each vertebral level. This technique offers the additional advantage of providing more rigid fixation, thus permitting less cumbersome post-operative splintage.

Other methods of fixation and correction may be required for more severe curvatures, or when abnormal vertebral pathology exists, as in congenital curvatures. These include: 1) anterior correction and fixation using the Zielke instrumentation; 2) fixation by metal rods secured to the vertebrae posteriorly by multiple-level sublaminar wiring (Luque technique); 3) posterior correction by devices that can be attached securely to the vertebrae by means of long pedicle screws (Cotrel-Dubousset instrumentation); 4) external correction by distraction between a screwed-on metal skull band (halo) above and a pelvic band below (halo-pelvic traction). The place of these various specialised techniques has not yet been finally established: they all carry a risk of neurological complications.

It must be emphasised that it is impossible to prevent the increase of a progressive scoliotic deformity by exercises alone, though these are an important adjunct to bracing, and useful in preserving mobility. The aim of all treatment must be to minimise progression, or to correct the deformity to an acceptable level at skeletal maturity. It is difficult and often impracticable to correct long-standing deformity in adults by any method.

SECONDARY STRUCTURAL SCOLIOSIS
In this group the spinal curvature is secondary to a demonstrable underlying abnormality.

Causes. The three commonest underlying causes are congenital abnormalities (especially hemivertebra), poliomyelitis with residual weakness of the spinal muscles (paralytic scoliosis), and neurofibromatosis.

Pathology. In *congenital hemivertebra* there is a sharp angulation at the site of the anomaly, with compensatory curves above and below (Fig. 138). Scoliosis following *poliomyelitis* is explained by unequal pull of the muscles on the two sides. The mechanism of scoliosis complicating *neurofibromatosis* is not clear; in this type the deformity may be very severe.

Clinical features. In most cases the visible deformity is the only symptom. The age of onset, site, nature, and severity of the curve vary with the underlying cause.

Complications. In exceptional cases of severe long-standing scoliosis the sharp angulation of the spinal cord over the apex of the deformity may cause interference with cord function, with consequent neurological manifestations leading in the worst cases to total paralysis below the level of the obstruction.

Treatment. In most cases treatment is along the lines suggested for idiopathic scoliosis.

COMPENSATORY SCOLIOSIS

Lumbar scoliosis is seen as a compensatory device when the pelvis is tilted laterally—as, for instance, when the lower limbs are unequal in length, or when there is a fixed abduction or adduction deformity at one or other hip. In such a case it is only by curving the lumbar spine through an angle equal to the pelvic tilt that the trunk can be held vertical. Usually there is no intrinsic abnormality of the spine itself, and the scoliosis disappears automatically when the pelvic tilt is corrected. In cases of many years' duration, however, the lumbar scoliosis may become fixed by adaptive shortening of the tissues on the concave side.

SCIATIC SCOLIOSIS

Sciatic scoliosis is a temporary deformity produced by the protective action of muscles in certain painful conditions of the spine.

Cause. In many cases the underlying cause is a prolapsed intervertebral disc impinging upon a lumbar or sacral nerve. But the deformity may also be observed in some cases of acute lumbago (p. 195), the pathogenesis of which is not entirely clear.

Pathology. The curve is in the lumbar region. The abnormal posture is assumed involuntarily in an attempt to reduce as far as possible the painful pressure upon the affected nerve or joint.

Clinical features. The predominant feature is severe back pain or sciatica, aggravated by movements of the spine (see prolapsed intervertebral disc, p. 190). The onset is usually sudden. The scoliosis is poorly compensated; so the trunk may be tilted over markedly to one side (see Fig. 162, p. 192). The curvature is not associated with rotation of the vertebrae.

Treatment. The treatment is that of the underlying condition.

KYPHOSIS

Kyphosis is the general term used to define excessive posterior curvature of the spinal column. The deformity may take the form of a long rounded curve ('round back'), or there may be a localised sharp posterior angulation ('hump back').

In the thoracic region there is normally a considerable posterior curvature: thoracic kyphosis exists only if this curve is excessive. In the cervical and lumbar regions there is normally an anterior curvature (lordosis): any reversal of this constitutes cervical or lumbar kyphosis.

Causes. Kyphosis is a manifestation of an underlying disorder of the spine. The causes are numerous. The following are the most important: 1) tuberculosis of the spinal column (Fig. 144); 2) wedge compression fracture of a vertebral body; 3) Scheuermann's kyphosis; 4) ankylosing spondylitis; 5) senile osteoporosis; and 6) destructive tumours of the spinal column (especially metastatic carcinoma).

Treatment. The treatment is that of the underlying condition. Often the deformity is best accepted unless it is unduly severe.

LORDOSIS

Lordosis is the opposite deformity to kyphosis. The term denotes excessive anterior curvature of the spinal column ('hollow back'). In practice, lordosis is seen only in the lumbar region, where a slight anterior curve is normal. Strictly, the term lordosis should be used only when this normal curve is exaggerated.

Causes. Spinal disorders tend to cause kyphosis or scoliosis rather than lordosis. In many cases lordosis is simply a postural deformity, predisposed to by lax muscles and heavy abdomen. Sometimes it is compensatory, balancing a kyphotic deformity above or below, or a fixed flexion deformity of a hip.

TUBERCULOSIS OF THE THORACIC OR LUMBAR SPINE
(Tuberculous spondylitis; Pott's disease)

Tuberculosis of thoracic or lumbar vertebral bodies is one of the commonest forms of skeletal tuberculosis, though it is now seen only rarely in Western countries.

Pathology. The infection begins at the anterior margin of a vertebral body, near the intervertebral disc (Fig. 143). The disc itself is usually involved at an early stage. The extent of the destruction varies widely from case to case. Commonly there is complete destruction of one intervertebral disc with partial destruction of the two adjacent vertebrae, most marked anteriorly (Fig. 144). But the changes may extend over several spinal segments; or, on the other hand, they may be confined to a single intervertebral disc, without evident bone involvement (Fig. 145). Anterior collapse of the affected vertebrae leads to an angular kyphosis (Figs 144, 146 and 147).

Abscess formation is usual. In the thoracic region pus collects around the spinal column, forming a fusiform paraspinal abscess (Fig. 147); or it may track towards the surface between ribs. From the lower thoracic or lumbar region pus tracks downwards behind the fascial sheath of the psoas muscle and generally bursts into the compartment behind the iliacus fascia to form

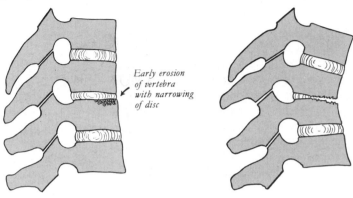

Early erosion of vertebra with narrowing of disc

Fig. 143   **Fig. 144**

Tuberculosis of the spine. The infection begins anteriorly near an intervertebral disc, which is soon destroyed (Fig. 143). It may spread to adjacent vertebrae, which collapse in front, with consequent angular kyphosis (Fig. 144).

a palpable abscess in the iliac fossa (psoas abscess). An abscess occasionally points posteriorly, or in the thigh. As in most instances of skeletal tuberculosis, the inflammation is low-grade and chronic rather than acute: hence the term 'cold abscess' for the quiet suppuration that is a common feature.

Secondary effects. An abscess or mass of granulation tissue encroaching upon the spinal canal may interfere with the spinal cord or with a spinal nerve. In cases of long-standing severe kyphosis the spinal cord is occasionally damaged by the bony ridge at the site of deformity.

Clinical features. The disease is commonest in young adults. One or more of the following symptoms may be present: 1) pain in the back; 2) stiffness of the back; 3) visible deformity of the back; 4) localised swelling (abscess); 5) weakness of legs or visceral dysfunction from involvement of the spinal cord.

On examination, the patient often looks ill. There may be visible or palpable angular kyphosis. There is local tenderness on firm palpation or percussion over the affected vertebrae. All spinal movements are greatly restricted and when they are attempted the spinal muscles go into protective spasm. An abscess may be detected over the thoracic wall or in the flank, iliac fossa, or upper thigh. Signs of spinal cord compression ('Pott's paraplegia') or of a nerve root lesion may be present. Tuberculous lesions are often manifest elsewhere.

Imaging. On *radiographic examination* the earliest signs are narrowing of an intervertebral space (Fig. 145) and local vertebral osteoporosis. Later, there is usually destruction of bone at the anterior margin of one or more of the vertebral bodies, leading to anterior collapse and wedge-shaped deformity of the affected vertebrae (Figs 146 and 147). An abscess shadow is nearly always visible: in the thoracic region it is seen as a fusiform paraspinal shadow (Fig. 147); in the lumbar region it is indicated by lateral bulging of the psoas outline, usually on one side. In the healing stage the bone outline in the area of destruction becomes sharper, and normal density is regained. Abscesses may become calcified. Computerised tomography (CT scanning) or magnetic resonance imaging (MRI) may be useful in defining the soft parts more clearly, especially if there are signs of spinal cord dysfunction. Ultrasound scanning is useful in delineating an abscess.

Fig. 145   **Fig. 146**

Figure 145—Early tuberculous lesion causing a narrowed lumbar disc space in a young adult. Narrowing of a disc space without osteophytic spurring of the vertebral margins always suggests infection. Figure 146—Severe tuberculous erosion of two lumbar vertebrae, with anterior collapse. The vertebra below also shows erosion at its upper anterior corner. One intervertebral disc is destroyed and the one above is much narrowed.

Investigations. The erythrocyte sedimentation rate is raised in the active stage. The Mantoux test is positive. Tubercle bacilli can sometimes be isolated from aspirated pus.

Diagnosis. Tuberculosis has to be distinguished: 1) from other causes of back pain with localised bony destruction or kyphosis (non-specific pyogenic spondylitis, ankylosing spondylitis, spinal tumours, Calvé's vertebral compression (eosinophilic granuloma), old compression fracture); and 2) from other causes of dysfunction of the spinal cord or cauda equina (prolapsed intervertebral disc; spinal tumour).

Important diagnostic features are: a history of contact with tuberculosis, or of previous tuberculous infection; restriction of *all* spinal movements by protective muscle spasm; abscess formation; the characteristic radiographic changes (including destruction of an intervertebral disc, which is not usual in cases of tumour and not marked in Calvé's disease); and the raised erythrocyte sedimentation rate.

Complications. These include: 1) chronic discharging sinus; 2) tuberculous infection of other organs, such as meninges, kidneys or lungs; and 3) interference with the spinal cord, causing weakness or paralysis in the lower limbs with or without sensory impairment or disturbance of bladder and bowel function ('Pott's paraplegia'). Paraplegia may arise early— that is, during the active stage of the disease—when it is caused by the pressure of pus or granulation tissue; or it may arise many years after healing has occurred, from mechanical impedance of the spinal cord where it is sharply angled at the site of a severe kyphos ('late onset paraplegia').

Prognosis. In most cases the outlook is good. In a few there is severe permanent kyphosis. There is a small risk of death from spread of the infection to other organs, or from the effects of paraplegia. The prognosis is worse in certain Asian and African countries where the disease tends to be florid, than in Britain, North America and the Antipodes where it is usually mild and responsive to treatment.

Treatment. Treatment of spinal tuberculosis is now much more often ambulatory than it

Fig. 147
Tuberculosis of the thoracic spine in a child. Note in the antero-posterior view the typical fusiform appearance of a paraspinal abscess, an almost constant feature of thoracic spinal tuberculosis. In the lateral view two vertebral bodies are seen partly collapsed in a wedge-shaped mass; the disc between them has been destroyed.

was in the past, largely because of the efficacy of antituberculous drugs. Nowadays treatment may entail only a brief stay in hospital—or indeed it may often be carried out entirely on an out-patient basis.

Treatment may be conservative or operative, depending upon the nature of the case and the facilities that are available.

Conservative treatment. Conservative management relies almost entirely upon anti-bacterial agents, continued uninterruptedly for nine to twelve months (see p. 120). Local treatment for the spine may be initially by plaster jacket or reinforced corset for relief of pain, though at many centres the back is left unsupported throughout. Once treatment has been instituted the patient is encouraged to be up and about. Adjuvant operation may be required in certain circumstances, mainly for the drainage of an abscess. 1) An abscess that is superficial should be either aspirated or drained by simple incision followed by immediate suture of the wound. 2) A paraspinal abscess in the thoracic region may be drained from the back by removing the head and neck of a rib and the adjacent transverse process (costo-transversectomy). With this regime, satisfactory healing may be expected in a high proportion of patients, though often with some residual kyphosis.

Operative treatment. The alternative management is by radical operation as recom-mended by Hodgson and Stock (1960) of Hong Kong. This may promote more rapid healing. The affected part of the spinal column is approached anteriorly and all diseased bone is excised. Thereafter the gap is bridged by bone grafts. Adjuvant antibacterial agents are given. By this method the duration of treatment is shortened and kyphosis may often be prevented or corrected.

Relief of paraplegia. If paraplegia from compression of the spinal cord does not show rapid improvement after the commencement of antibacterial therapy the spinal canal should be decompressed by operation. Occasionally this may be achieved by costo-transversectomy alone, particularly if a paraspinal abscess is the chief factor responsible for the compression. More reliably, it may be done by clearance of pus, necrotic tissue and diseased bone from the region of the spinal theca, either through an anterior approach or through a lateral route by unilateral excision of the pedicles of three or four vertebrae (lateral rhachotomy; antero-lateral decompression).

Assessment of cure. Signs of quiescence are: good general health; diminishing blood sedimentation rate; and arrest of the destructive process with hardening of the bony outlines as seen radiographically.

Comment

The choice between conservative treatment and radical operation depends to some extent upon the nature of the disease and also upon the orthopaedic facilities that are available in a particular country or district. In Britain and in most parts of Europe, in North America and in the Antipodes the disease tends to be relatively benign, and conservative treatment is usually appropriate. On the other hand in those parts of the world where the disease is often florid, particularly in the East, radical operation may sometimes be advisable, but only in centres where the necessary facilities and surgical skill are available.

PYOGENIC INFECTION OF THE THORACIC OR LUMBAR SPINE

(Pyogenic spondylitis; osteomyelitis of the spine)

Pyogenic infection of the spine is uncommon. It has often been confused with tuberculous spondylitis, which it may resemble clinically and radiographically.

Cause. It is caused by infection with the staphylococcus, streptococcus, pneumococcus, or occasionally with other bacteria such as the typhoid bacillus or other salmonella organisms, or brucella abortus.

Pathology. Organisms usually reach the spinal column through the general blood stream, from a septic focus elsewhere. Other possible routes are through the spinal venous plexus from a focus in the pelvis (Batson 1940), or through lymphatic channels from a neighbouring focus. As in tuberculous spondylitis, there is destruction of an intervertebral disc and erosion of the adjacent bone, with or without abscess formation. The spinal cord may be damaged by pressure, or by thrombosis of its vessels.

Clinical features. The clinical picture is inconstant: there are remarkable variations in the severity of the symptoms from case to case. The onset is often acute or subacute, and may be accompanied by pyrexia. In many respects the features are like those of tuberculous spondylitis—though usually more rapid in their course—the predominant findings being local pain and restriction of all movements by muscle spasm. A suppurative process elsewhere in the body is usually present or has recently subsided; or infection may follow operation for removal of displaced disc material, with consequent 'discitis'.

Radiographic features. Radiographs show local rarefaction or erosion of bone, diminution of disc space, and sometimes sub-ligamentous new bone formation. After healing, spontaneous bony fusion of affected vertebrae is often observed.

Investigations. The erythrocyte sedimentation rate is raised. Polymorphonuclear leucocytosis is to be expected. Serological studies can occasionally incriminate a particular organism, such as one of the salmonella group.

Diagnosis. Pyogenic infection has to be distinguished mainly from tuberculous spondylitis, which it may resemble closely. The relatively acute onset, history of pre-existing infection or septic focus, pyrexia, leucocytosis, and identification of the causal organism in pus, are the main diagnostic criteria.

Prognosis. If the infection is overcome, complete healing of the spinal lesion—often with bony fusion of affected vertebrae—is usual.

Treatment. Appropriate antibacterial drugs are given. The spine is rested, at first in bed, and later in a plaster jacket or by a suitable brace, until healing occurs. An abscess may require early drainage, especially if the spinal cord is threatened.

RHEUMATOID ARTHRITIS OF THE SPINAL JOINTS
(General description of rheumatoid arthritis, p. 111)

It has been noted above that rheumatoid arthritis often affects the cervical spine. Joints of the thoracic and lumbar spine may likewise be affected, but clinical manifestations are relatively uncommon. They consist in aching pain of a rather diffuse type, with impairment of spinal movements. The symptoms develop insidiously, without preceding injury. Examination of the limbs will usually reveal typical rheumatoid changes in several joints.

Imaging. *Radiographs* are not distinctive, but in cases of considerable duration there is rarefaction of the vertebrae with thinning of the inter-vertebral disc spaces. There may be erosion of the articular surfaces at the facet joints. *Radioisotope scanning* shows increased uptake in affected joints.

Treatment. This is along the lines recommended for rheumatoid arthritis of other joints (p. 115).

OSTEOARTHRITIS OF THE THORACIC AND LUMBAR SPINE
(Spondylarthritis; spondylarthrosis; spondylosis)

Osteoarthritis of the thoracic or lumbar intervertebral joints is found very commonly in those used to heavy work, but it is not necessarily accompanied by symptoms.

Cause. Predisposing factors are: 1) previous injury to the spinal joints; 2) previous disease involving the joints (for example, Scheuermann's kyphosis or an intervertebral disc lesion). In other cases the degenerative changes are simply a manifestation of increasing age or 'wear and tear'.

Pathology. The changes affect the central intervertebral (body-to-body) joints and the posterior intervertebral (facet) joints. One segment or several segments may be affected. In the central joints, which are affected first, there is degeneration with consequent narrowing of the intervertebral disc, and hypertrophy of bone at the joint margins leads to the formation of osteophytes (Fig. 148). In the posterior intervertebral (facet) joints the changes are those of osteoarthritis in any diarthrodial joint—namely, attrition of the articular cartilage and osteophyte formation (spurring) at the joint margins. These changes in the facet joints are probably the more important from a clinical point of view.

Secondary effects. Rarely, osteophytes encroach upon an intervertebral foramen sufficiently to interfere with the function of the issuing nerve. Thinning of the articular cartilage of the posterior intervertebral (facet) joints reduces the stability of the affected segment and predisposes to one type of spondylolisthesis (p. 197).

Clinical features. Spinal osteoarthritis can exist in quite marked degree without causing symptoms. But there is often a complaint of aching pain in the affected area, worse on activity and especially after stooping or lifting. Pain is often worse first thing in the morning, and there may be a feeling of stiffness when rising from a sitting position. In the lumbar region there is a tendency to acute exacerbations of pain, usually arising suddenly and lasting a few weeks (acute lumbago). These are possibly explained by strain or momentary subluxation of an unstable degenerate joint. Interference with a nerve in a narrowed intervertebral foramen leads to radiating pain in the distribution of the affected nerve (girdle pain or sciatica according to the level affected).

Fig. 148
Osteoarthritis of the lumbar spine. Marked narrowing of an intervertebral disc, with anterior osteophytes. Note also the slight posterior displacement of the upper vertebra. (See also Fig. 156).

On examination in the quiet phase, the objective findings are slight. Spinal movements may be moderately restricted, especially flexion; but there is no muscle spasm. If there is interference with a lumbar nerve root straight leg raising on the affected side is likely to be restricted. Apart from this, objective neurological signs are exceptional. During an acute exacerbation of pain there may be marked impairment of spinal movements, with muscle spasm (see acute lumbago, p. 195).

Radiographic features. The changes are most obvious in the central (body-to-body) intervertebral joints, which show narrowing of the inter-vertebral space and osteophyte formation (spurring) at the joint margins (Figs 148 and 156). Later the posterior intervertebral (facet) joints also show changes: there is narrowing of the joint space with sharpening of the margins of the facets. These changes are seen clearly only in oblique projections.

Diagnosis. Osteoarthritis has to be distinguished from other causes of back pain and from other causes of radiating nerve pain (girdle pain or sciatica) (Fig. 164, p. 193). It should be remembered that the demonstration of osteoarthritic changes in the radiographs does not necessarily mean that the arthritis is the cause of the patient's symptoms, for spinal osteoarthritis is common and often painless. The diagnosis is always presumptive rather than proved, and it is justified only when other possible causes have been excluded by careful consideration of the history, clinical examination and radiographs.

Treatment. This depends upon the severity of the disability. In mild cases treatment is unnecessary: explanation and reassurance suffice.

Thoracic spine. In osteoarthritis of the thoracic spine the symptoms are seldom severe, and if treatment is required a course of active spinal exercises to strengthen the posterior muscles is usually sufficient.

Lumbar spine. In lumbar osteoarthritis with moderate disability a well fitted surgical corset will usually afford adequate relief. Physiotherapy, mainly by exercises and passive mobilisation, may also be helpful. Heavy lifting and similar strains to the back should be strictly avoided. Rarely, if the pain from a localised lesion is bad enough to cause serious hardship, operative fusion of the affected segments of the spine may be required.

ANKYLOSING SPONDYLITIS
(Spondylitis ankylopoietica; Marie-Strumpell arthritis)

In ankylosing spondylitis there is chronic inflammation, progressing slowly to bony ankylosis, of the joints of the spinal column and occasionally of the major limb joints.

Cause. This is unknown. The condition is distinct from rheumatoid arthritis, although it is sometimes loosely termed 'rheumatoid spine'. There is a strong hereditary link to the HLA-B27 gene, and there is a relationship with certain types of sero-negative chronic juvenile arthritis in members of the family.

Pathology. The disease always begins in the sacro-iliac joints, whence it usually extends upwards to involve the lumbar, thoracic, and often the cervical spine. In the worst cases the hips or shoulders are also affected. The articular cartilage, synovium, and ligaments show chronic inflammatory changes and eventually they become ossified. After several years the inflammatory process becomes quiescent.

Clinical features. With few exceptions the disease is confined to men, and it nearly always begins between the ages of 16 and 25. The early symptoms are pain in the lower back and increasing stiffness. Later, the pain migrates upwards. Diffuse radiating pain down one or both lower limbs is also common. *On examination* the predominant finding is marked limitation of all movements in the affected area of the spine ('poker back'). When the thoracic region is involved chest expansion is markedly reduced—often to less than 2.5 centimetres (normal = 7.5 centimetres)—from ankylosis of the costo-vertebral joints: this is an important diagnostic feature. In a few cases the hips or shoulders are affected, with pain and limitation of movement.

Radiographic features. In the early stages there is fuzziness of both the sacro-iliac joints, so that the joint outline is no longer clearly defined (Fig. 149). Later, the sacro-iliac joints are completely obliterated and, if the disease progresses, the intervertebral joints in the lumbar, thoracic, and

Fig. 149

Ankylosing spondylitis. Characteristic fuzziness with loss of sharp outline of both sacro-iliac joints. Later, these joints undergo spontaneous bony fusion, and similar changes may creep upwards, sometimes affecting the whole of the spinal column.

Fig. 150

Ossification of the anterior longitudinal ligament in ankylosing spondylitis. In severe cases the spinal column may become rigid throughout its length.

sometimes even the cervical region undergo bony ankylosis, with prominent anterior bridging of the vertebral bodies (Fig. 150).

Investigations. The erythrocyte sedimentation rate is raised while the disease is active. In 90 per cent of cases the test for HLA-B27 antigen is positive.

Diagnosis. Ankylosing spondylitis has to be distinguished from other causes of back pain and sciatica (see Fig. 164). The marked limitation of spinal movement, the reduced chest expansion, the typical radiographic features, and the raised erythrocyte sedimentation rate are diagnostic.

Course and complications. The disease usually ceases to progress after ten or fifteen years, leaving permanent stiffness, the extent of which varies widely from case to case. Complications include fixed flexion deformity of the spine (Fig. 151), intercurrent respiratory infections, and iridocyclitis, which in severe cases may lead to blindness. There is also a relationship with Crohn's disease (regional ileitis), which may co-exist.

Treatment. Treatment is rather unsatisfactory, in that no method is known by which the disease process can be halted and spinal mobility preserved. In most cases the mainstay of treatment is a non-steroidal anti-

Figs 151 and 152
Figure 151—Patient with long-standing ankylosing spondylitis complicated by rigid flexion deformity. Figure 152—After corrective osteotomy in the lumbar region.

Fig. 151   Fig. 152

inflammatory agent—usually indomethacin or naproxen in the first instance. Steroid drugs are inappropriate except for ophthalmic complications. There may still be an occasional place for local radiotherapy for a particularly painful area, or for a related joint such as the shoulder, acromio-clavicular or sterno-clavicular joint, but this treatment is used very cautiously, if at all, because of the risk of delayed induction of leukaemia.

Apart from these measures, treatment should be directed towards preserving function. Activity rather than rest should be prescribed. Special exercises should be practised to make the most of such movement as remains. The patient should adopt the habit of sleeping flat upon his back on a firm mattress, with only a single pillow, to prevent increasing flexion deformity of the spine. If severe flexion deformity occurs through neglect of this precaution (Fig. 151) it may be corrected by wedge osteotomy of the spine in the lumbar region (Fig. 152).

SCHEUERMANN'S KYPHOSIS
(Adolescent vertebral osteochondritis; adolescent kyphosis)

Formerly termed *osteochondritis*, Scheuermann's disease is now regarded as unrelated to osteochondritis juvenilis (p. 96) and should no longer be so called. Basically, it seems to be an intrusion of part of the intervertebral disc

| Fig. 153 | Fig. 154 |

Scheuermann's vertebral kyphosis. Figure 153—In the active stage the upper and lower margins of the vertebral bodies are irregularly indented in front, and the corresponding parts of the ring epiphyses appear isolated. Figure 154—Radiograph of the lower part of the thoracic spine of a man aged 20 with established kyphosis from wedging of affected vertebrae.

into the vertebral end plate at multiple levels, mostly in the thoracic region. This leads to a rounded kyphosis. The cause and precise nature of the affection are uncertain. It is uncommon.

Pathology. The vertebral bodies ossify from three centres—a primary centre for the middle of the body, and secondary centres for the upper and lower surfaces. These secondary centres, known as the ring epiphyses, appear at about the time of puberty in the cartilaginous end plates that separate the vertebral bodies from the adjacent intervertebral discs. In Scheuermann's disease there is a disturbance of the normal development of the cartilage plates and ring epiphyses, possibly because they are damaged by bursting of the disc contents through the cartilage into the subjacent vertebral body (Fig. 153). The changes occur predominantly near the anterior margins of the vertebrae, where the greatest weight-thrust is borne. In consequence the disc is somewhat narrowed anteriorly, and through

Fig. 155 **Fig. 156**

Figure 155—Established Scheuermann's kyphosis, showing the characteristic curvature. Figure 156—The late effect of Scheuermann's adolescent kyphosis: slight wedging of several thoracic vertebral bodies with consequent rounded kyphosis and marked spurring of the contiguous corners of the vertebral bodies anteriorly, denoting osteoarthritis.

deficient growth of the affected part of the ring epiphysis the vertebral body becomes slightly wedge-shaped (Fig. 154). The deformity predisposes to the later development of osteoarthritis (Fig. 156).

Characteristically Scheuermann's disease affects several vertebrae in the thoracic region. Occasionally similar changes are confined to a single vertebra, and this localised form of the disease is as common in the lumbar as in the thoracic region.

Clinical features. The patient is usually 13 to 16 years old, and more often a boy than a girl. In the active stage there is pain in the thoracic spine, with 'round' back. After some months the pain subsides, leaving a rounded kyphosis of varying severity (Fig. 155). In later life there may be renewed pain from the development of osteoarthritis. *On examination* there is a slight or moderate rounded kyphosis in the thoracic region. In the active stage there is tenderness on firm palpation over the affected vertebrae.

Radiographic features. In the active stage of the disease the affected vertebral bodies show deep notched defects at their anterior corners, and the corresponding parts of the ring epiphyses may be irregular in shape and size (Fig. 154). The disc spaces are slightly narrowed but never totally destroyed. After healing, there is slight antero-posterior wedging of the affected vertebral bodies. Years later, osteoarthritic spurring of the anterior vertebral margins is observed (Fig. 156).

Diagnosis. In its characteristic form the affection is easily diagnosed from the history, clinical appearance, and radiographs. If localised to a single vertebra it may easily be confused with tuberculous spondylitis. Radiologically, the chief points of distinction are that in osteochondritis the margins of the notched defect in the vertebral body tend to be sclerotic rather than rarefied, and a paraspinal abscess shadow (almost a constant feature of thoracic spinal tuberculosis) is never seen. Furthermore, the erythrocyte sedimentation rate is not raised in Scheuermann's kyphosis.

Course and prognosis. The affection is self-limiting, the active stage lasting for one or two years. If the epiphyses become deformed, permanent wedging of the affected vertebrae, with consequent slight or moderate kyphosis, remains as a cosmetic blemish. Osteoarthritis often supervenes in later life but it is of little clinical significance.

Treatment. In a mild case treatment is often unnecessary. If pain is troublesome, support for the spine in extension, by a brace or plaster jacket, for four to six weeks may be advisable. This allows the pain to subside. Thereafter a spinal brace of Milwaukee type is worn for a further six months, and active exercises to strengthen the posterior spinal muscles are encouraged. In the worst cases—a small minority—operative correction may be considered. Operation entails excision of intervertebral discs, with interbody grafting, in the affected region of the spine, and it usually entails posterior instrumentation to provide correction and stability. It is a major procedure and clearly must not be undertaken without very careful assessment of every facet of the problem, since at best only 40 per cent of the deformity can be corrected.

CALVÉ'S VERTEBRAL COMPRESSION

(Vertebra plana; vertebral osteochondritis)

Whereas in Scheuermann's disease it is the vertebral ring epiphyses that are affected, Calvé's disease affects the central bony nucleus of a vertebral body. It is generally confined to a single vertebra. It is uncommon.

Fig. 157
Calvé's disease of vertebral body. The bony nucleus has shrunk into a thin dense wafer. The adjacent intervertebral discs are intact. The usual cause is eosinophilic granuloma.

Pathology. Mainly from its radiological features and from its benign course, Calvé's disease was in the past regarded as homologous with osteochondritis of other developing bony nuclei (p. 96), and it is possible that this is indeed the true explanation in some cases. Histological studies have shown, however, that in at least some instances the characteristic vertebral collapse has been caused by an *eosinophilic granuloma* (p. 56), and it is probable that this is the usual pathology.

In a typical case the bony nucleus of one of the vertebral bodies, usually in the thoracic region, becomes soft and is condensed into a thin wafer. Later, the bone may re-develop surprisingly well, but it is doubtful if it is ever restored quite to its full height. The intervertebral discs above and below are intact.

Clinical features. The affection occurs in children of 2 to 10 years of age. The complaint is of pain, usually in the thoracic region of the spine. *On examination*, there may be slight localised kyphosis. Percussion of the spinal column reveals deep tenderness in the affected region. Movements of the spine as a whole are impaired little, if at all.

Radiographic features. Radiographs show the characteristic extreme flattening of the affected vertebral body, which appears greatly increased in density (Fig. 157): it has been likened to a coin seen end on. The intervertebral disc spaces above and below are of normal depth.

Diagnosis. The radiographic appearance is distinctive. It serves to differentiate the condition from tuberculous disease or other infection, which always destroys the intervertebral disc.

Treatment. Calvé's disease is non-progressive, and in practice treatment is required only for as long as the symptoms last. If pain is severe the child should be kept recumbent in bed, but in most cases he may safely resume an active life without external support within a few weeks.

PROLAPSED LUMBAR INTERVERTEBRAL DISC

Herniation of part of a lumbar intervertebral disc is a common cause of combined back pain and sciatica.

Cause. Prolapse of a disc is often precipitated by injury. Spontaneous age-degeneration of the disc is probably an important predisposing factor.

Pathology. The discs between L.5 and S.1 and between L.4 and L.5 are those most often affected. Part of the gelatinous nucleus pulposus protrudes through a rent in the annulus fibrosus at its weakest part, which is postero-lateral (Figs 158–161); or sometimes the torn annulus itself protrudes backwards. If it is small, the protrusion bulges the pain-sensitive posterior longitudinal ligament, causing pain in the back. If it is large, the protrusion herniates through the posterior ligament and may impinge upon an issuing nerve to cause sciatic pain. The nerve affected is that which leaves the spinal canal at the interspace next below the site of the disc lesion. Thus the first sacral nerve is impinged upon by a prolapse between L.5 and S.1, the fifth lumbar nerve by a prolapse between L.4 and L.5, and so on. Natural healing is by shrinkage and fibrosis of the extruded disc material; not by its reposition within the disc.

Secondary effects. Progressive degeneration of the disc leads, after months or years, to osteoarthritis, with ultimate involvement of the posterior intervertebral (facet) joints as well as the central (body-to-body) joints.

Clinical features. In a typical case of disc prolapse at the L.4–L.5 or L.5–S.1 level the clinical picture is clearly defined. The patient is aged between 18 and 60. A few hours or days after jarring or straining the back he is seized, while twisting, stooping or coughing, with agonising pain in the lumbar region. He is hardly able to move. The acute pain gradually lessens in severity, but after a few days a radiating pain is felt in one or other buttock and down the back or side of the thigh to the calf and foot. Tingling or numbness is felt in the calf or foot. The pain is aggravated by coughing or sneezing.

On examination the patient with a fully developed acute attack stands either with a lumbar scoliosis (sciatic scoliosis) (Fig. 162) or with the normal anterior lumbar curve obliterated. Forward flexion is greatly restricted, as also may be extension. Lateral flexion, on the other hand, is usually free and painless—certainly to one side if not to both. Straight leg raising is restricted on the affected side, usually markedly—an important clinical sign. Careful tests may reveal slight muscle wasting or weakness in the distribution of the affected nerve, and the corresponding tendon jerk (knee jerk in L.3–L.4 lesions; ankle jerk in L.5–S.1 lesions) is impaired or absent.

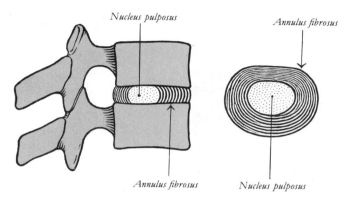

Fig. 158
A normal intervertebral disc seen in sagittal section (*left*)
and in horizontal section (*right*).

Fig. 159   **Fig. 160**   **Fig. 161**
Stages in prolapse of an intervertebral disc. Figure 159—The annulus fibrosus is torn but there has been no extrusion of the nucleus pulposus. Figure 160—Extrusion of nuclear material through the rent. The posterior longitudinal ligament is stretched but the protrusion has not reached the nerve. Figure 161—The protrusion is larger and the nerve is stretched over it. Sometimes a fragment of the torn annulus itself protrudes backwards.

Variations. Atypical cases are common. Thus a definite history of injury or strain is often lacking. The pain may begin gradually rather than suddenly. The symptoms may be confined to the back and never radiate to the lower limb (acute lumbago). On the other hand, the pain is sometimes felt predominantly in the limb and is relatively mild in the back. The severity of the pain varies greatly from case to case, and its exact distribution

Fig. 162
Sciatic scoliosis in a patient with prolapsed intervertebral disc. There is a temporary list to the left, assumed involuntarily to reduce the pressure on the trapped nerve at the site of the prolapse.

Fig. 163
Radiculograph showing a rare central herniation of a lumbar intervertebral disc at the L.4–5 level. The column of radio-opaque fluid is compressed, and there is failure to fill the L.5 nerve root sheaths on both sides.

depends upon the level of the disc prolapse: for instance, in the relatively uncommon cases of mid-lumbar (L.3–L.4) prolapse the pain radiates towards the groin and the front of the thigh rather than to the back of the thigh and leg.

In a severe case in which the prolapse is almost central there may be pressure upon the cauda equina, with consequent loss of bladder sensibility and retention of urine.

Imaging. *Radiographic features.* In a case of acute prolapsed disc plain radiographs do not show any abnormality, and the purpose of radiography is mainly to exclude other causes of back pain and sciatica. It is only when a disc has been deranged for many months or years that appreciable narrowing of the disc space and spurring of the joint margins (denoting secondary osteoarthritis) are observed.

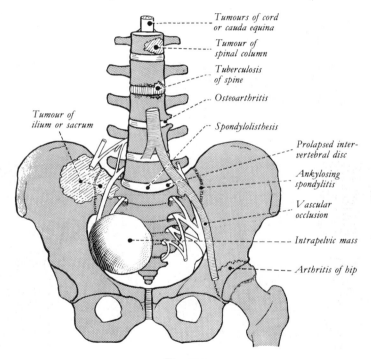

Fig. 164
Eleven causes of pain in the back or lower limb. All must be considered in differential diagnosis.

Radiculography may outline the disc protrusion, thus indicating its level (Fig. 163). This investigation, however, has been largely superseded by *magnetic resonance imaging*, which can show the intervertebral disc substance and the nerve roots: the bulging disc material can thus be visualised directly. *Discography* and *ascending spinal venography* have only an occasional place.

Investigations. Lumbar puncture reveals either normal cerebrospinal fluid or, commonly, a slight increase of protein content.

Correlation of pathology with clinical features. The initial injury or strain marks the time when the annulus fibrosus is torn or damaged. The nucleus pulposus is very gelatinous and an interval elapses before it becomes extruded. Bulging of the extruded material beneath the posterior longitudinal ligament corresponds to the stage of acute back pain. Herniation through the ligament with impingement against the adjacent nerve is responsible for the radiating limb pain and, in low lumbar lesions, the restriction of straight leg raising.

Diagnosis. Prolapsed intervertebral disc must be differentiated from other causes of pain in the back or leg (Fig. 164). The conditions with which it is most likely to be confused are: tuberculosis of the spine or sacro-iliac joints; intraspinal tumour; tumour of the spine or pelvis; spondylolisthesis; ankylosing spondylitis; osteoarthritis of the spine; arthritis of the hip; and occlusion of the aorta or of the iliac or femoral artery, with consequent

Fig. 165	**Fig. 166**
Plaster jacket used in the conservative treatment of prolapsed lumbar intervertebral disc.	Steel-reinforced surgical corset used for mild cases of prolapsed intervertebral disc and for certain types of chronic low back pain.

ischaemic pain in the proximal limb muscles on exercise. A dramatically sudden onset is always suggestive of a mechanical derangement and especially of a prolapsed disc, whereas pain that increases relentlessly without intermission suggests a progressive lesion, inflammatory or neoplastic. Although the clinical features are often highly suggestive, definitive diagnosis rests upon radiculography or magnetic resonance imaging.

Treatment. *Conservative treatment* is successful in relieving the symptoms in a high proportion of cases—probably at least nine out of ten. The principle is to provide rest for the lumbar spine. This is preferably secured by a plaster jacket (Fig. 165) or well fitted brace, which allows the patient to be up and about; but rest in bed is a commonly used alternative, and it is often combined with continuous or intermittent traction on the legs or pelvis. In either case rest for the spine must be continued for six to twelve weeks according to progress. Thereafter a less restrictive corset (Fig. 166) should be worn for several months if minor symptoms persist.

Intradiscal injection of chymopapain. Chymopapain is an enzyme with the property of dissolving fibrocartilaginous tissue. Injected into the disc substance, it causes partial dissolution of the nucleus pulposus and, in a favourable case, of protruding disc material. In the long term there is marked narrowing of the disc space as seen radiologically. Intradiscal injection of chymopapain is a method of treatment that has been slow in gaining acceptance, largely because the potential dangers were not at first fully assessed. It may be used in selected cases as a possible alternative to excision of the disc, with the advantage that operation is avoided.

In most reported series the success rate in cases that would otherwise entail operation is in the order of 80 per cent. Rarely, inadvertent leakage of the enzyme into the spinal canal has led to nerve damage and even death, but when the method is used with proper skill and with due precautions the risks are probably smaller than those of operation.

Operative treatment. Excision of the displaced disc material is indicated in the following circumstances: 1) when the sciatic pain is so excruciating from the beginning that it prevents sleep and leads to deterioration of the general health; 2) when severe sciatic pain is unrelieved by appropriate conservative treatment continued for at least eight weeks; 3) when severe neurological disturbance suggests massive prolapse with compression of the cauda equina. In this last condition operation must be carried out as an emergency procedure because the attendant impairment of bladder, bowel and sexual function quickly becomes irreversible.

At operation the disc is exposed from behind by retraction of the posterior spinal muscles away from the midline, excision of the ligamentum flavum and perhaps part of a lamina at the appropriate level, and gentle retraction of the theca. The protruded part of the disc forms an obvious rounded bulge, over which the emerging spinal nerve may be seen tightly stretched. The extruded material is removed, together with as much of the remaining nuclear tissue as can be pulled out from between the vertebral bodies. Many surgeons now favour excision by a magnification technique, through a cannula inserted through a small 'stab' incision.

ACUTE LUMBAGO

Lumbago is a symptom rather than a disease. In a typical attack of acute lumbago the patient is suddenly seized with agonising pain in the lumbar region of the spine, usually while stooping, lifting, turning, or coughing.

The pain is often so severe that any movement is difficult and the patient is 'stuck'. With rest, the pain gradually subsides, but in some cases the acute back pain is succeeded by sciatica, suggesting irritation of a lumbar or sacral nerve.

The pathogenesis of acute lumbago is not entirely clear. Indeed there may be more than one cause. Probably in many cases the underlying lesion is a prolapsed disc that has not yet been retropulsed far enough to interfere with a nerve root (Fig. 160). It is in these cases that sciatica may develop later, as the size of the prolapse increases. But other examples of acute lumbago are more convincingly ascribed to some other mechanical disorder, such as sudden nipping of synovial membrane in one of the facet joints, or momentary subluxation with consequent ligamentous strain, especially at an intervertebral joint that is unstable on account of disc degeneration or osteoarthritis. In such a case acute attacks of pain may recur at intervals of months or years, with intervals of relative freedom between the attacks.

Treatment should usually be to provide rest for the spine, either by recumbency or by a plaster jacket or surgical corset, as for a prolapsed intervertebral disc. Full recovery is often observed within one or two weeks. Because of the frightening severity of the pain confident reassurance may be needed.

SPONDYLOLYSIS

In spondylolysis there is a defect in the neural arch of the fifth (rarely the fourth) lumbar vertebra. There is loss of bony continuity between the superior and the inferior articular processes, the deficiency being bridged by fibrous tissue (Fig. 167). If this stretches or gives way, the consequent vertebral displacement constitutes one variety of spondylolisthesis (see below).

Fig. 167
Site of the defect in spondylolysis.
There is lack of bony continuity at
the isthmus of the neural arch (pars
interarticularis) on each side.

Though the defect was formerly regarded as congenital it is now widely believed that it may be caused by injury; or, more often, it may be the result of a stress fracture in childhood or adolescence.

Clinically, spondylolysis (the defect without displacement) is often symptomless, but it is sometimes a cause of deep lumbar back pain. *Radiographically*, the defect is usually best shown in oblique projections.

Treatment. This is often unnecessary. Aching may be relieved by a surgical corset. If pain is unusually troublesome an attempt may be made to close the defect in the pars interarticularis on each side by transfixing it with a screw and laying in slender bone grafts (Buck 1970); or alternatively, local fusion of the spine may be undertaken (see p. 200).

SPONDYLOLISTHESIS

(Lumbar spondylolisthesis)

Spondylolisthesis is the term applied to spontaneous displacement of a lumbar vertebral body upon the segment next below it. Displacement is usually forwards, but may be backwards (retrospondylolisthesis).

Cause. There are three predisposing factors: 1) congenital malformation of the articular processes (rare); 2) spondylolysis (a defect in the pars inter-articularis of the neural arch) (p. 196); and 3) osteoarthritis of the posterior (facet) joints.

Pathology. In the normal spine forward displacement of a vertebral body is prevented by engagement of its articular processes with those of the segment next below it. In spondylolisthesis there is a failure of this check mechanism, and the attachments of the intervertebral disc alone are not strong enough to hold the vertebral bodies in alignment.

In the first type of spondylolisthesis, the least common, there is a congenital basis for the displacement. The posterior intervertebral joints are unstable because the articular processes are congenitally malformed or even rudimentary; thus they form no bar to forward displacement of the spinal column (Fig. 168). This defect occurs most often at the lumbo-sacral joint. Displacement may be severe and, since the whole vertebra is displaced complete with its neural arch, the cauda equina may be trapped, with consequent severe neurological disturbance (Fig. 168).

In the second type, which is the best recognised, a defect in the neural arch of a vertebra allows separation of its two halves (see spondylolysis, p. 196, and Fig. 169). The body, with the pedicles and superior articular processes (and the whole of the spinal column above it), slips forwards, leaving behind the laminae and inferior articular processes (Fig. 169). The fifth lumbar is the vertebra usually affected, the fourth occasionally. Displacement may gradually increase, especially during adolescence, and it sometimes reaches a severe degree. There may be minor irritation of one of the issuing nerves, with consequent sciatica; but despite severe bony displacement serious interference with the nerves of the cauda equina is exceptional in this type of spondylolisthesis.

In the third type of spondylolisthesis, seen fairly commonly, the posterior intervertebral (facet) joints become unstable on account of osteoarthritis, with degeneration and thinning of the articular cartilage that is essential to a snug fit of the joint surfaces (Fig. 170). It may occur at any level in the lumbar spine—most commonly between the fourth and fifth lumbar vertebrae. In this type the vertebral displacement is occasionally backwards rather than forwards (see Fig. 148), but in either case displacement is never severe, and neurological disturbance is unusual.

The intervertebral disc at the site of vertebral slipping is inevitably damaged, and disc prolapse may occur.

Fig. 168
Spondylolisthesis secondary to congenital malformation of the articular processes at the lumbosacral joint. The cauda equina is trapped between the body of the sacrum and the lamina of the displaced fifth lumbar vertebra. In this type of spondylolisthesis neurological signs are to be expected.

Fig. 169
Spondylolisthesis due to defect of the neural arch of a vertebra, in this case affecting the fifth lumbar vertebra. The body and superior articular processes have slipped forwards, leaving the spinous process and inferior articular processes in normal relationship with the sacrum. (Radiographically the defect is seen best in oblique projections.)

Fig. 170
Spondylolisthesis secondary to osteoarthritis. Wearing down of the cartilage of the posterior intervertebral (facet) joints has permitted slight forward displacement of the fourth lumbar vertebra on the fifth. The condition may occur at any level in the lumbar spine.

Clinical features. The clinical features of spondylolisthesis are inconstant: they depend to some extent upon the nature of the causative lesion and upon the degree of displacement. Thus in spondylolisthesis from under-development of the articular processes (Fig. 168), and in that from a defect of the pars interarticularis (Fig. 169), the patient is usually an adolescent or a young adult, whereas displacement from degeneration of the facet joints in osteoarthritis (Fig. 170) is seen characteristically in patients beyond middle age. In some cases the deformity is entirely symptomless. When symptoms occur they take the form of chronic backache, with or without sciatica. The back pain is worse on standing.

On examination there is often a visible or palpable 'step' above the sacral crest, due to the forward displacement of the spinal column; but this is obvious only when the displacement is severe. Spinal movements are restricted only slightly, if at all. *Abdomen*: When displacement is severe the spinal column is projected forwards and the lumbar vertebral bodies may be palpable through the abdominal wall. *Lower limbs*: Minor irritation of a sciatic root is often evidenced by impairment of straight leg raising; but severe neurological disturbance is seldom observed except in the rare cases in which congenital malformation of the articular processes allows dislocation of the whole vertebra complete with its neural arch (Fig. 168).

Fig. 171
Oblique radiograph of the lower lumbar region of a patient with spondylolisthesis, showing a defect of the pars interarticularis of the neural arch of the fourth lumbar vertebra (centre of illustration). Oblique radiographs such as this are important in the differentiation of spondylolisthesis caused by a neural arch defect from the other two types of spondylolisthesis.

Radiographic features. Radiographs show the displacement. The lateral and oblique views will demonstrate whether or not there is a defect of the neural arch (Fig. 171).

Diagnosis. Spondylolisthesis is distinguished from other causes of back pain and sciatica by the radiographs.

Treatment. When spondylolisthesis is symptomless treatment is not required. *Non-operative treatment*: Moderate symptoms are often adequately relieved by a well fitted surgical corset (Fig. 166), and this should be tried before operation is considered. *Operation*: This is justified only when the disability (from back pain or neurological disturbance) is severe. The operation entails the release of stretched or compressed nerves, followed by fusion of the affected segments of the spinal column.

Spinal fusion. Fusion, or arthrodesis, of spinal segments is effected by bridging the vertebrae with bone grafts, usually obtained from the ilium but sometimes from the tibia or fibula. In *posterior fusion* the grafts are fitted between or alongside the spinous processes, superficial to the laminae. In *anterior fusion* blocks of bone are inlayed in deep slots cut in the vertebral bodies after excision of most of the intervertebral disc from the front. In *lateral fusion* bone grafts are wedged between the transverse processes or, in the case of the lumbo-sacral joint, between transverse processes above and the lateral masses of the sacrum below. Each method has its special applications, but the choice also depends largely on the surgeon's individual preference.

SPINAL STENOSIS
(Claudication of the cauda equina)

In the syndrome of spinal stenosis standing and walking beyond a certain duration are associated with increasingly severe pain in the gluteal region and lower limb on one or both sides, ascribed to cramping of nerves and their blood vessels in a constricted spinal canal.

Pathology. The dimensions of the spinal canal in the lumbar region show considerable variation between individuals. The cross-sectional shape of the canal also varies, it being sometimes rounded and sometimes almost triangular. Thus in some persons there is a congenital narrowing or constriction of the canal which, though providing adequate room for the cauda equina in the absence of other pathology, nevertheless allows little or no margin of safety, so that if the canal becomes further narrowed from secondary causes such as the formation of osteophytes about the facet joints, or bulging of an intervertebral disc, the normal functioning of nerves of the cauda equina will be impaired by lack of room and constriction of their blood supply. To some extent the constriction seems to be selective rather than uniform throughout the cauda equina, the nerves lying in the narrow lateral recesses of a triangular canal being particularly vulnerable. For a long time the impairment of nerve function is intermittent rather than permanent, being rapidly reversible when the patient assumes a sitting posture.

Clinical features. The clinical history is characteristic. The patient, often in middle age, complains that after walking for a matter of ten to fifteen minutes, he develops a heavy aching sensation in one or both lower limbs, and that this steadily increases to such an extent that eventually he is forced to sit down. In most cases similar symptoms develop when the patient stands for a while, even without walking. Relief is obtained only by sitting or by lying with the hips and knees drawn up in a sitting posture—it is not sufficient just to stop walking. Sitting relieves the symptoms within a few minutes because on flexion of the spine the canal is widened, and the patient can then resume walking or standing for a further period. *Examination* may reveal little abnormality, though frequently there are features to suggest degenerative change in the lumbar spine—for instance impairment of spinal mobility.

Imaging. *Plain radiographs* may give the impression that the spinal canal is narrower than usual and they may show further constriction of the canal by posterior osteophytes upon the margins of the vertebral bodies or in relation to the facet joints. *Radiculography* shows a block to the passage of radio-opaque fluid along the affected part of the lumbar spinal canal when the spine is straight. If the examination is repeated with the patient in a sitting posture, passage of fluid along the canal may be found to be restored. *Computerised tomography (CT scanning)* and *magnetic resonance imaging (MRI)* show very clearly the shape of the spinal canal, the dimensions of which may be measured and compared with the normal. They may also show bony or soft-tissue excrescences encroaching upon either a normal or a congenitally constricted canal.

Diagnosis. The spinal stenosis syndrome bears superficial resemblance to intermittent claudication from vascular disease. Confusion should be avoided, however, because of the important distinction that pain in spinal stenosis, unlike that from arterial disease, comes on not only with walking but also with standing, and is relieved only by sitting or by flexing the spine. Moreover, examination of the vascular system shows no abnormality. The diagnosis is best confirmed by radiculography, which shows the level of the constriction of the spinal canal.

Treatment. Mild symptoms may be controlled by appropriate modification of activities—for instance by using a bicycle instead of walking, and by the avoidance of prolonged standing. In the fully-established case, treatment should be by operation to decompress the spinal canal by removal of intruding osteophytes and enlargement of the lateral recesses at the level of the constriction. Decompression may have to be carried out over a number of segments, depending upon the longitudinal extent of the constriction as shown radiographically and by radiculography.

TUMOURS OF THE TRUNK AND SPINE

These tumours will be considered in two categories: 1) tumours that affect the spinal column or its contents—spinal cord or nerve roots; and 2) other tumours of the trunk.

TUMOURS IN RELATION TO THE SPINAL COLUMN, SPINAL CORD, OR EMERGING NERVES

Classification and pathology. As in the cervical region, tumours involving the spine or related nerves may arise: 1) in the spinal column itself; 2) in the meninges or, rarely, the spinal cord; 3) in the fibrous component of a peripheral nerve (neurofibroma); or 4) in adjacent soft tissues.

Tumours of the spinal column may be benign (for instance chondroma, giant-cell tumour, haemangioma, osteoblastoma) but are more often malignant. Such tumours may be primary (sarcoma, multiple myeloma, chordoma), but metastatic tumours predominate. A meningeal tumour (meningioma) is an occasional cause of compression of the spinal cord or cauda equina. Nerve compression may also be a consequence of a neurofibroma growing within the spinal canal.

Clinical features. The effects of these tumours vary according to their site and character. Broadly, the effects may be placed in three groups: 1) local destruction of the skeleton; 2) compression of the spinal cord; 3) interference with peripheral nerves.

Local destruction of the skeleton. The commonest cause is a malignant tumour of the bones of the spinal column (Fig. 172)—usually a metastatic carcinoma. The predominant symptom is pain, which is constant and increases relentlessly in its severity. Frequently there are associated neurological manifestations from involvement of the spinal cord or nerve roots. The local objective signs vary from case to case. Sometimes the tumour is palpable—as, for instance, a sacral tumour. Sometimes deformity, from collapse of the bony structure, is evident clinically; or there may be marked restriction of spinal movement, with protective muscle spasm.

Compression of the spinal cord. This may occur from tumours of the spinal cord itself or of its meninges, from tumours of nerves (neurofibroma), or from tumours of the bony spinal column. The clinical manifestations depend upon the exact location of the tumour. Typically, when the spinal cord is slowly compressed, initial root pain (girdle pain in thoracic involvement, lower limb pain in lumbar) is followed by lower motor neurone paresis at the segmental level corresponding to the site of the tumour, by progressive sensory and upper motor neurone paralysis below the lesion, and often by bladder or bowel dysfunction.

Interference with peripheral nerves. Peripheral nerves—especially the nerves of the cauda equina—may be involved by tumours of the nerves themselves (neurofibroma), by tumours of the spinal column (benign or malignant), or by tumours in the peripheral course of the nerves (for example, a tumour of a rib, or a tumour arising from or within the pelvis). The clinical features depend upon the particular nerve or nerves affected and upon the extent of the involvement. Typically, there will be constant, progressive, and ultimately severe pain along the course of the affected nerve, with sensory impairment, increasing motor weakness, and depression of reflexes in the distribution of the nerve. Retention of urine is usually a prominent feature of a tumour interfering with the cauda equina.

Fig. 172
Partial collapse of the second and fourth lumbar vertebrae in a patient with myelomatosis. Note that the intervertebral discs are not destroyed.

Imaging. *Plain radiographs* will usually help in discovering a tumour arising in the bones of the spinal column (Fig. 172), or eroding the bone from outside. In cases of vertebral destruction from tumour the adjacent intervertebral discs are typically preserved. This point helps in the distinction from erosion and collapse due to infection, in which the discs are destroyed at an early stage (compare Figs 145 and 172).

Radiographs of the chest may reveal a primary lung tumour or a metastasis; and radiographs of the rest of the skeleton may be helpful in the diagnosis of disseminated tumours such as multiple myeloma.

Myelography is indispensable if a tumour of the spinal cord or cauda equina is suspected. *Radioisotope scanning* may show evidence of a lesion before it is evident radiographically. *Computerised tomography* (CT scanning) is capable of showing even quite small tumours within the vertebrae. It may also help in the recognition of soft-tissue tumours in the spine or pelvis. *Magnetic resonance imaging* is even more helpful in showing the full extent of the tumour and the extent to which adjacent tissues have been infiltrated.

Diagnosis. The possibility of a tumour has to be borne in mind constantly in the differential diagnosis of back pain and lower limb pain, especially when associated with radiological signs of vertebral erosion or collapse or with neurological disturbance affecting the trunk, lower limbs or viscera (Fig. 164). Other causes of vertebral erosion or collapse include previous trauma, pathological fracture from rarefying disease of bone, tuberculous or pyogenic infection, and syphilis. Other causes of spinal cord or cauda equina disturbance include prolapsed intervertebral disc, severe angular deformity in scoliosis or kyphosis, tuberculous or pyogenic infection, osteoarthritis, spondylolisthesis, herpes zoster, and primary neurological diseases such as disseminated sclerosis and motor neurone disease.

A history of insidious onset, with relentless increase of symptoms without remission, always suggests the possibility of tumour. Careful search should always be made for a primary tumour elsewhere in the body.

OTHER TUMOURS OF THE TRUNK

TUMOURS OF THE STERNUM AND RIBS

The sternum and ribs contain abundant red marrow, favourable to the development of blood-borne metastatic tumours or of deposits in myelomatosis or the lymphomas. Histological examination of the sternal marrow (obtained by sternal puncture) is often of diagnostic importance in suspected metastasising tumours, for the material will often show tumour cells even in the absence of clinically evident metastases.

TUMOURS OF THE SCAPULA

The commonest tumour of the scapula is a chondroma. It grows outwards from the flat body of the bone and is therefore classed as an ecchondroma. It may attain a large size. Although it is often benign at first, there is a risk of malignant change, with the development of a chondrosarcoma. For that reason a chondroma that appears to be enlarging should always be excised with an adequate margin of healthy bone. A large part of the scapula can be removed without causing serious disability.

TUMOURS OF THE PELVIC GIRDLE

The pelvic bones, like the scapula, are sometimes the seat of a chondroma (ecchondroma). It may reach a large size, and there is risk of malignant change.

The considerable content of red marrow renders the pelvic bones liable to carcinomatous metastatic deposits, and they are also a common site of tumour deposits in myelomatosis.

CHRONIC LOWER LUMBAR LIGAMENTOUS STRAIN
(Postural back pain)

The terms *chronic ligamentous strain* and *postural back pain* are used to cover an ill defined group of affections characterised by persistent backache without demonstrable pathology. These conditions are common—in fact they form a considerable proportion of the cases of back pain seen in orthopaedic practice.

Cause. It is assumed that the spinal muscles fail in their function of protecting the deep ligaments in maintaining posture. Predisposing causes include childbirth, overweight, general flabbiness of muscle, and debilitating illness. A similar condition may follow 'whiplash' injury of the spine, common in occupants of a car struck from behind by another vehicle.

Pathology. No precise lesion is demonstrable.

Clinical features. The patient is nearly always a woman. She often dates the onset of pain from childbirth, sometimes from an operation, or from a debilitating illness; but equally often the onset is unexplained. The pain is characteristically in the lumbar or lumbo-sacral region. It tends to be worse on activities such as stooping. *On examination* there may be no abnormal physical signs but in many cases there is some restriction of spinal movement. *Radiographs* are normal.

Diagnosis. This depends upon the exclusion of demonstrable pathological lesions by careful clinical and radiographic examination. A history of long-continued lumbar backache, with a total lack of clinical or radiological abnormalities, should always suggest this group of affections.

Course and prognosis. Aching often persists for many years despite treatment. Nevertheless in most cases the condition is a source of nagging discomfort rather than a serious handicap to the normal activities of life.

Treatment. Often reassurance alone is required. When treatment is called for, the four methods available are: 1) physiotherapy; 2) manipulation; 3) external support; and 4) local injections of anaesthetic solution or of hydrocortisone. In young patients physiotherapy, in the form of active exercises to strengthen the spinal muscles, with or without heat and massage, should be tried for at least two months. If this is ineffective manipulation of the lumbar and sacro-iliac joints, with or without anaesthetic, is worth a trial: it may be followed by repeated longitudinal traction and muscle exercises.

If pain persists despite these measures, fitting with a surgical corset is advised. In elderly and flabby patients physiotherapy is seldom of benefit and early resort should be had to a reinforced corset (Fig. 166).

Local injections are often worth a trial in cases of persistent pain resistant to the measures described. Injections of a local anaesthetic solution, often combined with hydrocortisone, may be given directly into areas of local tenderness; or alternatively the injection may be into the extradural space of the spinal canal (epidural injection). The outcome of such injections is however often disappointing.

The prolonged use of analgesic drugs for this type of back pain should be discouraged, because of the risks of side effects or addiction.

COCCYDYNIA

In its widest sense, coccydynia includes any painful condition in the region of the coccyx. In practice, the term is restricted to the clinical entity in which persistent pain continues for many weeks or months after a local injury, despite the absence of demonstrable pathology. Eventually it is a self-limiting affection, though it may cause severe discomfort while it lasts—often for months.

Cause. Typically coccydynia develops after an injury—usually a fall on the 'tail'. Occasionally a history of injury is lacking.

Pathology. In some cases there is probably a strain of the sacro-coccygeal joint; in others the lesion is thought to be simply a contusion of the periosteum over the lower sacrum or coccyx. Rarely, a crack fracture of the coccyx or sacrum is demonstrated.

Clinical features. There is pain localised to the sacro-coccygeal area, worse when sitting. In severe cases there is also pain on defaecation. Usually the patient is free from pain when standing or lying. *On examination* there is localised tenderness over the sacro-coccygeal region. In some cases the pain can be reproduced by moving the coccyx. In the absence of a fracture, *radiographs* do not show any alteration from the normal.

Diagnosis. It is important to consider other causes of pain in this area, especially infections of the sacro-coccygeal joint and tumours of the sacrum or coccyx. Investigation should include rectal examination, and radiographs must always be obtained.

Treatment. In most cases treatment is not required. All that is necessary is to exclude serious organic disease, and then to reassure the patient that the condition is harmless and that it may be expected to resolve spontaneously if left alone. Various remedies have been advocated, including short-wave diathermy, manipulation, and injections of local anaesthetic or hydrocortisone; but none is uniformly successful. In the exceptional case of unusually severe and persistent pain the coccyx may be excised.

SENILE OSTEOPOROSIS

Although the symptoms of senile osteoporosis are mainly in the back, it is strictly a general affection of the skeleton and was described as such on page 65. The spinal features are aching pain, kyphosis, liability to compression fractures of vertebral bodies, and marked rarefaction of the bones of the spinal column.

DISORDERS OF THE SACRO-ILIAC JOINTS

Sacro-iliac lesions are a rather uncommon but nervertheless important cause of back symptoms or of referred pain in the lower limb. Of the various types of arthritis, ankylosing spondylitis is the best recognised. Tuberculous arthritis is seen mainly in developing countries.

ANKYLOSING SPONDYLITIS

Although ankylosing spondylitis usually affects a larger area of the spine it always begins in the sacro-iliac joints and the patient may present himself initially with sacro-iliac pain. The disease was described fully earlier in this chapter (p. 184). In a related condition, *sacro-iliitis*, the radiological changes resemble those of ankylosing spondylitis but the remainder of the spine is unaffected.

TUBERCULOSIS OF A SACRO-ILIAC JOINT

This is rarely seen in Western countries but it still occurs in countries where the standard of living is poor. The patient is a child or young adult. The condition is usually confined to one side, but it may be bilateral. As in tuberculous disease of other joints, there is destruction of articular cartilage and thickening of synovial membrane, often with erosion of bone and abscess formation.

Clinically, the main feature is pain behind the affected joint and in the iliac fossa or groin. A diffuse, ill localised pain may be referred down the lower limb. Examination shows restriction of lower spinal movements, and side-to-side compression of the pelvis aggravates the pain. An abscess is often palpable posteriorly or in the iliac fossa. *Radiographs* show local rarefaction, with loss of definition or 'fuzziness' of the joint outline.

Treatment is like that for tuberculosis of other joints (p. 120). Constitutional treatment is by rest and antibacterial drugs. Local treatment is by an initial period of rest in bed, or by support for the trunk and pelvis in a plaster hip spica. If there is an abscess it should be aspirated. When the acute pain has subsided some surgeons allow the patient up in a sacro-iliac support, whereas others advise operative fusion (arthrodesis) of the affected joint as a safeguard against recrudescence of the disease.

OTHER FORMS OF SACRO-ILIAC ARTHRITIS

Pyogenic arthritis may occur, but it is uncommon. Its general features conform with those of pyogenic arthritis elsewhere, as described on page 109.

Rheumatoid arthritis may affect the sacro-iliac joints in common with the other joints of the spine (p. 182)

Osteoarthritis of the sacro-iliac joints is uncommon and seldom, if ever, the cause of serious disability.

SACRO-ILIAC LIGAMENTOUS STRAIN

Sacro-iliac strain was formerly a common diagnosis in cases of pain localised predominantly in the upper gluteal region. It is now believed that in the vast majority of such cases the pain does not in fact originate in the sacro-iliac joint, but is referred to the gluteal region from a disorder in the lower lumbar spine—often an intervertebral disc lesion. Exceptionally, however, true sacro-iliac ligamentous strain occurs.

Clinically, the patient is usually adult. The symptoms are often noticed first after a major injury of the pelvis or after childbirth. The pain is accurately localised to the sacro-iliac joint, and there is a tendency also to referred diffuse aching in the thigh. The pain is aggravated by twisting the trunk. Examination reveals a good range of spinal movements with pain only at the extremes. Forcible stress applied to the sacro-iliac joints by firm lateral compression of the pelvis, or by extending one hip while the other is held fully flexed, reproduces the pain. There are no neurological signs. *Radiographs* show no abnormality. In traumatic cases *radioisotope scanning* may show increased uptake of the isotope in the region of the joint.

Treatment. Genuine sacro-iliac strain often responds to physiotherapy by local heat, massage and exercises, which may be supplemented by manipulation of the joint, with or without anaesthetic. If this fails, recourse is usually made to a surgical corset (Fig. 166, p. 194).

EXTRINSIC DISORDERS SIMULATING SPINAL DISEASE

ABDOMINAL DISORDERS

PEPTIC ULCER

The pain of peptic ulcer is often felt in the back as well as in the epigastrium. Exceptionally, it is felt entirely in the back or beneath the left costal margin, when it may simulate girdle pain referred along a thoracic spinal nerve.

VISCEROPTOSIS

Dragging of pendulous viscera upon the posterior abdominal wall is a contributory cause of backache. Flabbiness of the back muscles, with consequent ligamentous strain, is usually present as well. The pain from both conditions may be relieved by fitting a combined abdominal and lumbosacral support.

RENAL OR PERIRENAL INFECTIONS

Rarely, a carbuncle of the kidney or a perinephric abscess is confused with a back condition. The usual features are pain in the back and loin, general malaise, pyrexia, and leucocytosis.

RENAL CALCULUS

The pain may be felt chiefly in the back, though it is always towards the loin rather than in the midline. The pain is often aggravated by jarring movements—for instance, riding on a jolting bus or stepping from a pavement. There may be a history of haematuria or of attacks of colic. Spinal movements are unaffected. Radiographs may reveal the calculus; but in cases of doubt intravenous pyelography should be performed.

Biliary calculus and cholecystitis
Pain beneath the right costal margin from a gall-bladder lesion is easily confused with girdle pain referred along an intercostal nerve from a spinal condition.

PELVIC DISORDERS

Intrapelvic tumour
A tumour or other mass within the pelvis may interfere with the sacral plexus or its branches, causing pain which is generally of sciatic distribution. It may thus simulate sciatica arising from a spinal cause such as a prolapsed intervertebral disc or spinal tumour (Fig. 164, p. 193). A pelvic mass will usually be palpable on rectal examination, which should form part of the routine investigation in cases of radiating lower limb pain. Computerised tomography or magnetic resonance imaging may be helpful in diagnosis.

Gynaecological disease
The importance of gynaecological disorders as a cause of back pain has been exaggerated. In point of fact, there is no reasonable ground for attributing significant back symptoms to gynaecological causes unless a major intrapelvic disorder is demonstrable. It is often observed, however, that back pain from any cause tends to be exacerbated before and during menstruation.

LOWER LIMB DISORDERS

Arthritis of the hip
The pain from arthritis of the hip sometimes simulates sciatic pain referred from a spinal lesion. Characteristically, hip pain is referred from the groin down the front of the thigh towards the knee. Irritation of the fourth lumbar nerve root by a spinal lesion causes pain in a somewhat similar distribution. The best safeguard against error is to examine the movements of the hip joint in every case of radiating lower limb pain.

VASCULAR DISORDERS

Arterial occlusion
It should always be remembered that occlusion of the aorta, of the iliac arteries or of their major branches may be associated with ischaemic muscle pain on exercise which, from its distribution in the lower back or buttocks, may easily be confused with back pain or sciatica caused by a prolapsed intervertebral disc or other spinal lesion, and in particular with spinal stenosis (p. 200). The important clue to the correct diagnosis is the history of onset of pain only during exercise, with rapid relief when the exercise is stopped. In such a case the femoral or popliteal pulse will usually be weak or absent; but it should be noted that the posterior tibial and dorsalis pedis

pulses may be easily palpable even when there is complete occlusion at or near the aortic bifurcation. Plain radiographs may show calcification of the aorta or iliac vessels, and arteriography will show the site and extent of the occlusion.

AORTIC ANEURYSM

It is important to note that severe pain in the back may be a presenting symptom in a patient with a leaking aortic aneurysm or with a dissecting aneurysm.

References and bibliography, page 403.

11. The shoulder region

The mechanics of the shoulder are rather complex. The shoulder 'joint' in fact comprises three components—the gleno-humeral joint or shoulder joint proper, the acromio-clavicular joint, and the sterno-clavicular joint. The gleno-humeral joint allows a free range of abduction, flexion and rotation, under the control of the scapulo-humeral muscles. The other two joints together allow 90 degrees of rotation of the scapula upon the thorax and a moderate range of antero-posterior gliding of the scapula, under the control of the cervico-scapular and thoraco-scapular muscles.

Disorders of the shoulder include most varieties of arthritis; but it is notable that osteoarthritis—common in most joints—is rare in the gleno-humeral joint. As if to make up for this, the shoulder exhibits several affections peculiar to itself—notably tears of the musculo-tendinous cuff, the painful arc syndrome, and 'frozen' shoulder. Together these form a large proportion of shoulder disabilities.

Pain in the shoulder and arm is notoriously prone to misinterpretation, and special care is required to differentiate intrinsic pain arising in the shoulder from extrinsic pain referred from the cervical spine, the thorax, or the abdomen.

SPECIAL POINTS IN THE INVESTIGATION OF SHOULDER SYMPTOMS

History

Characteristics of shoulder pain. It is important to find out the precise location and distribution of the pain. True shoulder pain is seldom confined to the shoulder itself. Typically, it radiates from a point near the tip of the acromion down the lateral side of the upper arm to about the level of the deltoid insertion. It is unusual for true shoulder pain to extend below the elbow.

Pain arising in the acromio-clavicular joint or sterno-clavicular joint is localised to the joint itself and does not radiate down the limb.

Referred pain in the shoulder region. The pain referred from an irritative lesion of the brachial plexus often extends from the base of the neck, over the top of the shoulder, and thence into the arm. Unlike true shoulder pain, it frequently radiates below the elbow into the forearm or hand, and it may be accompanied by paraesthesiae—often described as 'pins and needles' or 'a numb feeling'. Pain may also be referred to the shoulder from a lesion in the thorax or upper abdomen.

Exposure
The patient must be stripped to the waist. The examination is conducted most easily with the patient standing; alternatively he may sit upon a high stool. For the greater part of the examination the surgeon stands behind the patient, so that he may observe more easily the position of the scapula.

Steps in routine examination
A suggested plan for the routine examination of the shoulder is summarised in Table VI.

Movements at the shoulder
In examining shoulder movements it is important to determine how much of the movement occurs at the gleno-humeral joint and how much is contributed by rotation of the scapula. An accurate distinction between the two types of movement can be made only by grasping the lower half of the scapula so that its movements can be detected (Fig. 173). In the normal shoulder about half the range of abduction occurs at the gleno-humeral joint and half by scapular rotation. Disorders of the shoulder generally cause restriction of gleno-humeral movement rather than of scapular movement.

Table VI
Routine clinical examination in suspected disorders of the shoulder

1. LOCAL EXAMINATION OF THE SHOULDER REGION

Inspection
Bone contours alignment
Soft-tissue contours
Colour and texture of skin
Scars or sinuses

Palpation
Skin temperature
Bone contours
Soft-tissue contours
Local tenderness

Movements
Distinguish between true gleno-humeral movement and scapular movement during abduction, flexion, extension, lateral rotation, and medial rotation
? Pain on movement
? Muscle spasm
? Crepitation on movement

Power
Cervico-scapular and *thoraco-scapular muscles* (controlling scapular movement)—Test elevation of scapula, retraction of scapula, abduction-rotation of scapula.
Scapulo-humeral muscles (controlling movement at gleno-humeral joint)—Abduction, adduction, flexion, extension, lateral rotation, medial rotation

Acromio-clavicular joint
Examine for swelling, increased warmth, tenderness, pain on movement, and stability

Sterno-clavicular joint
Examine for swelling, increased warmth, tenderness, pain on movement, and stability

2. EXAMINATION OF POTENTIAL EXTRINSIC SOURCES OF SHOULDER SYMPTOMS

This is important if a satisfactory explanation for the symptoms is not found on local examination. The investigation should include: 1) the neck, with the brachial plexus; 2) the thorax, with special reference to the heart and pleura; and 3) the abdomen, for subdiaphragmatic lesions.

3. GENERAL EXAMINATION

General survey of other parts of the body.

Stand behind the patient. *Abduction:* Instruct the patient to try to raise both arms sideways from the body so that the palms of the hands meet above the head. Measure the range, and observe what proportion of the movement takes place at the gleno-humeral joint and how much is contributed by rotation of the scapula upon the thorax. *Flexion:* Instruct the patient to raise the arms forwards towards the vertical. Again observe (by means of the hand upon the scapula) what proportion of the movement occurs at the gleno-humeral joint. *Extension:* Ask the patient to raise the elbows backwards. *Lateral (external) rotation:* The elbows are held in to the sides and are flexed 90 degrees (Fig. 174): the forearms then serve as convenient

Fig. 173
Examining shoulder abduction. One hand grasps the scapula while the other steadies the elbow. In this way the proportion of the total range contributed by gleno-humeral movement and by scapular rotation can be assessed.

Fig. 174
Examining shoulder rotation. The elbow is supported by the examiner's hand and flexed to the right angle to eliminate forearm rotation. The forearm thus serves as a pointer to indicate the range of rotation at the shoulder.

pointers to indicate the angle of rotation (normal range = 80 degrees). *Medial (internal) rotation:* Instruct the patient to place the back of his hand in contact with his lumbar region and to carry the elbow forwards (normal range = 110 degrees).

Estimation of muscle power
In estimating the power of the shoulder muscles two groups must be distinguished: 1) the cervico-scapular and thoraco-scapular muscles; and 2) the scapulo-humeral muscles.

Fig. 175
Examination for weakness of the serratus anterior. If the serratus anterior is weak or paralysed winging of the scapula occurs when the arm is raised from the side or pushed forward against resistance.

The cervico-scapular and thoraco-scapular muscles. These control movements of the scapula. Estimate the power of each group in turn and compare on the two sides. *Elevators of the scapula* (levator scapulae, upper fibres of trapezius): Instruct the patient to shrug the shoulders against the resistance of the examiner's hands. *Retractors of the scapula* (rhomboids and middle fibres of trapezius): Instruct the patient to brace the shoulders back. *Abductor-rotators of the scapula* (serratus anterior, with middle and lower fibres of trapezius): Instruct the patient to push horizontally forwards with the hand against a wall (Fig. 175) or simply to raise the arm from the side. If the serratus anterior is weak winging of the scapula (backward projection of its vertebral border) will be observed (Fig. 175).

The scapulo-humeral muscles. These control movements of the gleno-humeral joint. Estimate the power of each muscle group, testing in turn the abductors, adductors, flexors, extensors, lateral rotators, and medial rotators. If the patient has lost the power to initiate active gleno-humeral movement from the dependent position, determine whether he can maintain abduction when the limb has been raised with assistance to 90 degrees. Ability to *sustain* abduction but not to *initiate* it is characteristic of isolated rupture of the supraspinatus tendon (see Figs 184 and 185, p. 220).

The acromio-clavicular and sterno-clavicular joints

The clavicle may be regarded as a link, jointed at each end, connecting the scapula to the sternum (Fig. 176). Movement of the scapula must occur about a fulcrum at one or both ends of this link. In the normal shoulder movement of the scapula, with consequent movement at the acromio-clavicular and sterno-clavicular joints, occurs mainly: 1) during elevation of the arm above 90 degrees; and 2) when the shoulders are braced backwards or drawn forwards.

Fig. 176
The mechanics of scapular rotation. The clavicle serves as a link, jointed at each end, by which the scapula is held away from the sternum. Full rotation of the scapula entails movement both at the acromio-clavicular joint and at the sterno-clavicular joint.

To examine the acromio-clavicular and sterno-clavicular joints stand in front of the patient. Examine the joints on each side for deformity, swelling, increase of local temperature, local tenderness, and pain on movement—especially at the extremes of elevation of the arm and backward bracing of the shoulders. Observe whether there is any tendency to subluxation or dislocation of the joint on movement.

Radiographic examination

Gleno-humeral joint. The routine shoulder film is a plain antero-posterior projection with the limb in the anatomical position. When additional information is required a special axillary projection with the arm abducted 90 degrees (giving a lateral view of the humerus), or stereoscopic films, should be obtained. Further films showing the upper end of the humerus in varying degrees of rotation are sometimes informative. *Arthrography*, after injection of radio-opaque fluid into the joint, will show whether or not the capsule is intact.

Acromio-clavicular joint and sterno-clavicular joint. Special projections are used to show each of these joints.

Other imaging techniques

Radioisotope scanning, computerised tomography and *magnetic resonance imaging* must each be considered in appropriate circumstances.

Extrinsic sources of shoulder and arm pain

In many cases in which the main complaint is of pain in the shoulder or arm there is no local abnormality, the symptoms being referred from a lesion elsewhere. Thus pain over the shoulder is a common symptom in affections of the neck, especially when the brachial plexus or its roots are involved. Shoulder pain is also a feature of irritative lesions in contact with the diaphragm, either in the thorax or in the abdomen. The possibility of such extrinsic lesions must always be considered in the investigation of shoulder pain.

Fortunately, with careful interrogation and clinical examination there is little difficulty in distinguishing intrinsic from extrinsic lesions. The important point is that intrinsic lesions of the shoulder always give rise to local physical signs that are readily demonstrable on examination. If the shoulder is clinically normal it is improbable that it is the seat of disease, and attention should be directed towards possible sources of referred pain.

CLASSIFICATION OF DISORDERS OF THE SHOULDER REGION

DISORDERS OF THE SHOULDER (GLENO-HUMERAL) JOINT

Arthritis

Pyogenic arthritis
Rheumatoid arthritis
Tuberculous arthritis
Osteoarthritis
'Frozen' shoulder

Painful arc syndrome (including
  calcified deposit in tendon)
Rupture of long tendon of biceps

Mechanical derangements

Recurrent dislocation
Complete tear of tendinous
  (rotator) cuff

Miscellaneous

Tenosynovitis of long tendon of
  biceps

DISORDERS OF THE ACROMIO-CLAVICULAR JOINT

Osteoarthritis
Persistent dislocation or
  subluxation

DISORDERS OF THE STERNO-CLAVICULAR JOINT

Arthritis
Persistent or recurrent dislocation

DISORDERS OF THE SHOULDER (GLENO-HUMERAL) JOINT

PYOGENIC ARTHRITIS OF THE SHOULDER

(General description of pyogenic arthritis, p. 109)

Pyogenic arthritis of the shoulder is uncommon. It occurs most often in children, in whom infection may spread to the shoulder from a focus of osteomyelitis in the upper metaphysis of the humerus (p. 231).

The clinical features resemble those of pyogenic arthritis of other joints. The onset is rapid and is accompanied by pyrexia; and the shoulder is swollen, abnormally warm, and restricted in movement. Treatment follows the lines suggested on page 110.

RHEUMATOID ARTHRITIS OF THE SHOULDER

(General description of rheumatoid arthritis, p. 111)

The shoulder is commonly affected by rheumatoid arthritis, though less commonly than the more peripheral joints such as hands, wrists and feet. Often both shoulders are affected simultaneously with other upper limb joints, with consequent serious impairment of function.

As in other superficial joints, the main clinical features are local pain and stiffness, increased warmth, swelling from synovial thickening, and impairment of movement. There is wasting of the deltoid muscle, with consequent flattening of the shoulder contour (Fig. 177). Radiographs show rarefaction of bone, narrowing of the cartilage space, and eventually erosion of bone at the joint margins (Fig. 178).

Fig. 177   **Fig. 178**

Rheumatoid arthritis of the shoulder. In Figure 177 note the marked flattening of the contour from muscle wasting. The radiograph in Figure 178 shows rarefaction of the bones, with narrowing of the joint space from loss of articular cartilage.

Treatment. This is mainly that for rheumatoid arthritis in general, as described on page 115. Exercises are important in maintaining a useful range of movement.

Operative treatment. Replacement arthroplasty may be appropriate if the disability is very severe. A two-piece ball and socket prosthesis with the convex component of metal and the concave component of plastic is fitted and retained in position with acrylic cement. Relief of pain is often good initially, but active movement beyond a very restricted range is not usually to be expected because of associated degeneration of the tendinous (rotator) cuff. As with replacement of other joints, there is a risk of gradual loosening of the prosthesis; so the operation is not to be undertaken lightly.

TUBERCULOUS ARTHRITIS OF THE SHOULDER

(General description of tuberculous arthritis, p. 117)

Tuberculous arthritis of the shoulder has become a rare disease in Western countries. It occurs much less commonly than tuberculosis of the spine, hip, and knee.

Fig. 179
Advanced tuberculous arthritis of the shoulder. Note the loss of articular cartilage and the marked erosion of bone at the joint surfaces.

The pathological and clinical features correspond to those of tuberculous arthritis in any major joint. Pain is usually the predominant symptom, and examination may reveal diffuse swelling with increased warmth, and marked restriction of true gleno-humeral movement. An abscess may form.

Radiographs in the early stages show diffuse rarefaction throughout the gleno-humeral area. Later, the cartilage space is narrowed and the underlying bone may be eroded (Fig. 179). In a doubtful case synovial biopsy may be necessary to establish the diagnosis.

Treatment follows the lines of that for other tuberculous joints (p. 120), with anti-tuberculous drugs as the mainstay. In a favourable case in which treatment has been begun early, good recovery of function is to be hoped for. If in a florid case there is marked destruction of cartilage or bone, permanent elimination of the joint by arthrodesis may be advisable (see Fig. 15, p. 29).

OSTEOARTHRITIS OF THE SHOULDER

(General description of osteoarthritis, p. 120)

Unlike most other joints, the shoulder is seldom affected by osteoarthritis. When it is affected there is usually a clear predisposing factor, such as previous injury or disease, avascular necrosis of the humeral head, or senility. The rarity of osteoarthritis of the shoulder is explained by its freedom from pressure stresses.

Pathology. The articular cartilage is worn away. The underlying bone becomes eburnated and at the joint margins it hypertrophies to form osteophytes.

Clinical features. The patient is usually elderly: osteoarthritis is exceptional in the shoulders of younger patients. The main complaint is of pain in the shoulder and down the upper arm. *On examination* there is no increase of local skin temperature and no synovial thickening. But a soft swelling due to effusion of fluid into the joint is common. Movements are restricted.

Fig. 180
Osteoarthritis of the shoulder in an old woman. Note loss of articular cartilage, marginal osteophytes and sclerosis at the joint surfaces. Osteoarthritis is uncommon in the shoulder.

Radiographs show narrowing of the cartilage space; the joint outlines are clear-cut and often show some sclerosis; there is 'spurring' from osteophyte formation at the joint margins (Fig. 180).

Treatment. In many cases treatment is unnecessary once the nature of the affection has been explained. If treatment is called for, conservative measures should usually be relied upon; short-wave diathermy, massage, and gentle exercises are often helpful. If there is a large effusion it should be aspirated. Only exceptionally would operation be justified: if it were, replacement arthroplasty (see under rheumatoid arthritis, p. 214) would usually be advised, but arthrodesis might occasionally be appropriate.

'FROZEN' SHOULDER

(Adhesive capsulitis; periarthritis)

'Frozen' shoulder is a common but ill understood affection of the gleno-humeral joint, characterised by pain and uniform limitation of all movements but without radiographic change, and with a tendency to slow spontaneous recovery under appropriate treatment.

Cause. This is unknown. There is no evidence of infection. Injury is an inconstant factor and its significance is doubtful.

Pathology. This is not fully understood. It is believed that there is a loss of resilience of the joint capsule, with adhesions between the synovial folds. Whatever their nature, the changes are reversible, for in most cases the joint is eventually restored to normal or almost so.

Clinical features. The patient complains of severe aching pain in the shoulder and upper arm, of gradual and spontaneous onset. *On examination* the only finding is uniform impairment of all gleno-humeral movements—abduction, flexion, extension, rotation—which are often reduced to about a quarter or half of their normal range. In a severe case much of the shoulder movement that remains is contributed by scapular movement, which is unimpaired. *Radiographs* do not show any abnormality.

Diagnosis. The characteristic feature of 'frozen' shoulder is the uniform limitation of all gleno-humeral movements without evidence of inflammatory or destructive changes.

Course. There is a tendency towards spontaneous recovery, usually within six to twelve months. The pain subsides first, leaving gleno-humeral joint stiffness, which thereafter gradually resolves with active use of the limb. If movements are not practised deliberately some permanent restriction of movement may remain.

Treatment. In the early, acutely painful stage the arm is rested in a sling, which is removed for short periods each day to permit gentle assisted shoulder exercises. Generally, non-steroidal anti-inflammatory drugs should be prescribed in addition to conventional analgesics. When the pain lessens, active exercises are intensified and continued for weeks or months until full movement is regained. If mobilisation is very slow after the pain has abated the shoulder may be manipulated gently under anaesthesia.

It is important to warn the patient at the beginning that recovery may take many months, but at the same time to give assurance that eventually recovery is likely to be complete.

RECURRENT ANTERIOR DISLOCATION OF THE SHOULDER

Traumatic dislocation of the shoulder is liable to cause structural changes in the gleno-humeral joint which predispose to repeated dislocations. Rarely, dislocation may occur repeatedly in a patient with unduly lax ligaments, in the absence of trauma.

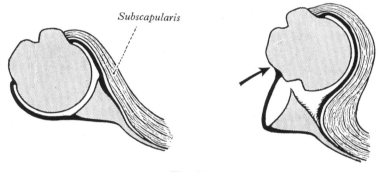

Subscapularis

Fig. 181

Horizontal section of left shoulder showing the pathology of recurrent dislocation. The diagram on the left shows the normal condition. In the right-hand diagram the humeral head is shown dislocated forwards. It has stripped the capsule from the margin of the glenoid, creating a pocket in front of the neck of the scapula into which the humeral head is displaced. Note that the humeral head has been dented by the sharp glenoid margin, producing the typical defect of the articular surface.

Pathology. This is twofold (Figs 181 and 182). 1) The capsule, and with it the glenoid labrum, is stripped from the anterior margin of the glenoid rim but retains an attachment farther down the neck of the scapula, where it becomes continuous with the periosteum. Thus there is created an intra-capsular 'pocket' in front of the glenoid margin, into which the humeral head may be displaced (Fig. 181). 2) The articular surface of the humeral head is dented postero-laterally, probably by the initial violence (Figs 181 and 182). The consequent defect in the contour of the articular surface allows the head to slip over the front of the glenoid when the arm is in lateral rotation, abduction and extension. The dislocation is anterior, and it must be emphasised that the humeral head always remains within the capsule, in contradistinction to non-recurrent dislocation, in which the humeral head is displaced through a rent in the capsule (Strachan 1980).

Fig. 182   **Fig. 183**

Figure 182—Typical defect of articular surface of humeral head, found in most cases of recurrent dislocation of the shoulder. Figure 183—Radiographic appearance with the arm in 80 degrees of medial rotation. The defect is seen in profile at the upper and outer quadrant of the humeral head.

Clinical features. Nearly always, recurrent dislocation follows an initial violent dislocation, often in a heavy fall. Thereafter dislocation recurs with trivial violence, characteristically during combined abduction, lateral rotation and extension (for example, in putting on a coat). *On examination* no clinical abnormality is apparent.

Radiographic features. Routine radiographs with the limb in the anatomical position do not show any abnormality, but special profile views taken with the arm in 60–80 degrees of medial rotation show the characteristic bony defect of the humeral head (Fig. 183). Arthrography may be of value in demonstrating the site and extent of a capsular defect.

Treatment. Conservative treatment is not effective. If dislocation recurs frequently operation is justified. The most reliable methods are the Bankart operation, in which the capsule is re-attached to the front of the glenoid margin; and the Putti-Platt operation, in which the subscapularis tendon is shortened by overlapping or 'reefing' in order to limit lateral rotation.

RECURRENT ANTERIOR DISLOCATION FROM LIGAMENTOUS LAXITY

Whereas in most cases of recurrent anterior dislocation of the shoulder the pathology comprises stripping of the anterior capsule from the glenoid rim and postero-lateral denting of the humeral head, as described above, there is a separate small proportion of patients in which these changes are not present. Instead, there is general laxity of the ligaments about the shoulder, with a voluminous capsule that allows subluxation or even full dislocation of the humeral head to occur without preceding injury. Such patients can often displace the humerus voluntarily and with increasing ease, and displacement may often be either anterior or posterior. The humeral head always remains within the lax capsule, and there is no capsular rupture.

Treatment. These patients should be dissuaded from repeatedly demonstrating their ability to subluxate or dislocate the joint, which can sometimes become an obsessive neurosis or at least a 'party trick'. If operation is called for, a bone-block operation, by which the area and depth of the glenoid fossa are increased by a suitably shaped bone graft, is generally to be recommended.

RECURRENT POSTERIOR DISLOCATION

Posterior dislocation of the shoulder is much less common than anterior dislocation. Often the cause is an electric shock or an epileptiform convulsion, and it is not uncommon for both shoulders to be dislocated together. The dislocation is prone to become recurrent. The pathology is analogous to that of recurrent anterior dislocation: 1) the capsule, glenoid labrum and periosteum are stripped from the back of the neck of the scapula; and 2) the humeral head is dented supero-medially. Dislocation occurs on abduction and medial rotation.

Operative repair may be effected by reefing the infraspinatus tendon on the lines of the Putti-Platt reefing of the subscapularis for anterior dislocation. An alternative method is to deepen the glenoid socket by screwing a suitably shaped block of iliac bone to the back of the neck of the scapula (bone-block operation).

Like recurrent anterior dislocation, recurrent posterior dislocation may sometimes occur spontaneously, without previous injury, in a patient with ligamentous laxity.

COMPLETE TEAR OF TENDINOUS (ROTATOR) CUFF

(Torn supraspinatus)

It is important to distinguish complete tears of the tendinous cuff[1] from incomplete tears. The clinical effects are different. Whereas an incomplete tear is one cause of the 'painful arc syndrome' (p. 221), a complete tear impairs seriously the ability to abduct the shoulder.

Cause. The tendon gives way under a sudden strain, usually caused by a fall. Age-degeneration of the tendon is a constant predisposing factor.

Pathology. The tear is mainly of the supraspinatus tendon, but it may extend into the adjacent subscapularis or infraspinatus tendons. The tear is close to the insertion of the tendons and usually involves the capsule of the joint, with which the tendons are blended. The edges of the rent retract, leaving a gaping hole which establishes a communication between the shoulder joint and the subacromial bursa (Fig. 184). In general, it may be said that a tendon that ruptures is usually already degenerate: thus rupture occurs mainly in the elderly.

Clinical features. The patient is usually a man over 60: only occasionally is a younger patient affected. After a strain or fall he complains of pain at the tip of the shoulder and down the upper arm, and of inability to raise the arm.

---

[1]The term *tendinous cuff* denotes the supraspinatus tendon together with the adjoining flat tendons that are blended with it—namely, the infraspinatus behind and the subscapularis in front. They form a cuff over the shoulder that has also been termed, inaccurately, the *rotator cuff*. Distally, the tendons forming the cuff blend with the capsule of the shoulder.

On examination there is local tenderness below the margin of the acromion. When the patient attempts to abduct the arm no movement occurs at the gleno-humeral joint but a range of about 45–60 degrees of abduction

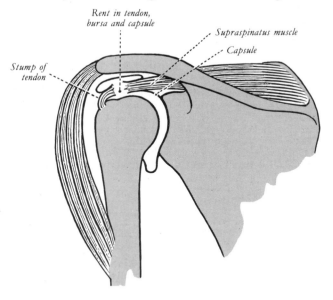

Fig. 184
Tear of supraspinatus shown diagrammatically. Note that the subacromial bursa communicates with the shoulder joint through the rent.

Fig. 185   **Fig. 186**
Complete tear of tendinous cuff (torn supraspinatus). Figure 185—Active abduction from the resting position is possible only by scapular rotation, the deltoid being unable to initiate gleno-humeral abduction without the help of the supraspinatus. Figure 186—When the limb is raised passively beyond the horizontal abduction can be sustained actively by the deltoid.

can be achieved, entirely by scapular movement (Fig. 185). There is, however, a full range of passive movement; and if the arm is abducted with assistance beyond 90 degrees the patient can sustain the abduction by deltoid action (Fig. 186). Thus the essential and characteristic feature in cases of torn supraspinatus tendon is inability to initiate gleno-humeral abduction. The usual explanation is that the early stages of abduction demand the combined action of the deltoid muscle, which supplies the main motive force, and the supraspinatus, which stabilises the humeral head in the glenoid fossa (like the workman's foot against a ladder that is being raised from the ground).

Diagnosis. Complete tear of the tendinous cuff must be distinguished from other causes of impaired gleno-humeral abduction, especially the painful arc syndrome and paralysis of the abductor muscles (as from poliomyelitis or nerve injury). Inability to initiate gleno-humeral abduction, with power to sustain abduction once the limb has been raised passively, is characteristic of a widely torn supraspinatus. In the painful arc syndrome the power of abduction is retained but the movement is painful. In a case of complete tear *arthrography* will show a communication between the joint and the subacromial bursa. The tear may also be well demonstrated by ultrasound scanning.

Treatment. In old patients operation should usually be avoided, because the degenerate state of the tendon makes satisfactory repair impracticable: the disability tends to become gradually less noticeable, and indeed the power of active abduction (by deltoid action alone) may sometimes be regained despite the persistence of a large tear.

In younger patients operation should usually be undertaken to suture the rent in the tendon. Thereafter passive movements may be begun within a few days but attempts to lift the arm actively should be deferred for four weeks, when provisional healing of the tendon may be expected to have occurred. The results of operation are not uniformly satisfactory, probably because of the poor quality of the degenerate tendon.

PAINFUL ARC SYNDROME
(Supraspinatus syndrome)

This is a clinical syndrome characterised by pain in the shoulder and upper arm during the mid-range of gleno-humeral abduction, with freedom from pain at the extremes of the range. The syndrome is common to five distinct shoulder lesions.

Cause. The pain is produced mechanically by nipping of a tender structure between the tuberosity of the humerus and the acromion process and coraco-acromial ligament.

Pathology. Even in the normal shoulder, the clearance between the upper end of the humerus and the acromion process is small in the range of abduction between 45 and 160 degrees. If a swollen and tender structure is present beneath the acromion it is liable to get nipped during the arc of movement in which the clearance is small (Fig. 188), with consequent pain. In the neutral position and in full abduction the clearance is greater and pain is less marked or absent (Figs 187 and 189).

Five primary lesions can give rise to the syndrome (Fig. 190). In general, though, these labels only represent variations of a process of degeneration which is the underlying defect.

| Fig. 187 | Fig. 188 | Fig. 189 |

Mechanical basis of the painful arc syndrome. The black spot represents any tender lesion near the supraspinatus insertion. Figure 187—With the arm dependent, the lesion is free from pressure. Figure 188—With the arm in mid-abduction the lesion is nipped between the humerus and the acromion. Figure 189—At full elevation the lesion is again free from pressure.

| Fig. 190 | Fig. 191 |

Figure 190—Five causes of the painful arc syndrome. The clinical features are the same in each. 1. Incomplete tear of supraspinatus. 2. Supraspinatus tendinitis. 3. Calcified deposit in supraspinatus. 4. Subacromial bursitis. 5. Crack fracture of greater tuberosity. Figure 191—Painful arc syndrome. The middle arc of abduction is painful whereas the extremes are painless.

1) *Minor tear of supraspinatus tendon.* Tearing or strain of a few degenerate tendon fibres causes an inflammatory reaction with local swelling, but power is not significantly impaired as it is after a complete tear of the tendinous cuff.

2) *Supraspinatus tendinitis.* In this condition there is believed to be an inflammatory reaction provoked by degeneration of the tendon fibres.

3) *Calcified deposit in supraspinatus tendon.* A white chalky deposit forms within the degenerate tendon, and the lesion is surrounded by an inflammatory reaction. Pain occurs when the calcified material bursts into the surrounding tissues.

4) *Subacromial bursitis.* The bursal walls are inflamed and thickened from mechanical irritation.

5) *Injury of greater tuberosity.* A contusion or undisplaced fracture of the greater tuberosity is a frequent cause.

Clinical features. Whatever the primary cause, the clinical syndrome has the same general features, though they vary in degree. With the arm dependent pain is absent or minimal. During abduction of the arm pain begins at about 45 degrees and persists through the arc of movement up to 160 degrees (Fig. 191). Thereafter the pain lessens or disappears. In descent from full elevation pain is again experienced during the middle arc of the range: often the patient will twist or circumduct the arm grotesquely in an effort to get it down with the least pain. The severity of the pain varies from case to case. In cases of calcified deposit in the supraspinatus tendon the pain may be so intense that the patient is scarcely able to move the shoulder and is driven to seek emergency treatment.

Fig. 192
To show the radiological distinction between a calcified deposit and bone. A calcified deposit has a homogeneous texture, and it differs in that respect from an avulsed fragment of bone, which would show trabeculation. (See also Fig. 5, p. 12.)

Radiographic features. These vary with the underlying cause. Plain radiographs will reveal a fracture of the greater tuberosity or a calcified deposit (Fig. 192). A calcified deposit is distinguished radiologically from an avulsed fragment of bone by the fact that it is homogeneous and does not show the trabeculation characteristic of bone.

Diagnosis. Painful arc syndrome is sometimes confused with arthritis of the acromio-clavicular joint, which also causes pain during a certain phase of the abduction arc. But in acromio-clavicular arthritis the pain begins later in abduction (not below 90 degrees) and increases rather than diminishes as full elevation is reached.

Differentiation between the five primary causes of the syndrome is aided by the history and by radiography. A history of injury suggests a strain of the supraspinatus tendon or a lesion of the greater tuberosity, whereas a spontaneous onset suggests tendinitis, calcified deposit or subacromial bursitis. As noted, radiography will confirm or exclude a fracture or a calcified deposit (Fig. 192).

Treatment in the acute case. In mild cases treatment is often unnecessary. When treatment is called for, the method used should depend upon the primary cause of the syndrome. In most cases non-operative measures are successful, but operation is sometimes required.

Calcified deposit in supraspinatus tendon. In cases of moderate severity treatment is by rest in a sling and short-wave diathermy or ultrasound therapy, with mobilising exercises when the pain begins to subside. If the pain is intense, as it sometimes is in these cases, immediate relief can be gained by removing the toothpaste-like deposit through an aspiration needle or through an incision into the tendon. Sometimes pain is so severe that intervention becomes almost an emergency measure.

Contusion or crack fracture of greater tuberosity. Reliance should be placed on active use and mobilising exercises.

Strain of supraspinatus, supraspinatus tendinitis, and *subacromial bursitis.* Most of these cases respond to short-wave diathermy and mobilising exercises.

Treatment in the chronic case. In cases of painful arc syndrome in which severe symptoms persist despite a full trial of efficient conservative treatment operation may be required. The acromion process, or preferably its anterior third, is excised with the coraco-acromial ligament to prevent the possibility of further nipping of inflamed tissue between it and the upper end of the humerus.

RUPTURE OF LONG TENDON OF BICEPS

The long tendon of the biceps is one of several tendons in the body that are prone to rupture without violent stress or injury. (Others are the supra-spinatus tendon and the tendon of extensor pollicis longus.)

Cause. The tendon will not rupture under ordinary stresses unless it is already weak. The predisposing factor is age-degeneration, probably accelerated by oft-repeated friction and angulation at the point where the tendon enters the bicipital groove of the humerus.

Clinical features. The patient is usually a man past middle age. While lifting or pulling with the arm he feels something give way in the region of the front of the shoulder. There is only moderate discomfort, and often the patient neglects to seek early advice. Later he may notice an unusual bulge of the muscle in front of the arm.

On examination soon after the rupture, there is slight tenderness over the bicipital groove of the humerus. When the patient contracts the biceps muscle, as in flexing the elbow or supinating the forearm against resistance, the belly of the long head is seen to bunch up into a short round mass like a ball. There is surprisingly little weakness of elbow flexion or of supination.

Treatment. The disability is usually so slight that operation is not required. When repair is considered necessary, it is sufficient to suture the distal stump of the tendon to the walls of the bicipital groove; the proximal stump is ignored.

TENOSYNOVITIS OF LONG TENDON OF BICEPS

(Biceps tendinitis)

This is an uncommon and rather minor affection characterised by pain and local tenderness in the region of the bicipital groove of the humerus and the long tendon of the biceps. It is generally ascribed to frictional irritation of the tendon within its groove, but it may be associated with degeneration of the tendinous cuff.

Clinical features. The complaint is of pain in the front of the shoulder, worse on active use of the arm. Examination reveals local tenderness in the course of the long tendon of the biceps in the bicipital groove of the humerus. The pain can often be exacerbated by moving the shoulder while the tendon is tautened by forced supination of the forearm.

Treatment. Excessive use of the shoulder should be avoided. Physiotherapy by ultra-sound, interferential therapy or short-wave diathermy is worth a trial. Failing this, a local injection of hydrocortisone may be advised.

DISORDERS OF THE ACROMIO-CLAVICULAR JOINT

OSTEOARTHRITIS OF THE ACROMIO-CLAVICULAR JOINT

Though not common, acromio-clavicular osteoarthritis is seen much more often than is osteoarthritis of the gleno-humeral joint. Pathologically, there are degeneration and attrition of articular cartilage, and spurs of bone (osteophytes) are formed at the joint margins.

Clinical features. There is pain, localised accurately to the acromio-clavicular joint and aggravated by strenuous use of the limb—especially in overhead work. *On examination* irregular bony thickening of the joint margins due to osteophytes may be felt. There is no soft-tissue thickening and no increase of local skin temperature. The total range of shoulder movements is not appreciably decreased, but the local acromio-clavicular pain is exacerbated at the extremes of movement, especially on elevation of the arm: the arc of movement below 90 degrees is painless, but above 90 degrees pain develops and persists throughout the remainder of the arc of full elevation (compare painful arc syndrome, p. 221).

Radiographs show narrowing of the cartilage space and marginal osteophytes.

Treatment. Often treatment is not needed. Overhead work should be avoided. In severe cases operation is justified: it should take the form of excision of the lateral end of the clavicle, the conoid and trapezoid ligaments being preserved.

PERSISTENT ACROMIO-CLAVICULAR DISLOCATION OR SUBLUXATION

Persistent upward displacement of the lateral end of the clavicle is a common sequel to traumatic dislocation or subluxation of the acromio-clavicular joint. In most cases the displacement is slight and causes no symptoms. Exceptionally there is pain, worse during full elevation of the arm. *On examination* the lateral end of the clavicle is unduly prominent, and a distinct step can be felt between it and the surface of the acromion.

Treatment. Usually treatment is unnecessary. Overhead work should be avoided. Rest in a sling for a few days is sufficient to relieve a temporary exacerbation of pain brought on by over-use of the arm. If disabling pain persists, operation is advised. A simple and effective method is to excise the lateral end of the clavicle.

DISORDERS OF THE STERNO-CLAVICULAR JOINT

ARTHRITIS OF THE STERNO-CLAVICULAR JOINT

The sterno-clavicular joint is occasionally the seat of pyogenic arthritis, rheumatoid arthritis or tuberculous arthritis. Each of these follows the general pattern described in Chapter 7. None in common, and further description is not required here. Other forms of arthritis are rarely encountered in this joint.

PERSISTENT OR RECURRENT DISLOCATION OF THE STERNO-CLAVICULAR JOINT

Forward dislocation of the medial end of the clavicle may be permanent, or it may recur on certain movements of the limb. Often, but not always, there is a history of precipitating injury. The symptoms are slight: there is a prominence in the region of the joint, with mild local pain. Recurrent displacement of the clavicle in and out during movements of the arm may be an annoying disability. *On examination* the medial end of the clavicle, when displaced, is easily felt as a prominent forward projection. In recurrent dislocation the clavicle can be felt to click out of joint when the shoulders are braced back, and to go back into position when the shoulders are arched forwards.

Radiographs reveal the displacement, when present. It is difficult to show the joint clearly and special projections are necessary.

Treatment. In many cases treatment is unnecessary. Non-operative treatment is ineffective. Operation is occasionally justified: the displacement is reduced and the clavicle is held in place by constructing a new retaining ligament from the tendon of the subclavius muscle or from a strip of fascia.

EXTRINSIC DISORDERS SIMULATING SHOULDER DISEASE

Pain in the shoulder or arm often has no local cause, but is referred from an extrinsic lesion. Such a possibility must always be considered in differential diagnosis.

DISORDERS OF THE BRACHIAL PLEXUS OR ITS ROOTS

The pain caused by pressure upon the brachial plexus or its roots is commonly attributed erroneously to an affection of the shoulder. Such pain varies in its precise distribution according to the site and nature of the lesion. Usually it radiates from the base of the neck, across the top of the shoulder, and down the front, side or back of the arm; thence it extends into the forearm, and often into the hand and fingers. Thus in its typical form the pain from a nerve lesion in the neck differs from the pain of a shoulder lesion, which typically does not extend below the elbow.

Affections that may cause referred symptoms in the distribution of the brachial plexus include prolapsed cervical intervertebral disc, osteoarthritis of the cervical spine, cervical rib, herpes zoster, and tumours involving the spinal cord or the component nerves of the brachial plexus. These conditions were described in Chapter 9.

DISORDERS OF THE UPPER ARM

Shoulder pain typically radiates distally and is often felt near the insertion of the deltoid muscle. Pain arising locally at this site, for instance from a lesion in the shaft of the humerus, may thus be confused with pain arising at the shoulder itself. Radiographs including the upper half of the humerus will usually help to make the distinction.

DISORDERS WITHIN THE THORAX

ANGINA PECTORIS

In a small proportion of cases of angina pectoris the pain is felt predominantly in the shoulder region (usually on the left side). Other features are invariably present to suggest a cardiac origin, and the shoulder shows no clinical abnormality. If the history and findings are elicited with care there is little difficulty in distinguishing cardiac pain from true shoulder pain.

PLEURISY

Basal pleurisy is sometimes a cause of shoulder pain, which is explained by irritation of phrenic nerve endings, with referred pain in the distribution of the cutaneous branches of the same cervical roots (mainly C.4). The shoulder is clinically normal, and the other features of the chest condition are usually sufficiently clear to indicate its true nature.

TUMOUR

Pancoast's apical lung carcinoma is a well known cause of radiating shoulder and upper limb pain, from involvement of the lower trunks of the brachial plexus. Chest radiography is diagnostic.

DISORDERS WITHIN THE ABDOMEN

CHOLECYSTITIS

This is a cause of referred pain in the right shoulder, from irritation of the phrenic nerve endings under the diaphragm. The associated abdominal symptoms and signs, and the lack of clinical abnormality in the shoulder, should prevent diagnostic errors.

SUBPHRENIC ABSCESS

This also is an occasional cause of referred shoulder pain. Constitutional symptoms and pyrexia, with normal clinical findings in the shoulder, exonerate the shoulder from blame.

References and bibliography, page 403.

12. The upper arm and elbow

Apart from injury, disorders of the upper arm and elbow region are generally straightforward and present few special problems. They conform to the general descriptions of bone and joint diseases that were given in Part 2. Thus the humerus is subject to the ordinary infections of bone, and occasionally to bone tumours—especially metastases. The elbow is liable to every type of arthritis, though none is particularly common. After the knee, it is the joint most often affected by osteochondritis dissecans and loose body formation. The ulnar nerve lies in a vulnerable position at the back of the medial epicondyle, and the possibility of impairment of nerve function complicating disease or injury of the joint should always be remembered. Replacement arthroplasty of the elbow is undertaken increasingly, but compared with those of hip and knee arthroplasty the results still leave much to be desired, especially from the point of view of the longevity of the new joint.

SPECIAL POINTS IN THE INVESTIGATION OF UPPER ARM AND ELBOW SYMPTOMS

History
The interrogation follows the usual lines suggested in Chapter 1. It is important to ascertain the exact site and distribution of the pain, and its nature. Pain arising locally in the humerus is easily confused with pain arising in the shoulder, which characteristically radiates to a point about half-way down the outer aspect of the upper arm. Elbow pain is localised fairly precisely to the joint, though a diffuse aching pain is often felt also in the forearm. When the ulnar nerve is interfered with behind the elbow the symptoms are mainly in the hand.

In the elbow, a history of previous injury, perhaps long ago in childhood, is often significant. Injuries in this region are notoriously liable to have late effects in the form of impaired movement, deformity, arthritis, loose body formation, or interference with the ulnar nerve.

Exposure
The whole length of the upper limb must be uncovered. The opposite limb must be similarly exposed for comparison.

Steps in routine examination
A suggested plan for the routine clinical examination of the upper arm and elbow is summarised in Table VII.

Table VII
Routine clinical examination in suspected disorders
of the upper arm and elbow

1. LOCAL EXAMINATION OF THE ARM AND ELBOW

Inspection
Bone contours and alignment
Soft-tissue contours
Colour and texture of skin
Scars or sinuses

Palpation
Skin temperature
Bone contours
Soft-tissue contours
Local tenderness

Movements (active and passive)
Humero-ulnar joint:
Flexion
Extension
Radio-ulnar joint:
Supination
Pronation
? Pain on movement
? Crepitation on movement

Power
Flexors
Extensors
Supinators
Pronators

Stability
Lateral ligament
Medial ligament

The median nerve
Sensory function
Motor function (opponens action)
Sweating

The radial nerve
Sensory function
Motor function (extension of wrist,
thumb and fingers)

The ulnar nerve
Sensory function
Motor function
Sweating

2. EXAMINATION OF POTENTIAL EXTRINSIC SOURCES OF ARM PAIN

This is important if a satisfactory explanation for the symptoms is not found on local examination. The investigation should include: 1) the neck, with the brachial plexus; and 2) the shoulder.

3. GENERAL EXAMINATION

General survey of other parts of the body. The local symptoms may be only one manifestation of a widespread disease.

Movements at the elbow
The elbow joint has two distinct components: the hinge joint between the humerus above and the ulna and radius below, allowing flexion-extension movement; and the pivot joint between the upper ends of the radius and ulna, allowing rotation of the forearm. It should be remembered that free rotation of the forearm is dependent not only upon an intact superior radio-ulnar joint; it demands also free mobility between the radius and ulna throughout their length, and distally at the inferior radio-ulnar joint. *Flexion-extension:* The normal range is from 0 to 155 degrees.[1] *Supination-pronation:* Rotation movements must be tested with the

---

[1]0 = the anatomical position, with the arm straight.

elbow flexed to a right angle, to eliminate rotation at the shoulder (Fig. 193). The normal range is 90 degrees of supination (palm up) and 90 degrees of pronation (palm down). If the range of rotation is restricted possible causes must be sought in the forearm and wrist as well as in the elbow.

Fig. 193
Examining rotation of the forearm. The elbow is flexed 90 degrees to eliminate rotation at the shoulder.

The ulnar nerve

Because of the vulnerability of the ulnar nerve in its course behind the elbow, tests of ulnar nerve function should be carried out as part of the routine examination of the elbow. Examine for sensibility in the little finger and medial half of the ring finger, and test the ulnar-innervated small muscles of the hand for wasting or weakness: a simple test is to ask the patient to spread the fingers and to bring them together again forcibly, to prevent a card gripped between the middle and ring fingers from being withdrawn. Note whether the skin in the territory of the ulnar nerve sweats equally with the rest of the hand.

The median and radial nerves

The integrity of the median and radial nerves should also be tested. Criteria of integrity of the median nerve are volar sensibility in the lateral three and a half digits, and active power of opposition of the thumb. Integrity of the radial nerve is demonstrated by ability to dorsiflex the wrist and to extend the digits at the metacarpo-phalangeal joints. A distal lesion, affecting the posterior interosseous division of the nerve, may leave wrist extension intact while impairing extension of the digits.

Imaging

Radiographic examination. Radiographs of the humerus must always include antero-posterior and lateral projections, and they should take in both the shoulder joint and the elbow.

Routine radiographs of the elbow comprise an antero-posterior projection with the elbow straight and a lateral projection with the joint semiflexed. In special circumstances additional oblique or tangential projections may be helpful. A radiograph of the forearm bones and of the inferior radio-ulnar joint is also required when rotation of the forearm is impaired.

Other imaging techniques. Radioisotope scanning with ^{99m}technetium may be helpful in appropriate circumstances. CT scanning and magnetic resonance imaging have an occasional place.

Extrinsic sources of pain in the upper arm

Pain in the upper arm is commonly referred from a lesion elsewhere—particularly from the shoulder, and from the neck when the brachial plexus or its roots are involved. Shoulder pain usually radiates from the tip of the acromion process to about the middle of the outer aspect of the arm, but it does not extend below the elbow. In contrast, nerve pain from interference with the brachial plexus often extends throughout the length of the arm and forearm into the hand and fingers; and frequently there are accompanying paraesthesiae in the form of tingling, numbness, or 'pins and needles'.

CLASSIFICATION OF DISORDERS OF THE ARM AND ELBOW

DISORDERS OF THE UPPER ARM

Infections
Acute osteomyelitis
Chronic osteomyelitis

Tumours
Benign tumours of bone
Malignant tumours of bone

Cystic lesions
Simple bone cysts

DISORDERS OF THE ELBOW

Deformities
Cubitus valgus
Cubitus varus
Arthritis
Pyogenic arthritis
Rheumatoid arthritis
Tuberculous arthritis
Osteoarthritis
Neuropathic arthritis
Haemophilic arthritis

Mechanical derangements
Osteochondritis dissecans
Loose body formation

Extra-articular disorders
Tennis elbow
Olecranon bursitis
Friction neuritis of the ulnar nerve

DISORDERS OF THE UPPER ARM

ACUTE OSTEOMYELITIS
(General description of acute osteomyelitis, p. 69)

Osteomyelitis is less common in the upper limb than in the lower. Nevertheless the humerus is a well recognised site of haematogenous infection—especially its upper metaphysis.

Pathology. Except in time of war the humerus is seldom infected directly by organisms introduced from without, for compound fractures are rare. Infection is usually haematogenous, from a focus elsewhere in the body. This type of infection occurs mainly in children, and it usually begins in a metaphysis of the bone—more often the upper metaphysis than the lower. Since both the upper and the lower metaphyses are partly enclosed within the capsule of the shoulder and of the elbow respectively, a metaphysial infection is liable to spread directly to the adjacent joint, causing pyogenic arthritis (see Fig. 51, p. 71).

Clinical features. There is constitutional illness, with pyrexia. Locally, there is severe pain at the site of infection. *On examination* there is intense and well localised tenderness over the affected area—usually near one end of the bone. Later, there may be swelling and increased warmth, and a fluctuant abscess may form. The adjacent joint is commonly swollen from an effusion of fluid ('sympathetic' effusion), even if the joint itself is not involved in the infection. In the absence of joint infection, however, movements are restricted only slightly, if at all.

Imaging. *Radiographs* do not show any abnormality at first. After about two weeks there are often localised rarefaction and subperiosteal new bone formation (Fig. 194), but these changes may be slight. *Radioisotope scanning* shows increased uptake in the affected area.

Fig. 194
Acute osteomyelitis of upper end of humerus. Radiograph four weeks after onset showing marked rarefaction of the bone, with patchy areas of destruction and much subperiosteal new bone formation.

Investigations. Blood culture is often positive in the incipient stage. There is a marked polymorphonuclear leucocytosis. The erythrocyte sedimentation rate is increased.

Treatment. This is the same as for acute osteomyelitis elsewhere (p. 73). It is mainly by rest and antibacterial therapy, with drainage of the subperiosteal abscess when appropriate.

CHRONIC OSTEOMYELITIS
(General description of chronic osteomyelitis, p. 74)

As in other bones, chronic pyogenic osteomyelitis of the humerus is nearly always a sequel to acute osteomyelitis that has been neglected or has responded poorly to treatment. The bone is thickened, often throughout its whole length, and there may be a persistent or intermittent purulent discharge from a sinus, or recurrent flare-ups with local pain and induration. *Radiographs* show irregular thickening with patchy areas of sclerosis and cavitation, and sometimes a sequestrum.

Treatment was described on page 76.

TUMOURS OF BONE

BENIGN TUMOURS
(General description of benign bone tumours, p. 80)

GIANT-CELL TUMOUR (OSTEOCLASTOMA)

Giant-cell tumour is uncommon in the humerus, but when it does occur the usual site is at the upper end, where it often extends close up to the articular surface. The tumour occurs chiefly in young adults, and its general characteristics are like those of giant-cell tumour of bone at other sites (p. 80).

Treatment. The high risk of recurrence after simple curettage and bone grafting has to be balanced against the likely disability after radical excision of the whole of the upper end of the humerus. Each case must be considered on its merits, but if the tumour is large there is much to be said for radical local excision of the affected part of the bone and replacement by a custom-made metal prosthesis.

MALIGNANT TUMOURS
(General description of malignant bone tumours, p. 84)

Primary malignant tumours of bone are much less common in the upper limb than in the lower, and examples are seen only infrequently. Metastatic tumours, by comparison, are common, especially in the proximal part of the humerus (Fig. 195).

Fig. 195
Metastatic tumour in the humerus from primary carcinoma of the lung. This is a common site for metastatic tumours, which often lead eventually to pathological fracture.

OSTEOSARCOMA (Osteogenic sarcoma)

The upper metaphysis of the humerus is the favourite site in the upper limb for this highly malignant tumour. It occurs only exceptionally at the lower metaphysis. The tumour affects children or young adults and has the usual characteristics of such tumours, destroying the metaphysial region and bursting out through the cortex to invade the adjacent soft tissues. It metastasises early through the blood stream, notably to the lungs.

Treatment. The treatment of osteosarcoma was discussed on page 89. Osteosarcoma in the upper limb has to be considered separately from the same tumour in the lower limb, where the great majority of cases occur. Amputation is much less acceptable in the upper limb, especially in a disease in which the chance of lasting cure is in any case slender. Thus in the upper limb there is a strong case, whenever it is practicable, for advising radical local excision or radiotherapy, with adjuvant chemotherapy, in preference to amputation. In this difficult field each individual case has to be considered on its merits, and treatment should be carried out only at special centres where it can be based on an adequate breadth of experience.

EWING'S TUMOUR
This occurs occasionally in the shaft of the humerus but it is very uncommon. In its behaviour it conforms to the general description given in Chapter 5.

MULTIPLE MYELOMA
The tumour foci in myelomatosis (p. 92) develop readily in the proximal half of the humerus, which contains abundant vascular marrow.

METASTATIC TUMOURS
Carcinomatous deposits from tumours of the lung, breast, prostate, kidney, and thyroid are common in the humerus. They usually occur near the upper end of the shaft, where there is much vascular marrow. Such metastases are a common cause of pathological fracture in the upper limb. A typical example is shown in Figure 195.

BONE CYST

Bone cysts were described on page 99. The humerus is the commonest site of simple bone cyst, which occurs especially in children or adolescents, and at the upper end of the bone. The cyst replaces the normal bone structure and may thus lead to pathological fracture. As a general rule, small cysts may simply be kept under observation. A large cyst should first be aspirated and injected with corticosteroid solution. Only if this is unsuccessful should the cyst be curetted and packed with bone chips. A fracture may sometimes require internal fixation.

DISORDERS OF THE ELBOW

CUBITUS VALGUS

The normal elbow, when fully extended, is in a position of slight valgus— usually 10 degrees in men and 15 degrees in women. This is known as the carrying angle. If the angle is increased, so that the forearm is abducted excessively in relation to the upper arm, the deformity is known as cubitus valgus (Fig. 196).

Cause. Cubitus valgus is usually a consequence of previous disease or injury in the elbow region. The most frequent causes are: 1) previous fracture of the lower end of the humerus or of the capitulum, with mal-union; and 2) interference with epiphysial growth on the lateral side, from injury or infection.

Clinical features. Apart from the visible deformity there are no symptoms unless secondary effects develop.

Secondary effects. The most important sequel of cubitus valgus is interference with the function of the ulnar nerve. When valgus deformity is marked, the nerve is angled sharply round the prominent medial part of the joint, and repeated friction may lead to fibrosis of the nerve trunk. Symptoms develop insidiously over a long period: there are tingling and blunting of sensibility in the ulnar distribution in the hand, with weakness and wasting of the ulnar-innervated small hand muscles (p. 243).

Fig. 196
Cubitus valgus (left elbow). The deformity predisposes to friction neuritis of the ulnar nerve.

Treatment. Slight uncomplicated deformity is best left alone. If angulation is severe, correction by osteotomy near the lower end of the humerus is justified. If the function of the ulnar nerve is impaired the nerve should be transposed from its post-humeral groove to a new bed at the front of the elbow.

CUBITUS VARUS

Cubitus varus is the opposite deformity to cubitus valgus. The carrying angle, or normal angle of valgus at the fully extended elbow, is decreased or reversed.

Cause. The causes are similar to those of cubitus valgus: 1) previous fracture with mal-union (especially supracondylar fracture of the humerus); and 2) interference with epiphysial growth on the medial side.

Clinical features. There are usually no symptoms other than the visible deformity, which may be embarrassing, especially to a child.

Treatment. Minor degrees of deformity can safely be left uncorrected. If the angulation is severe it may be corrected by osteotomy through the lower end of the humerus.

PYOGENIC ARTHRITIS OF THE ELBOW

(General description of pyogenic arthritis, p. 109)

Pyogenic arthritis is usually an acute infection with suppuration, but it may occur in subacute or even in chronic form.

Pathology. As with other joints, organisms reach the elbow in three ways: 1) through the blood stream (haematogenous infection); 2) through a penetrating wound; or 3) from an adjacent focus of osteomyelitis in the humerus, radius, or ulna. The last-mentioned route is the most common, and the arthritis is simply an extension into the joint of an infection of the humerus, facilitated by the location of the lower metaphysis of the humerus within the elbow joint (see Fig. 51, p. 71).

Clinical features. The symptoms and signs correspond to those described for pyogenic arthritis elsewhere (p. 109). The onset is acute or subacute, with pain and swelling of the elbow. There is constitutional illness, with pyrexia. The elbow is swollen, partly from fluid, partly from synovial thickening. The overlying skin is warmer than normal. All movements are limited by pain and muscle spasm. *Radiographs*, normal at first, may later show diffuse rarefaction and loss of cartilage space. Radioisotope scanning shows increased uptake of the isotope in the affected area.

Treatment. This is by aspiration or surgical drainage combined with systemic and local antibiotics, as described on page 110.

RHEUMATOID ARTHRITIS OF THE ELBOW

(General description of rheumatoid arthritis, p. 111)

One or both elbows are commonly affected in rheumatoid arthritis, usually in conjunction with several other joints.

Pathology. The pathological changes are like those of rheumatoid arthritis elsewhere. Beginning as a chronic inflammatory thickening of the synovial membrane, it tends later to involve the articular cartilage, which may eventually be almost totally destroyed. The subchondral bone may also be eroded (Fig. 197).

Clinical features. As in other joints, the main symptoms are pain, swelling from thickening of the synovial membrane, abnormal warmth of the overlying skin, and impairment of movement, particularly of rotation of the forearm. In the later stages there is commonly a fixed flexion deformity.

Fig. 197
Destruction of the joint surfaces of the elbow in a case of severe rheumatoid arthritis of long duration.

Imaging. *Radiographic examination:* At first there are no changes. Later, there is diffuse rarefaction in the area of the joint. In long-established cases the cartilage space is lost and there may be some erosion of the bone ends (Fig. 197).

Radioisotope scanning shows increased uptake of isotope in the region of the joint.

Treatment. Primary treatment is along the lines suggested for rheumatoid arthritis in general (p. 115).

Operative treatment. If extensive destruction of the articular cartilage leads to persistent disabling pain, operation must be considered. If pain is largely at the lateral side of the joint the simple operation of excision of the head of the radius, with limited synovectomy, often gives good relief. Replacement arthroplasty, by the fitting either of a hinged prosthesis with long stems cemented into the humerus and ulna, or by replacement only of the articular surfaces by metal and plastic liners, is still in a stage of development. Whereas favourable short-term results are being achieved, the outlook for the longer term is not yet clear. There is still an occasional place for the older technique of excision arthroplasty, especially as a salvage procedure, and rarely for arthrodesis.

TUBERCULOUS ARTHRITIS OF THE ELBOW
(General description of tuberculous arthritis, p. 117)

Tuberculous arthritis is much less common in the elbow than it is in the large weight-bearing joints such as the hip and knee.

The pathological and clinical features of joint tuberculosis were described on page 117, and further description is not required here. Biopsy may be required to establish the diagnosis.

Treatment. As for other tuberculous joints, the mainstay of treatment is antibacterial therapy, as described on page 120. *Local treatment:* Initial treatment is by immobilisation in plaster for two to four months while the disease is overcome. Thereafter treatment depends upon the damage sustained by the joint. If there is no evidence of destruction of articular cartilage or bone there is a good chance that the joint has been saved, and active elbow movements may be encouraged.

Operation. If the elbow remains painful, with radiological evidence of destruction of cartilage and bone, operation may be required. A choice has to be made between replacement arthroplasty (see under rheumatoid arthritis, p. 236), which is applicable only when the disease has become quiescent, excision arthroplasty and arthrodesis.

OSTEOARTHRITIS OF THE ELBOW
(General description of osteoarthritis, p. 120)

Osteoarthritis seldom occurs in an elbow that was previously normal. In nearly every case a predisposing factor has been present for several years. This is usually a damaged articular surface from previous fracture involving the joint, or from osteochondritis dissecans.

Fig. 198
Osteoarthritis of the elbow. Note the narrowed cartilage space and pointed osteophytes at the joint margins. In this case osteoarthritis was secondary to osteochondritis dissecans occurring many years before.

Clinical features. There is slowly increasing pain in the elbow, worse on heavy use of the limb. The patient may also notice that movement is impaired. In some cases there are attacks of sudden locking, suggesting the presence of a loose body in the joint. There is often a history of previous injury or disease involving the elbow—for instance, osteochondritis dissecans. *On examination* there is palpable thickening at the joint margins, from osteophytes. Flexion and extension are impaired but rotation is often full. There is coarse crepitation on movement.

Radiographs show narrowing of the cartilage space and pointed osteophytes at the joint margins (Fig. 198). Loose bodies (formed from detached osteophytes or from flakes of articular cartilage) may be present.

Treatment. In most cases treatment is not required once the nature of the trouble has been explained to the patient. When treatment is called for conservative measures are tried first. A course of mild analgesic medication may be prescribed. Heavy use of the elbow should be avoided or reduced. Physiotherapy in the form of short-wave diathermy may be worth a trial. Exceptionally operation is advisable. Thus if a loose body has caused symptoms of locking it may be removed with excellent prospects of relief; and if the arthritis is predominantly in the lateral (humero-radial) half of the joint excision of the head of the radius is often helpful. In osteoarthritis, in contrast to rheumatoid arthritis, the more radical operation of replacement arthroplasty is hardly ever required.

NEUROPATHIC ARTHRITIS OF THE ELBOW

(General description of neuropathic arthritis, p. 126)

In neuropathic arthritis (Charcot's osteoarthropathy) of the elbow the joint becomes disorganised in consequence of a loss of sensibility to pain. It is a rare form of arthritis.

Cause. The usual underlying cause of the disease in the elbow is syringomyelia, but any other affection that leads to loss of sensibility (e.g. diabetic neuropathy) may be responsible.

Fig. 199
Neuropathic arthritis of the elbow. There is marked absorption of bone, with pathological dislocation. The underlying cause was syringomyelia.

Pathology. The protective mechanism which prevents the normal joint from being damaged by everyday stresses fails because the ligaments are insensitive to pain. A vicious circle is established: repeated unrecognised injuries impair the stability of the joint and thereby render it more liable to further injury. The ultimate result is gross disorganisation.

Basically, the changes consist in degeneration and attrition of the joint surfaces, sometimes with coincident massive hypertrophy of bone at the joint margins. Pathological dislocation may occur (Fig. 199).

Clinical features. The main symptoms are swelling and a feeling of weakness due to instability. In the early stages pain may not be entirely absent, but in general lack of pain is a striking feature. *On examination* there is marked thickening and irregularity of the bone ends. The joint is abnormally lax, and lateral mobility is often pronounced. Clinical evidence of the underlying condition (usually syringomyelia) will be found. *Radiographs* show a disorganised joint, often with much destruction of bone (Fig. 199). *Investigations* should be directed towards establishing the nature of the underlying neurological disorder.

Treatment. This is mainly that of the underlying disorder. If the elbow is severely disorganised it should be protected by a right-angled brace of plastic or leather. Operation is usually inappropriate.

HAEMOPHILIC ARTHRITIS OF THE ELBOW
(General description of haemophilic arthritis, p. 125)

Haemophilic arthritis affects the elbow more often than any other joint except the knee. As in other joints, the main feature is intra-articular haemorrhage, often recurrent, with consequent irritation and, later, degeneration of the joint.

The clue to the diagnosis is a history of previous bleeding or of a haemophilic tendency in the family. Haemarthrosis without major injury should always arouse suspicion of haemophilia. A prolonged blood clotting time is an important confirmatory finding.

Treatment (for fresh haemarthrosis). If antihaemophilic factor is available it should be given in adequate dosage and the joint should be aspirated. The elbow is supported by crepe bandages and a light plaster splint. Gentle exercises are resumed after two weeks. If antihaemophilic factor is not available reliance must be placed on splintage, without aspiration. In this event, particularly after repeated haemarthrosis, permanent damage with fibrosis of the synovial membrane and the formation of intra-articular adhesions must be expected in the long term.

OSTEOCHONDRITIS DISSECANS OF THE ELBOW
(General description of osteochondritis dissecans, p. 130)

After the knee, the elbow is the most frequent site of osteochondritis dissecans. The disorder is characterised by necrosis of part of the articular cartilage and of the underlying bone, with eventual separation of the fragment to form an intra-articular loose body (Fig. 200).

Cause. The precise cause is unknown. Impairment of blood supply to the affected segment of bone and cartilage by thrombosis of an end artery has been suggested. Injury probably plays a part.

Pathology. The part of the elbow affected is nearly always the capitulum of the humerus. The necrotic segment of articular surface varies in size; commonly its surface area is about a centimetre in diameter and its depth less than half a centimetre. A line of demarcation forms between the avascular segment and the surrounding normal bone and cartilage, and after an interval of months the avascular segment separates as a loose body (sometimes two or three), leaving a shallow cavity in the articular surface which is ultimately filled with fibrous tissue. The damage to the joint surface predisposes to the later development of osteoarthritis.

Clinical features. In the early stages, before the fragment has separated, the symptoms are those of mild mechanical irritation of the joint—namely, aching after use and intermittent swelling. *On examination* at this stage there is often an effusion of clear fluid into the joint, and there is slight limitation of flexion or extension.

When a loose body has separated, the main features are recurrent painful locking of the elbow and subsequent effusion of fluid.

Radiographic features. In the early stages there is an area of irregularity on the affected subchondral bone, usually of the capitulum. Later a shallow cavity, whose margins are demarcated clearly from the bone within it, is seen (Fig. 200). Eventually the bony fragment separates from the cavity and lies free within the joint, usually in the lateral compartment.

Fig. 200
Osteochondritis dissecans. A fragment of the capitulum is separating. This is the typical site of osteochondritis dissecans in the elbow.

Treatment. Operation is delayed until the fragment of bone and cartilage is ripe for separation or has actually separated. The fragment is then removed.

LOOSE BODIES IN THE ELBOW

Causes. There are four important causes of loose bodies in the elbow: 1) osteochondritis dissecans (one to three bodies); 2) osteoarthritis (one to three bodies); 3) fracture with separation of a fragment (one to three bodies); and 4) synovial chondromatosis (fifty to five hundred bodies).

Pathology and clinical features. *Osteochondritis dissecans* was described on page 239 and *osteoarthritis* on page 237.

Loose body after fracture. A fragment may rarely be detached from the capitulum. Sometimes the medial epicondyle is detached and sucked into the joint, retaining its attachments to the flexor muscles.

Synovial chondromatosis (osteochondromatosis). This is a rare disease of synovial membrane in which numerous synovial villi become pedunculated and transformed into cartilage; eventually they are detached to form a large number of loose bodies, many of which become calcified (Fig. 201).

Clinical features. Many so-called loose bodies are 'silent'—that is, they cause no symptoms. Often in such cases the fragment is not in fact loose, but has soft-tissue attachments that prevent its moving about the joint.

The characteristic symptom of a freely movable loose body is sudden locking of the elbow during movement, with sharp pain. The joint is usually unlocked after an interval, either spontaneously or by the patient's manoeuvres. Several hours later the joint swells. The symptoms subside within a few days, but repeated attacks are to be expected.

Examination in the stage of swelling shows the joint to be distended with fluid—a clear, pale, straw-coloured effusion. Between attacks a loose body may sometimes be felt. There is often a history or clinical evidence to suggest the cause of the loose body formation.

Fig. 201
Multiple loose bodies in the elbow. A case of synovial chondromatosis.

Radiographs show the loose body or bodies (Fig. 201) and usually indicate the nature of the primary condition.

Treatment. Symptomless loose bodies may usually be safely left alone; but if a loose body causes locking it should be removed by operation.

TENNIS ELBOW
(Epicondylitis)

'Tennis elbow' is a common and well defined clinical entity. It is an extra-articular affection characterised by pain and acute tenderness at the origin of the extensor muscles of the forearm.

Cause. It is believed to be caused by strain of the forearm extensor muscles at the point of their origin from the bone. Although it sometimes occurs after playing tennis, other activities are more often responsible.

Pathology. No pathology has been demonstrated. Hypothetically, it is assumed that there is incomplete rupture of aponeurotic fibres at the muscle origin, which is a region plentifully supplied by nerve endings. The elbow joint itself is unaffected.

Clinical features. There is pain at the lateral aspect of the elbow, often radiating down the back of the forearm.

On examination there is tenderness precisely localised to the front of the lateral epicondyle of the humerus (Fig. 202). Pain is aggravated by putting the extensor muscles on the stretch—for example, by flexing the wrist and fingers with the forearm pronated. Movements of the elbow are full. *Radiographs* do not show any alteration from the normal.

Course. If left alone the symptoms eventually subside spontaneously, but they may persist for as long as two years or more.

Treatment. In mild cases the patient is often willing to await spontaneous recovery once the harmless nature of the affection has been explained. Treatment is unpredictable in its results and no method can be relied upon in every case.

Conservative treatment. Initially, trial may be made of a course of non-steroidal anti-inflammatory drugs. In most cases, however, treatment will be by the injection of hydrocortisone, preferably with local anaesthetic solution, into the point of greatest tenderness. This method is often successful, but only if the injection is made precisely into the tender spot (Fig. 202). This is not always done easily, and consequently it may

Fig. 202
In tennis elbow the point of greatest tenderness is at the front of the lateral epicondyle, not over its greatest prominence. To be curative, injection must be made precisely at the point of greatest tenderness.

sometimes be necessary to repeat the injection on one or two occasions at two-weekly intervals. In a successful case the pain is often exacerbated for twenty-four hours or so after the injection, before it begins gradually to disappear.

Operative treatment. If severe disability fails to respond to conservative treatment, operation is well worth-while. The extensor origin is stripped from its attachment to the lateral epicondyle and allowed to fall back into place. Hypothetically, this completes the detachment of pain-sensitive fibres from the bone and allows healing to occur.

OLECRANON BURSITIS

The bursa behind the olecranon process is liable to traumatic bursitis, septic bursitis, and gout.

In *traumatic bursitis* ('student's elbow') the bursa is distended with clear fluid (Fig. 203). Treatment at first should be by aspiration, followed by the injection of hydrocortisone into the bursa. If the swelling recurs the bursa should be excised.

Septic bursitis is treated by incision to secure adequate drainage.

Fig. 203
Olecranon bursitis.

In *gouty bursitis* there is acute or subacute inflammation, and whitish deposits of sodium biurate (tophi) may be visible through the walls of the bursa. If the symptoms are troublesome the bursa may be excised.

FRICTION NEURITIS OF THE ULNAR NERVE

The ulnar nerve is vulnerable where it lies in the groove behind the medial epicondyle of the humerus. Its function may be interfered with either by constriction or by recurrent friction while in tension. Constriction is usually secondary to osteoarthritis, with encroachment of osteophytes upon the ulnar groove. Friction under tension occurs when the carrying angle of the elbow is increased (cubitus valgus, p. 234). This latter type is often a late sequel of a supracondylar fracture of the humerus sustained in childhood ('tardy ulnar palsy'). In both cases the nerve undergoes fibrosis, and unless the mechanical fault is relieved without undue delay the changes may eventually become irreversible.

Clinical features. The patient complains of numbness or tingling in the ulnar distribution, and often of clumsiness in performing fine finger movements, as for instance in such activities as playing musical instruments.

On examination in the fully developed condition the following signs are present: *Sensory*—There is blunting or loss of sensibility along the ulnar border of the hand and in the little finger and medial half of the ring finger. *Motor*—There are wasting and weakness of the ulnar-innervated small hand muscles. *Sweating*—The skin in the ulnar territory is drier than normal because sweating is impaired. In doubtful cases nerve conduction studies may be carried out on the ulnar nerve, to detect any slowing of impulses at the elbow level.

Treatment. Whenever the ulnar nerve is interfered with by a lesion at the elbow operation should be undertaken. The operation will consist in decompression of the nerve by division of the overlying aponeurosis of the flexor carpi ulnaris; or, if deformity is present, by transposing the nerve to a new bed at the front of the elbow.

References and bibliography, page 403.

13. The forearm, wrist and hand

So much in everyday life depends upon the efficient working of the hand, and so great is the practical and economic consequence of its disablement, that the care of the diseased or injured hand has become one of the most vital branches of orthopaedic surgery. It is also one of the most fascinating.

Hand surgery is an art and a science in itself. Indeed it has already become a distinct speciality, demanding a knowledge and experience not only of orthopaedic surgery but also of plastic surgery, microvascular surgery, and neurology.

In the treatment of hand disorders the primary emphasis should always be on restoration of function. Keen judgment is often called for in deciding between the claims of rest and of movement. It should be remembered that the hand tolerates immobilisation badly. Whereas the wrist may be immobilised for many weeks or even months with impunity, to immobilise injured or diseased fingers for a long time is to court disaster in the form of permanent joint stiffness. Although rest may be essential in the early days after a hand injury or in the acute stage of an infection, active finger exercises must be insisted upon as soon as that stage has passed. It is wise to accept it as a general rule that fingers should never be immobilised for longer than two, or at most three, weeks.

SPECIAL POINTS IN THE INVESTIGATION OF FOREARM, WRIST AND HAND COMPLAINTS

History
It should be remembered that symptoms in the hand are often caused by disorders of the neck (with involvement of the brachial plexus or its roots) and sometimes by disorders at the elbow. Enquiry should always be made into any previous injury or other trouble with the neck or with the upper extremity as a whole.

Exposure
For the local examination the whole forearm should be uncovered to well above the elbow. The sound limb should be exposed likewise for comparison.

245

Steps in clinical examination
A suggested routine of clinical examination is summarised in Table VIII.

Movements at the wrist
Like the elbow, the wrist comprises two distinct components: 1) the radio-carpal joint (including the intercarpal joints), allowing flexion, extension, adduction and abduction; and 2) the inferior radio-ulnar joint, allowing supination and pronation. The movements at each component must be examined independently.

The radio-carpal joint. The normal range of flexion is 80 degrees and of extension 90 degrees. The range of adduction, or ulnar deviation, is about 35 degrees, and of abduction, or radial deviation, about 25 degrees. It is impracticable to measure the movements of the intercarpal joints individually, and it is simplest to regard them as integral parts of the radio-carpal joint.

A rapid and reasonably accurate method of comparing the range of flexion-extension movement on the two sides is as follows: *To judge the range of extension*: The patient places the palms and fingers of the two hands in contact in the vertical plane and lifts the elbows as far

---

Table VIII
Routine clinical examination in suspected disorders
of the forearm, wrist, and hand

---

1. LOCAL EXAMINATION OF THE FOREARM, WRIST, AND HAND

Inspection
Bone contours
Soft-tissue contours
Colour and texture of skin
Scars and sinuses

Palpation
Skin temperature
Bone contours
Soft-tissue contours
Local tenderness

Movements (active and passive)
At the wrist:
Radio-carpal joint—Flexion-extension; adduction-abduction
Inferior radio-ulnar joint—Supination and pronation
At the hand:
Carpo-metacarpal joint of thumb— Flexion-extension; adduction-abduction; opposition

Metacarpo-phalangeal joints—Flexion-extension; adduction-abduction
Interphalangeal joints—Flexion-extension

Power
Power of each muscle group in control of:
1) wrist movement; 2) thumb and finger movement; and 3) gripping

Stability
Tests for abnormal mobility

Nerve function
Tests of sensory function, motor function and sweating in distribution of median, ulnar and radial nerves

Circulation
Arterial pulses, warmth and colour, capillary return, cutaneous sensibility.

---

2. EXAMINATION OF POSSIBLE EXTRINSIC SOURCES OF FOREARM AND HAND SYMPTOMS

This is important if a satisfactory explanation for the symptoms is not found on local examination. The investigation should include: 1) the neck and thoracic inlet, with special reference to the brachial plexus; 2) the upper arm; and 3) the elbow.

---

3. GENERAL EXAMINATION

General survey of other parts of the body. The local symptoms may be only one manifestation of a more widespread disease.

as he can while keeping the 'heels' of the hands together (Fig. 204). The angle between hand and forearm is easily compared on the two sides. *To judge the range of flexion*: The manoeuvre is reversed. The patient places the backs of the hands together, with the fingers directed vertically downwards, and lowers the elbows as far as he can (Fig. 204). The angle between hand and forearm is compared on the two sides.

Fig. 204
A simple method of comparing the range of extension and flexion at the two wrists. Note the obvious impairment at the left wrist.

The inferior radio-ulnar joint. The normal range is 90 degrees of supination and 90 degrees of pronation. To determine the range accurately the patient's elbows must be flexed to a right angle in order to eliminate rotation at the shoulder (see Fig. 193, p. 230).

It must be emphasised that impaired rotation does not necessarily denote an abnormality of the wrist: it may equally well be caused by a disorder of the elbow or of the forearm.

Movements of the hand
Movements of the hand occur mainly at three groups of joints: 1) the carpo-metacarpal joint of the thumb; 2) the metacarpo-phalangeal joints; and 3) the interphalangeal joints.

Carpo-metacarpal joint of thumb. This joint allows movement in five directions: flexion, or movement of the thumb metacarpal medially in the plane of the palm; extension, or movement of the thumb metacarpal laterally in the plane of the palm; adduction, or movement of the metacarpal towards the palm in a plane at right angles to it; abduction, or movement of the metacarpal away from the palm in a plane at right angles to it; and opposition, or rotation of the metacarpal to bring the thumb nail into a plane parallel with the palm (Figs 205 and 206).

Fig. 205   **Fig. 206**
To show the difference between flexion of the thumb across the palm (Fig. 205) and true opposition (Fig. 206). In opposition the thumb metacarpal is rotated so that the thumb nail lies in a plane parallel with the palm.

Metacarpo-phalangeal joints of thumb and fingers. These joints allow flexion-extension movement through 90 degrees (the range is variable in the thumb), and a small range of abduction from, and adduction to, the midline of the middle finger.

Interphalangeal joints of thumb and fingers. These are true hinge joints, allowing only flexion and extension.

Power
Test the power of each movement in turn. In the hand this examination demands considerable patience, for each muscle group must be tested individually. Thus in the thumb it

is necessary to test the abductors, the adductor, the extensors (longus and brevis), the flexors (longus and brevis), and the opponens. In the fingers test the flexors (profundus and superficialis), the extensor digitorum and extensor indicis, the interossei and the lumbricals. *Grip*: Test the power of grip, which demands the combined action of the flexors and extensors of the wrist and the flexors of the fingers and thumb.

Nerve function
The state of the median, ulnar and radial nerves is determined by tests of sensory function, motor function, and sweating. Intact function of the median nerve is indicated by ability to oppose the thumb to the little finger (see Figs 205 and 206). Intact ulnar nerve function is shown by ability to spread the fingers apart and to bring them together again to grip a card between the middle and ring fingers. An index of radial nerve function is the ability to extend the thumb and to extend the fingers at the metacarpo-phalangeal joints.

Circulation
The state of the circulation is assessed from the condition of the arterial pulses, the warmth and colour of the digits, the capillary return at the nail beds, and cutaneous sensibility. It should be remembered that sensibility to touch in the fingers is a most useful index of the adequacy of the circulation. Nerves require a blood supply to enable them to conduct impulses, and if the circulation is interrupted sensibility is quickly lost.

Extrinsic sources of forearm and hand symptoms
It is sometimes difficult to determine whether symptoms and signs in the forearm or hand are caused by a local disorder or whether they are referred from a more proximal lesion. This difficulty arises mainly in neurological conditions. For instance, the symptoms of compression of the median nerve in the carpal tunnel may be mimicked closely by a prolapsed cervical disc, and the symptoms of constriction of the ulnar nerve at the elbow may likewise be confused with those from a low cervical disc lesion or a cervical rib. When symptoms in the hand are not satisfactorily explained by the local condition a search must be made for a possible cause in the neck, upper arm, or elbow.

Imaging
Radiographic examination. Routine radiographs should include antero-posterior and lateral projections of the forearm, wrist and hand. For detailed study of the carpal bones additional oblique projections are required.

If it is suspected that the symptoms may be referred from the neck or proximal part of the limb, radiographs of the appropriate part should be obtained.

Other techniques of imaging. *Radioisotope scanning* (p. 16) may be helpful in appropriate circumstances.

CLASSIFICATION OF DISORDERS OF THE FOREARM, WRIST AND HAND

DISORDERS OF THE FOREARM

Infections of bone
Acute osteomyelitis
Chronic osteomyelitis

Tumours of bone
Benign tumours
Malignant tumours

Miscellaneous
Volkmann's ischaemic contracture
Frictional tenosynovitis crepitans

ARTICULAR DISORDERS OF THE WRIST AND HAND

Deformities
Madelung's deformity
(dyschondrosteosis)

Rheumatoid arthritis
Osteoarthritis

Arthritis
Pyogenic arthritis

Miscellaneous
Kienböck's disease

EXTRA-ARTICULAR DISORDERS ABOUT THE WRIST AND HAND

Infections
Acute infections of the fascial
spaces
Chronic infective tenosynovitis

Neurological disorders
Compression of the median nerve
in the carpal tunnel

Tumours
Tumours of bone
Tumours of soft tissue

Miscellaneous
Ganglion
Dupuytren's contracture
Rupture or severence of tendons
De Quervain's tenovaginitis
Digital stenosing tenovaginitis

DISORDERS OF THE FOREARM

ACUTE OSTEOMYELITIS
(General description of acute osteomyelitis, p. 69)

Acute osteomyelitis is rather uncommon in the forearm bones. As in other sites, the infection may be blood-borne (haematogenous) or it may be introduced from without, usually in consequence of a compound fracture. The haematogenous type occurs mainly in children. It affects the radius more often than the ulna, and the lower metaphysis rather than the upper (see Fig. 54, p. 72). The upper metaphyses of both radius and ulna are partly or wholly within the capsule of the elbow; so an infection of the metaphysis may spread directly to the joint to cause pyogenic arthritis. At the wrist, in contrast, the metaphysis of the radius is wholly outside the capsule, so direct spread of infection to the joint is unlikely. The lower metaphysis of the ulna is partly within the capsule.

The clinical features and treatment are like those of acute osteomyelitis elsewhere.

CHRONIC OSTEOMYELITIS
(General description of chronic osteomyelitis, p. 74)

As in other bones, chronic osteomyelitis of the radius or ulna follows an acute infection.

Treatment. In most cases treatment should follow the usual lines, reliance being placed on rest and antibacterial drugs for non-suppurative flares of infection, and on thorough drainage operations and sequestrectomy for persistent purulent discharge.

BONE TUMOURS IN THE FOREARM

BENIGN TUMOURS

(General description of benign tumours of bone, p. 80)

Any type of benign tumour may occur in the forearm bones. Only chondroma and giant-cell tumour require further mention here.

CHONDROMA

Chrondromata of long bones occur chiefly in multiple form, in the condition known as dyschondroplasia, Ollier's disease or multiple chondromatosis (p. 49). Their special significance in the forearm lies in the fact that the tumours may interfere with the normal growth of the affected bone. If growth is retarded in one bone but proceeds normally in its partner marked curvature of the bones is to be expected, and it may cause ugly deformity, as seen commonly in dyschondroplasia.

Treatment. Severe deformity from uneven growth of the radius and ulna should be corrected by osteotomy, combined when necessary with excision of the lower end of the ulna, or sometimes of the head of the radius.

GIANT-CELL TUMOUR (OSTEOCLASTOMA)

The lower end of the radius is one of the common sites in the upper limb for the development of a giant-cell tumour, which though classed as benign may show invasive tendencies. The lower end of the ulna is also susceptible. The tumour extends into the former epiphysial region close up to the articular surface (see Fig. 70, p. 81).

Treatment. If the lower end of the ulna is the part affected the bone should be excised up to a point well proximal to the tumour. The resulting disability is negligible. If the tumour is in the lower end of the radius radical excision and replacement by a suitable bone graft is to be recommended. A graft obtained from the upper part of the fibula is suitable because its shape matches that of the original bone. Ideally, the graft should be taken with the supplying artery and veins, which are anastomosed to suitable vessels in the recipient area by a microsurgical technique.

MALIGNANT TUMOURS

(General description of malignant tumours of bone, p. 84)

The radius and ulna are seldom affected by malignant bone tumours, whether primary or metastatic. When osteosarcoma does occur in the forearm the lower end of the radius is the usual site.

VOLKMANN'S ISCHAEMIC CONTRACTURE

This is a flexion deformity of the wrist and fingers from fixed contracture of the flexor muscles in the forearm.

Cause. It is caused by ischaemia of the flexor muscles, brought about by injury to, or obstruction of, the brachial artery near the elbow; or by tense oedema of the soft tissues of the forearm constrained within an unyielding fascial compartment.

Pathology. The effects of sudden occlusion of the brachial artery vary. In a few cases gangrene of the fingers will follow. More often, the collateral circulation is sufficient to keep the hand alive, but not to nourish adequately the flexor muscles of the forearm or the main peripheral nerve trunks. The ischaemia that follows tense oedema in the anterior fascial compartment of the forearm, a consequence of severe injury in the region, has similar effects. Necrosis of muscle fibres of the forearm flexor group—especially the flexor digitorum profundus and flexor pollicis longus—with subsequent fibrosis and shortening, is the essential feature of Volkmann's contracture. It is often associated with temporary or permanent ischaemic paralysis of the peripheral nerves, especially the median nerve.

Fig. 207
To show how a supracondylar fracture of the humerus may damage the brachial artery, with risk of gangrene or ischaemic contracture. Over-tight plaster or dressings may have the same result.

Any major fracture in the elbow region or upper forearm may lead to arterial occlusion. That most commonly responsible is a supracondylar fracture of the humerus with displacement, the brachial artery being severed or contused by the sharp lower end of the main shaft fragment (Fig. 207). Contusion alone is sufficient to interrupt the flow of blood, because the artery goes into spasm and its lumen may be occluded by thrombosis.

Progressive oedema within the closed anterior fascial compartment of the forearm—for instance after fracture of the forearm bones—is commonly responsible for obstruction of the arterial flow (compartment syndrome).

In some cases the cause of the vascular obstruction is an over-tight plaster or bandage.

Clinical features. The condition is commonest in children. After sustaining a supracondylar fracture of the humerus or some other injury in the elbow region or forearm the child complains of severe pain in the forearm.

On examination in the incipient stage, the fingers are white or blue, and cold. The radial pulse is absent. Active finger movements are weak and painful. Passive extension of the fingers is especially painful and restricted. There may or may not be evidence of interruption of nerve conductivity—

namely, anaesthesia of the fingers and paralysis of the small muscles of the hand.

In the established condition, which develops gradually within a few weeks of the injury, there is a striking flexion contracture of the wrist and fingers, from shortening of the fibrotic forearm flexor muscles (Fig. 208). Sensory

Fig. 208
Typical appearance of the hand in established Volkmann's ischaemic contracture.

and motor paralysis of the hand may persist as complicating factors, but they do not form an essential feature of Volkmann's contracture as such.

Fig. 209   **Fig. 210**

In Volkmann's contracture the wrist can be partly extended if the fingers are flexed (Fig. 209), and the fingers can be partly extended if the wrist is flexed (Fig. 210): but the shortened fibrotic flexor muscles prevent extension of wrist and fingers together.

Diagnosis. In the incipient stage absence of the radial pulse, with marked unwillingness to extend the fingers because of pain, should always arouse suspicion of Volkmann's contracture. If there are also anaesthesia and paralysis of the hand the diagnosis is practically certain. In the established condition the history and clinical features make the diagnosis clear.

Volkmann's ischaemic contracture bears no real resemblance to Dupuytren's contracture (p. 273), for it affects the wrist as well as all the joints of the fingers, and there is no palpable thickening in the palm. Moreover the contracture is demonstrably brought about by shortening of the flexor muscles, because if the wrist is flexed passively to relax the flexor tendons the range of extension at the finger joints is increased. Conversely, if the tendons are relaxed by flexing the fingers fully the range of wrist extension is increased (Figs 209 and 210).

Treatment. In the *incipient stage* the problem is that of dealing with a sudden occlusion of the brachial artery or obstruction to the blood flow within a tightly congested fascial compartment. The case must be handled as an emergency, because the effects of occlusion become irreversible after about six hours. The following action must be taken. *First step*: All splints, plaster, and bandages that might be obstructing the circulation are removed. In the case of a fracture, gross displacement of the fragments is corrected as far as possible by gentle manipulation and a well padded plaster splint is applied. Likewise if the elbow is dislocated it must be reduced without delay. Heat cradles or hot bottles are applied over the other three limbs and trunk to promote general vasodilation.

If these measures fail to bring about a return of adequate circulation within half an hour, the next step is taken. *Second step*: At operation the anterior fascia of the forearm is exposed and split longitudinally throughout its length to open the fascial compartment, allowing the muscles to bulge through the gap. The brachial artery is then explored. If there is occlusion from kinking or spasm of the artery an attempt is made to relieve it by freeing the vessel and applying papaverine. If this fails, the artery may be distended by the injection of saline between clamps. In the last resort, the artery may have to be opened and damaged intima removed; or the damaged length of artery may be excised and continuity restored by a vein graft. These procedures are best accomplished by magnification techniques, by a surgeon with wide experience of vascular surgery.

In the **established stage** restoration to normal is impossible: reconstructive surgery at best can only improve what function remains. The choice of treatment depends upon the circumstances of each case. In a mild case acceptable function may be restored by intensive exercises guided by a physiotherapist: such cases are however exceptional. In more severe cases the muscle shortening may be counteracted by shortening of the forearm bones or by detachment and distal displacement of the flexor muscle origin (muscle slide operation).

In selected cases with severe muscle infarction, however, the best results are probably obtained by excision of the dead muscles and subsequent transfer of a healthy muscle (for example, a wrist flexor or a wrist extensor) to the tendons of flexor digitorum profundus and of flexor pollicis longus to restore active flexion of the digits. These muscle transfers may be combined, in appropriate cases, with arthrodesis of the wrist. When the median nerve is irreparably damaged by ischaemia nerve grafting is sometimes successful in restoring limited nerve function.

ACUTE FRICTIONAL TENOSYNOVITIS

(Peritendinitis crepitans; paratendinitis crepitans; repetitive stress syndrome)

This is an easily recognised clinical condition common in young adults whose occupations demand repetitive movements of the wrist and hand.

Cause. It is attributed to friction between the tendons and the surrounding paratenon, from over-use of the hand. It is entirely distinct from infective tenosynovitis.

Pathology. The tendons most often affected are those of the deep muscles at the back of the forearm, especially the extensors of the thumb and the radial extensors of the wrist. There is a mild inflammatory reaction about the tendon and its coverings, with local swelling and oedema.

Clinical features. After unusually active use of the wrist or hand over a period of days or weeks pain is felt at the back of the wrist and lower forearm, and swelling is noticed. The pain is aggravated by use of the hand.

On examination there is localised swelling in the line of the affected tendons—usually the extensors of the thumb or wrist. If the examiner's hand is placed over the swelling while the patient flexes and extends the wrist and digits a characteristic fine crepitation is felt: it is caused by the fibrin-covered tendon gliding within the inflamed paratenon. This typical crepitation is diagnostic of frictional tenosynovitis.

Treatment. Initially, a trial should be made of local injection of hydrocortisone. If this is unsuccessful, the wrist should be immobilised in plaster of Paris for three weeks, the fingers being left free. This affords sufficient rest to allow the inflammation to resolve. Excessive use of the fingers and thumb should be avoided for two months.

COMMENT

The condition described above is a distinct clinical entity with incontrovertible evidence of organic pathology. In recent years the label 'repetitive stress syndrome' has been applied, too often, to a range of rather vague and purely subjective symptoms affecting the hand, or sometimes the whole arm, in persons occupied for long periods in repetitive tasks such as keyboard operation and computer work. In many such cases it is difficult to separate a genuine physical disability (if it exists at all) from the psychological or 'functional' overlay that is often a prominent feature of such conditions.

ARTICULAR DISORDERS OF THE WRIST AND HAND

MADELUNG'S DEFORMITY
(Radio-ulnar dyschondrosteosis)

Madelung's deformity (radio-ulnar dyschondrosteosis) is a congenital sub-luxation or dislocation of the lower end of the ulna, from malformation of the bones. Although it is seemingly a localised disorder there may be minor generalised abnormalities of bone structure, often with short stature.

A similar wrist deformity is more often caused by disease or injury, such as a fracture of the lower end of the radius with upward displacement of the lower fragment.

Fig. 211
Relative shortening of radius with sub-luxation of inferior radio-ulnar joint, radial deviation of the hand and prominent head of ulna (Madelung's deformity).

The deformity varies in degree from a slight prominence of the lower end of the ulna at the back of the wrist, to complete dislocation of the inferior radio-ulnar joint with marked radial deviation of the hand (Fig. 211). The more severe types of deformity may be associated with congenital absence or hypoplasia of the radius.

Treatment. If the disability justifies operation the lower end of the ulna should be excised. In a severe case, with marked radial deviation of the hand, it may be necessary also to fuse the radius (or ulna, if the radius is absent) to the carpus in order to gain satisfactory correction.

PYOGENIC ARTHRITIS OF THE WRIST AND HAND
(General description of pyogenic arthritis, p. 109)

Pyogenic arthritis of the wrist is uncommon. Infection may be haemato-genous, or it may be introduced through a penetrating wound. Spread from a focus of osteomyelitis is rare, partly because osteomyelitis itself is uncommon in the forearm bones, and partly because the lower metaphysis of the radius is entirely outside the capsule of the joint. (The lower metaphysis of the ulna is partly intracapsular (see Fig. 51, p. 71).)

In the hand, any of the small joints may be infected by pyogenic organisms. The distal interphalangeal joints of the digits are prone to infection spreading from a suppurative lesion in the adjacent pulp space, or from a penetrating wound. These infections often cause permanent damage to the joint, with impairment of movement or even rigid ankylosis.

Clinical features. The symptoms and signs are those of pyogenic arthritis of any superficial joint: acute onset with constitutional illness, pain and swelling about the joint, increased local warmth, and marked impairment of movement.

Radiographic features. In the early stages radiographs do not show any alteration from the normal. Later, if the infection persists, there is diffuse rarefaction, with loss of cartilage space and possibly some destruction of bone (Figs 212 and 213).

Fig. 212   **Fig. 213**

Figure 212—Pyogenic arthritis of the wrist. *Left*—Initial radiograph, with no apparent abnormality. *Right*—Four weeks after onset. Note the rarefaction and the slight but significant narrowing of the spaces between the bones (normally occupied by articular cartilage), indicating destruction of articular cartilage. Figure 213—Pyogenic arthritis with destruction of the interphalangeal joint of the thumb, following a penetrating injury.

Treatment. Appropriate antibiotic therapy is begun. The joint is immobilised on a splint in a position of function. If suppuration occurs the joint is aspirated or drained by incision, and the appropriate antibiotic drug is injected into it. When the infection has been overcome active movements are encouraged.

RHEUMATOID ARTHRITIS OF THE WRIST AND HAND

(General description of rheumatoid arthritis, p. 111)

Rheumatoid arthritis commonly affects the wrists and hands and is a major cause of serious loss of function and of ugly deformity. Usually many or all of the joints of the hand are affected, though occasionally the disease may begin in a single joint. Affected joints are swollen from synovial thickening, and movement is restricted. In the later stages articular cartilage and the underlying bone are eroded, and the fingers tend to deviate medially (ulnar drift), with dorsal prominence of the metacarpal heads (Fig. 214). *Radiographs* do not show any abnormality at first. Later, there is diffuse rarefaction of the bones. Later still, in progressive disease, destruction of cartilage leads to narrowing of the joint space (Fig. 215), and the subchondral bone may be eroded.

Fig. 214   **Fig. 215**

Figure 214—Typical appearance of hand in long-established rheumatoid arthritis of wrist, metacarpo-phalangeal and interphalangeal joints. Figure 215—The radiograph shows loss of cartilage space in many of the joints, with erosion of subchondral bone. Note also the ulnar deviation of the fingers.

Important though these joint changes are in rheumatoid disease of the hand, equally serious disability may be caused by involvement of the soft tissues. These soft-tissue changes may take several forms, the most important of which are: 1) chronic tenosynovitis; 2) rupture of tendons; and 3) contracture of intrinsic muscles.

Chronic tenosynovitis. Masses of greatly thickened vascular synovial tissue envelop the flexor or the extensor tendons over the wrist or in the hand. A secondary effect of such swelling in front of the wrist is that the median nerve may be compressed in the carpal tunnel.

Rupture of tendons. Both the extensor and the flexor tendons are liable to spontaneous rupture, from softening or fraying where they lie within inflamed synovial sheaths.

Contracture of intrinsic muscles. Fixed contracture of the intrinsic muscles of the hand may follow fibrosis induced by the disease. It leads to inability to flex the interphalangeal joints fully when the metacarpo-phalangeal joint is held extended.

Treatment. Management of these complex disabilities of the hand is difficult and often unsatisfactory. The tendency of the disease to progress during months or years of activity means often that the hand becomes seriously crippled. Nevertheless much can be done in some cases to retard the progress of the disease and to prevent or correct deformity, either by conservative treatment alone or by conservative treatment combined with operation.

Conservative treatment. The general plan of treatment is like that for rheumatoid arthritis as a whole (p. 115). It will usually include the administration of non-steroidal anti-inflammatory drugs: cortisone and related steroids should be avoided if possible because of their undesirable side effects. Physiotherapy is of value: it should take the form of warm water baths, with mobilising exercises and encouragement in active use of the hand. During an acute exacerbation the wrist joint may be immobilised temporarily on a splint of plaster of Paris or of plastic, but immobilisation is never advised for the joints of the fingers.

Operative treatment. In carefully selected patients operation can be a valuable adjunct to conservative treatment, though it can never replace it. It should never be undertaken lightly, but only after careful deliberation and full discussion with the patient. However, operation is often more rewarding when carried out in the fairly early stages of the disease, before deformity from changes in the joints and soft tissues has become fixed and irreversible. Depending upon the nature of each individual case, operation may take one or more of the following forms.

Synovectomy. Excision of masses of thickened synovial tissue from tendon sheaths or from joints may slow down the destructive progress of the disease.

Fig. 216
Flexible silicone rubber prosthesis used for arthroplasty of metacarpo-phalangeal joint.

Arthroplasty. When the metacarpo-phalangeal or interphalangeal joints are badly disorganised arthroplasty by the insertion of a flexible silicone-rubber ('Silastic') prosthesis may sometimes be appropriate (Fig. 216). But the patient must be prepared to cooperate in a long programme of rehabilitation afterwards. The improvement gained is often cosmetic rather than functional. The benefit is not always lasting, because of breakage or loosening of the prosthesis.

Arthrodesis. For selected joints that are painful, stiff, deformed or unstable, arthrodesis in the position of most useful function is sometimes the best solution to the problem.

Tendon repair or replacement. Ruptured tendons may be repaired by suture or by grafting when practicable, or their lost function may be compensated by a tendon transfer operation (p. 33).

Release of tight intrinsic muscles. Impaired finger movement and grasp from fixed contracture of the intrinsic muscles can be improved by partial division of the aponeurotic insertion of the muscles into the extensor expansion at the back of each finger.

OSTEOARTHRITIS OF THE WRIST
(General description of osteoarthritis, p. 120)

Although uncommon compared with osteoarthritis of the hip or knee, osteoarthritis of the wrist is a well recognised sequel to certain injuries and diseases affecting the joint.

Cause. Although it is essentially a wear-and-tear process osteoarthritis seldom develops in a wrist that was previously normal. The wear and tear is nearly always accelerated by previous injury to, or disease of, the joint surfaces. The commonest predisposing factors are comminuted fracture of the lower end of the radius with involvement of the articular surface,

Fig. 217
Osteoarthritis of the wrist caused by an ununited fracture of the scaphoid bone. Note the diminished cartilage space, sclerosis, and spurring of bone at the joint margins, mainly at the radial side of the wrist.

fracture of the scaphoid bone complicated by avascular necrosis of the distal fragment, dislocation of the lunate bone, Kienböck's disease of the lunate bone, and long-established rheumatoid arthritis.

Pathology. The predominant change is degeneration and wearing away of the articular cartilage lining the joint surfaces. The changes eventually involve all the carpal joints as well as the radio-carpal joint.

Clinical features. Months or years after one of the predisposing conditions mentioned, the patient notices gradually increasing pain and stiffness of the wrist, worse on activity. *On examination* the wrist is slightly thickened from bony irregularity, but the swelling is not marked. The skin temperature is normal. Movements are markedly restricted, and painful if forced at the extremes.

Radiographic features. Radiographs show narrowing of the cartilage space and sharpening or spurring of the bone at the joint margins. The underlying causative condition (for example, an ununited fracture of the scaphoid bone) is usually evident (Fig. 217).

Treatment. In mild cases the condition is best left alone, especially if the patient can avoid subjecting the wrist to heavy stress. When active treatment seems necessary, a choice must be made between conservative and operative methods. Conservative treatment can only diminish the symptoms; it can never remove them. Nevertheless it is usually worth a trial. The most useful method is to provide support for the wrist by a brace made from moulded leather or plastic (Fig. 218).

Fig. 218
Polythene wrist support. A splint such as this is sometimes used in the
conservative treatment of osteoarthritis of the wrist.

Operative treatment sometimes becomes necessary when the disability is severe. The only reliable method is by total arthrodesis of the wrist, with ablation of the radio-carpal and all the intercarpal joints. The inferior radio-ulnar joint and the triangular fibrocartilage are left undisturbed; so rotation of the forearm is preserved.

OSTEOARTHRITIS OF THE JOINTS OF THE HAND

The metacarpo-phalangeal joints and the interphalangeal joints of the hand are frequently the site of osteoarthritis in the elderly. Such manifestations are relatively unimportant and in most cases treatment is not required. Commonly involved are the carpo-metacarpal joint of the thumb (trapezio-metacarpal joint) (Fig. 219) and the distal interphalangeal joints (Fig. 220).

OSTEOARTHRITIS OF THE TRAPEZIO-METACARPAL JOINT

This is a common affection in women beyond middle age but it may also occur in younger persons, especially when there has been previous injury such as a fracture of the base of the first metacarpal bone involving the joint. The arthritis may seriously impair the function of the thumb.

Clinical features. There is pain, localised to the trapezio-metacarpal joint, on using the thumb. The disability slowly increases over the years until activities like sewing or knitting become virtually impossible.

On examination the trapezio-metacarpal joint is prominent and slightly thickened. Active or passive movements of the thumb metacarpal cause pain. The range of movement at this joint varies widely even in normal individuals; so its measurement is of little practical value, though comparison with the opposite hand may be a guide to the extent to which movement is impaired.

Radiographs show narrowing of the cartilage space and sharpening or spurring of bone at the joint margins (Fig. 219). In many cases the joint is subluxated.

Fig. 219   **Fig. 220**

Figure 219—Osteoarthritis of the trapezio-metacarpal joint. Note the marked narrowing of the cartilage space and the large osteophytes. Figure 220—Typical Heberden's nodes, a characteristic feature of degenerative arthritis of the interphalangeal joints.

Treatment. In the early stages the condition is best left alone. Conservative treatment is generally disappointing, though sometimes the injection of hydrocortisone into the joint may give worth-while temporary relief.

Operative treatment. If the symptoms become disabling operation is advisable. The choice lies between arthroplasty and arthrodesis. Arthroplasty is done simply by excising the trapezium, allowing the resulting gap to fill with fibrous tissue. It gives results that are very satisfactory for the usual elderly sufferer from this disorder and should usually be the method of choice. The use of a prosthetic implant is better avoided. If heavy use is to be demanded of the hand in a young person (as in the case of a labourer, for example), arthrodesis of the trapezio-metacarpal joint is sometimes preferred.

OSTEOARTHRITIS OF INTERPHALANGEAL JOINTS

This leads to pain and stiffness especially in the distal interphalangeal joints. Characteristically the formation of osteophytes is a prominent feature, with the appearance of ugly swellings known as Heberden's nodes (Fig. 220).

KIENBÖCK'S DISEASE

(Osteochondritis of the lunate bone)

Kienböck's disease is an uncommon affection of the lunate bone characterised by temporary softening, fragmentation, and liability to deformation. It tends to predispose to the later development of osteoarthritis of the wrist.

Cause. The precise cause is unknown. A disturbance of blood supply, possibly from thrombosis of a nutrient vessel, is believed to be the essential factor, but how it comes about is not clear. Repeated injury (for example, using the front of the wrist to drive a chisel in carpentry, or operating a pneumatic road drill) has sometimes been noted in the case history, but a causative connection is not fully established.

Pathology. In its behaviour the disease resembles osteochondritis of developing epiphysial centres in children (p. 96), such as Perthes' disease: in effect, it is a form of avascular necrosis. The bone becomes granular in texture, small dense fragments being interspersed with softened areas. In this state the bone eventually crumbles, and under the pressure imposed by muscle action and use of the wrist it gradually becomes compressed into a thin saucer-shaped mass. The overlying cartilage dies. After about two years the bone texture is restored to normal, but the bone remains deformed and lacks a smooth cartilaginous covering. The bone behaves like a piece of grit in a bearing and leads gradually to the development of osteoarthritis of the wrist.

Clinical features. There is pain in the wrist, most marked at the centre of the joint over the lunate area. The pain is worse during active use of the wrist. Because of the pain, the strength of grip is impaired.

On examination there is discomfort on pressure over the lunate bone. An important sign is that movements of the wrist are substantially restricted and cause pain if forced.

Fig. 221
Kienböck's disease of the lunate bone. Note the increased density, fragmentation and beginning compression of the bone.

Radiographs are diagnostic. In the early stages the lunate appears slightly more dense than the surrounding bones, and if its depth is compared with that of the lunate bone of the sound wrist it is seen to be reduced, though only slightly at first (Fig. 221). Later, the bone has a fragmented appearance, small areas of increased density being scattered through it, and the flattening of the bone becomes obvious. Later still, signs of osteoarthritis of the wrist are evident.

Treatment. Treatment is often rather unsatisfactory. It must depend upon the duration of the symptoms and the degree of damage to the wrist. In the earliest stage, when radiographic changes are only just perceptible, there is probably a place for protecting the wrist in plaster for two or three months in the hope that the condition will resolve through revascularisation of the bone. But once the disease is clearly established surgical treatment is recommended. If the wrist is free from arthritis it is probably best to excise the lunate bone and replace it with a metal prosthesis. This probably gives better results than excision alone, without replacement, but the long-term results are nevertheless uncertain.

In late cases, if osteoarthritis is already present, excision of the lunate bone is of no avail. Treatment should then be the same as for osteoarthritis of the wrist (p. 260).

EXTRA-ARTICULAR DISORDERS ABOUT THE WRIST AND HAND

ACUTE INFECTIONS OF THE FASCIAL SPACES OF THE HAND

Acute infections of the hand account for a considerable proportion of the work of a casualty department or emergency room and are of great importance in industrial medicine. Unless they are treated efficiently they can lead to prolonged or even permanent disability, with impairment of working capacity.

Classification. If minor superficial infections are excluded there are six types to be considered: 1) nail-fold infection (paronychia); 2) pulp-space infection (whitlow, felon); 3) other subcutaneous infections; 4) thenar space infection; 5) mid-palmar space infection; 6) tendon sheath infection.

Cause. All types are caused by infection with pyogenic bacteria. The usual causative organism is the staphylococcus aureus, but the streptococcus and occasionally other bacteria may be responsible. Minor injury such as a prick, abrasion or blister usually provides the route by which infection can enter. Manual work in dirty conditions is clearly a factor that favours infection.

Pathology. The organisms reach the tissue planes by direct implantation from outside, often as the result of a trivial injury such as a prick or abrasion. They set up an acute inflammatory reaction which in many cases goes on to suppuration. Without effective treatment, infection may spread to adjacent tissue planes; occasionally it may give rise to spreading lymphangitis or to septicaemia.

Surgical anatomy. A knowledge of the anatomy of the fascial spaces[1] of the hand is indispensable for the correct treatment of hand infections.

The nail fold and subungual space. The subcuticular plane beneath the nail fold is potentially continuous, at the base and sides of the nail, with the subungual space deep to the nail. Infection beginning in the nail fold may therefore easily spread under the nail (Fig. 222), and the resulting abscess cannot be drained effectively unless part of the nail is removed.

The pulp space. The interval between the front of the distal phalanx and the skin is traversed by tough fibrous partitions, which subdivide the space into numerous fat-filled cells (like the cells of a honeycomb) disposed at right angles to the skin surface (Fig. 222). Infection occurring in this tough tissue is virtually within a closed compartment: tissue pressure rises rapidly and accounts for early throbbing pain.

Other subcutaneous spaces. Infection may occur in the subcutaneous plane at any point in the hand. Common sites are the middle or proximal segment of a finger, and the web

---

[1]The term 'space' as used in this connection is a misnomer. It refers to the interval or plane between adjacent tissues, and in the normal hand it is only a potential space.

spaces between the digits. Less common sites are the palm of the hand and the dorsum of the hand. These superficial spaces are clearly demarcated from the deep palmar spaces next to be described, and must not be confused with them.

The thenar space. This lies deeply under the lateral (radial) half of the hollow of the palm. It is the interval between the adductor pollicis muscle behind and the flexor tendon of the index finger and the first and second lumbrical muscles in front. Medially it is separated from the mid-palmar space by a fibrous septum that extends deeply from the fascia on the

Fig. 222

Diagrammatic section showing the site of suppuration in nail-fold infection (paronychia) and in pulp-space infection (whitlow). In nail-fold infection the pus is beneath the cuticle and may extend under the nail, as shown. In pulp-space infection the pus lies in the tough fibro-fatty tissue immediately in front of the distal phalanx.

Fig. 223   **Fig. 224**

Figure 223—Technique of drainage of paronychial abscess. For the mildest infections it is sufficient to raise the cuticle alone without incising it; but better drainage is secured by a vertical incision through the cuticle, on one or both sides. When pus has extended beneath the nail it is necessary also to remove the proximal third of the nail (shaded area). Figure 224—Incision for drainage of pulp abscess. The incision is deepened across the pulp, in front of the phalanx, and the abscess cavity is cleared out under direct vision.

deep surface of the flexor tendons to the fascia covering the interossei and adductor pollicis muscle (Figs 225 and 226). The space is prolonged forwards into the delicate sheath that surrounds the first lumbrical muscle. It sometimes communicates also with the second lumbrical canal. The lumbrical canals thus provide a potential communication between the subcutaneous web spaces and the thenar space: in practice, however, it is rare for infection to spread along this route.

The mid-palmar space. This lies under the medial (ulnar) half of the hollow of the palm. It is the interval between the interossei and metacarpal bones behind and the flexor tendons (in their sheaths) of the middle, ring, and little fingers in front (Fig. 225). Laterally, it is separated from the thenar space by the fibrous septum already described. The space is prolonged forwards into the sheaths of the second, third, and fourth lumbrical muscles (Fig. 226). Again, despite the potential communication between a web space and the mid-palmar space along the lumbrical canals, web-space infection very seldom spreads deeply to involve the palm.

The flexor tendon sheaths. Distinction must be made between the tough fibrous sheaths, which exist only in the digits, and the flimsy synovial sheaths, which line the fibrous sheaths and, in the case of the thumb and little finger, extend proximally into the palm. In acute infections of the tendon sheaths (acute infective tenosynovitis) the pus is within the

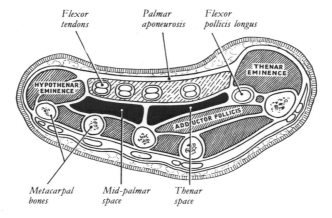

Fig. 225

The deep palmar spaces—the thenar space and the mid-palmar space—shown in diagrammatic transverse section.

Fig. 226   **Fig. 227**

Figure 226—Surface marking of the deep palmar spaces. The thenar space is continuous with the first lumbrical canal and the mid-palmar space with the second, third, and fourth lumbrical canals. Figure 227—Incisions for drainage through the web spaces.

synovial sheath and it is confined only by the limits of the sheath. The flexor sheaths of the index, middle, and ring fingers end proximally at the level of the transverse palmar skin crease (Fig. 228). The sheaths of the thumb and little finger extend proximally through the palm to end 2 or 3 centimetres above the level of the wrist. The proximal part of the sheath for the thumb is known as the radial bursa. The sheath for the little finger opens out proximally into the ulnar bursa, which encloses the grouped tendons of flexor digitorum superficialis and flexor digitorum profundus (Fig. 228).

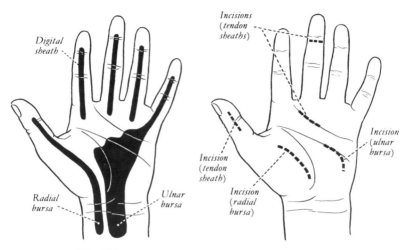

Fig. 228   **Fig. 229**

Figure 228—The synovial flexor sheaths. Whereas the sheaths for the index, middle and ring fingers end proximally at the bases of the fingers those for the thumb and little finger extend upwards to become continuous with the radial bursa and the ulnar bursa respectively. Figure 229—Incisions for drainage and irrigation of tendon sheaths and bursae.

Clinical features. In general, the symptoms of acute hand infections are local pain (often with throbbing), swelling and loss of function. There is often some degree of constitutional disturbance, with pyrexia.

On examination there are obvious swelling, redness of the skin (except in deep infections), and marked local tenderness over the site of the infection. Special features of the individual lesions are described in the following pages.

Principles of treatment. Before suppuration has occurred, the aim of treatment is to abort the infection and avoid the need for operation. The essentials of this expectant treatment are rest for the hand, elevation of the limb, and antibiotic drugs. In a minor case it may be sufficient to support the hand in a sling, but in a severe case rest is best assured by a light plaster back-splint, and elevation may be maintained by suspending the limb in a roller towel attached above the side of the bed. The question of antibiotics is difficult because the sensitivity of the organism is not at first known. Flucloxacillin is usually given, often in conjunction with ampicillin. Regrettably, patients are not often seen early enough to permit success from this expectant treatment.

When suppuration has already occurred, as indicated by severe throbbing pain, intense local tenderness, pyrexia, and loss of function, the abscess should be drained surgically without further delay. After adequate drainage has been secured the wound may be packed lightly open with vaselined gauze for two days. Thereafter, dry dressings are used and active finger exercises are encouraged.

COMMENT
There has been much discussion on the technique of surgical drainage for hand infections. It is necessary to emphasise certain general principles. These are as follows. First, the operation must be done under favourable conditions and without undue hurry. Anaesthesia may be general or regional (nerve block), but it should allow time for deliberate exploration of the abscess under a tourniquet, so that its full extent can be ascertained. Secondly, the incision must be adequate to allow complete emptying of the abscess. Thirdly, the incision must not endanger important underlying structures. Fourthly, the incision must be so sited that the resulting scar is innocuous. Within the limits imposed by these principles there is often more than one way of performing the actual drainage operation.

SPECIAL FEATURES OF INDIVIDUAL LESIONS

NAIL-FOLD INFECTION (paronychia). This is one of the commonest but least serious types of hand infection. *Clinical features*: There are pain, redness, and swelling at one or both sides of the nail fold and at the base of the nail. There is local tenderness over the reddened area. If suppuration has extended deep to the nail there is marked tenderness on pressure upon the nail. *Complications*: These are: 1) extension to the pulp space; and 2) chronic paronychia, following inadequate treatment of the acute infection. *Treatment*: In this type of infection conservative measures are often successful if begun within a few hours of the onset. When local suppuration has occurred the subcuticular abscess is drained by raising the cuticle from the nail or by raising it as a short flap after incising it vertically at one or both corners (Fig. 223). If pus has extended under the nail the proximal third of the nail must also be removed.

PULP-SPACE INFECTION (whitlow). This is almost as common as nail-fold infection. *Clinical features*: The pulp is swollen, tense and tender. Severe throbbing pain, with exquisite localised tenderness, suggests that suppuration is present. *Complications*: These are: 1) osteomyelitis of the terminal phalanx, often leading to necrosis and sequestration of its distal half; 2) pyogenic arthritis of the distal interphalangeal joint; and 3) very rarely, spread of infection to the flexor tendon sheath (suppurative tenosynovitis). *Treatment*: Conservative measures are seldom successful except in the earliest stages. Surgical drainage is effected well by a lateral incision just in front of the plane of the terminal phalanx (Fig. 224); it is deepened transversely across the pulp of the finger but should not extend proximally beyond a point half a centimetre distal to the terminal skin crease lest the flexor tendon sheath be inadvertently opened. An alternative method is to incise directly into the pulp over the centre of the abscess, a technique that is to be preferred if the abscess is already threatening to point at the surface.

SUBCUTANEOUS INFECTIONS (other than pulp-space infections). These infections are common. *Clinical features*: The infection may arise in any part of the hand or fingers. Common sites are the middle or proximal segment of a finger, and the web spaces. There is localised swelling with redness and tenderness. In many cases the infection has spread through the skin from a subcuticular infection or blister. Care must be taken not to confuse subcutaneous infections with the deep space infections. *Complications*: These are: 1) sloughing of skin over the lesion; and 2) spread to the deep space or to the flexor tendon sheaths. *Treatment*: Surgical drainage is by a short incision appropriately placed to reach the abscess without harming important structures or leaving an awkward scar. In the case of a web-space infection the incision should not divide the skin fold of the web: a short transverse incision in the palm just proximal to the skin fold is adequate (Fig. 227).

THENAR SPACE INFECTION. This is a very uncommon lesion. It may arise by extension from a subcutaneous lesion or a tendon sheath infection. *Clinical features*: The radial half of the palm is ballooned out and the swelling extends to the dorsal aspect of the web between thumb and index finger. *Treatment*: Drainage is by an incision at the dorsal aspect of the first web space (Fig. 227).

MID-PALMAR SPACE INFECTION. This is also uncommon. It usually arises by extension from a subcutaneous lesion or a tendon sheath infection. *Clinical features*: The ulnar half of the palm is ballooned out. Movements of the fingers are restricted and painful. *Treatment*: Drainage can be established through the web space between the middle and ring fingers or through that between the ring and little fingers (Fig. 227).

TENDON SHEATH INFECTION. This is rare, but important because prompt treatment is essential if the function of the finger is to be preserved. *Clinical features*: The finger is swollen throughout its length, and acutely tender over the flexor tendon sheath. It is held semiflexed and the patient is unwilling to extend it because of pain. *Complications*: These are: 1) necrosis of the tendons and adhesions between tendon and sheath, causing permanent stiffness of the finger in semi-flexion; and 2) spread of infection to involve the radial bursa (from the flexor sheath of the thumb), or the ulnar bursa (from the sheath of the little finger). *Treatment*: Systemic antibiotic therapy is begun immediately. The sheath is opened at its proximal end in the palm and at its distal end (Fig. 229), and irrigated with antibiotic solution through a fine tube passed along the sheath; the tube is withdrawn and the wounds are packed lightly open.

If the radial bursa or the ulnar bursa is infected it must be drained and irrigated through an additional incision in the palm (Fig. 229).

CHRONIC INFECTIVE TENOSYNOVITIS

(Including compound palmar ganglion)

Chronic inflammation of tendon sheaths in the lower forearm and hand may occur in response to low-grade infection. It is entirely distinct from acute tenosynovitis and is not preceded by it. It is now uncommon in Britain.

Cause. In most cases it is caused by infection with the tubercle bacillus. Sometimes other organisms are responsible. A similar condition may complicate rheumatoid arthritis without demonstrable bacterial infection (see p. 256).

Pathology. The flexor tendon sheaths in the lower forearm and hand are those most commonly affected; less often the lesion is confined to the extensor sheaths. The affected sheaths are greatly thickened and show the changes of chronic inflammation. In most cases there is histological evidence of tuberculosis. The sheaths often contain an excess of fluid and there may be collections of small fibrinous bodies. The tendons themselves are affected only slightly.

Fig. 230
Compound palmar ganglion. The swellings in the palm and at the front of the wrist are continuous deep to the flexor retinaculum, and fluctuation can be elicited between them.

Clinical features. There is a gradual onset of swelling, with mild aching pain, in the region of the affected tendon sheaths—usually the flexor sheaths of the lower forearm and hand. The function of the fingers and thumb is impaired.

On examination the swelling is confined to the line of the tendon sheaths. Characteristically it affects the lowest 5 or 6 centimetres of the front of the forearm and the proximal part of the palm (Fig. 230). Sometimes the flexor sheaths of the fingers and thumb are also swollen, giving the digits a fusiform appearance. In many cases fluctuation can be elicited between the forearm swelling and the swelling in the palm. This clinical sign depends upon the presence of fluid within the tendon sheaths, and it is not always found. The fully developed condition, with swelling in forearm and palm and fluctuation between the two, constitutes *compound palmar ganglion.*

At first the range of movements of the fingers and thumb is impaired only slightly, if at all. Later, there is moderate restriction of flexion and extension of the digits, with corresponding loss of function. A tuberculous lesion may be discovered elsewhere in the body.

Diagnosis. Persistent swelling of gradual onset in the line of the tendon sheaths in the lower forearm and hand always suggests chronic tenosynovitis. Fluctuation between the forearm swelling and the palmar swelling provides strong corroborative evidence. If an active tuberculous lesion is found elsewhere in the body it is reasonable to infer that the tenosynovitis is also tuberculous.

Treatment. In mild cases in which the function of the fingers and thumb is not impaired conservative treatment is advised. The wrist and forearm are immobilised in plaster of Paris for two months, the fingers being left free. In tuberculous cases a course of the appropriate antibacterial drugs is given (see p. 120).

In severe or intractable cases operation is recommended. It consists in excising thoroughly all the thickened and oedematous synovial membrane. After operation finger movements are encouraged and practised daily under the supervision of a physiotherapist. A useful range of finger movement is usually restored, but permanent inability to flex the fingers fully into the palm may have to be accepted.

BONE TUMOURS IN THE HAND

BENIGN TUMOURS
(General description of benign tumours of bone, p. 80)

The only bone tumour that requires special mention here is the benign chondroma.

Fig. 231
Multiple enchondromata in the metacarpals and phalanges.

CHONDROMA

A chondroma or benign cartilage tumour occurs in two forms: *enchondroma*, which grows within the bone and expands it; and *ecchondroma*, which grows mainly outwards from the surface of the bone. Both types are prone to occur in the metacarpals and phalanges of the hand. The tumour may be solitary, but in the condition known as dyschondroplasia, multiple chondromatosis or Ollier's disease the tumours may affect many bones in the hand as well as any of the long bones, pelvic bones or scapula, and they may cause ugly swelling and deformity of the fingers (Fig. 231). Malignant transformation is hardly known in a solitary chondroma of a bone of the hand, but it is a possibility in cases of multiple chondromatosis.

Treatment. If small, the tumour should be treated expectantly. Operation is required only if it is found to be enlarging. Large tumours should be excised, the bone substance being restored, if necessary, by grafts of cancellous bone. If the tumours are multiple excision should be advised only for any one or more that may be causing trouble.

MALIGNANT TUMOURS

(General description of malignant tumours of bone, p. 84)

Malignant tumours of the bones of the hand are uncommon. Mention is required only of chondrosarcoma and of metastatic carcinoma.

CHONDROSARCOMA
Rarely, this may arise in a previously existing benign chondroma, especially in the multiple form of chondromatosis (dyschondroplasia; Ollier's disease).

CARCINOMA
A carcinoma, especially from the lung, rarely metastasises to a phalanx, destroying the bone. It may simulate closely an infective lesion, and the correct diagnosis may be overlooked at first.

SOFT-TISSUE TUMOURS IN THE HAND

(General description of soft-tissue tumours, p. 104)

Special mention must be made of an unusual tumour that is seldom encountered outside the hand—namely, the giant-cell tumour of tendon sheath (localised nodular tenosynovitis).

GIANT-CELL TUMOURS OF TENDON SHEATH
This is a benign tumour, but it sometimes recurs locally unless it is removed entire. It arises from the sheath of a tendon, or from the fibrous expansion of an extensor tendon in a finger. As it enlarges it burrows between the tissue planes, taking the line of least resistance. Eventually it may form a bulky mass which almost surrounds the finger like a collar. On section the tumour is fleshy; histologically it is composed of cells of many forms, including round cells, giant cells of foreign-body type, xanthoma cells containing cholesterol, and fibroblasts.

Treatment. The tumour should be excised entire.

COMPRESSION OF MEDIAN NERVE IN CARPAL TUNNEL

(Carpal tunnel syndrome)

Constriction of the median nerve as it passes beneath the flexor retinaculum is a common cause of discomfort in the hand, especially in middle-aged or elderly women.

Cause. Any space-occupying lesion within the carpal tunnel may be responsible. Recognised causes are chronic inflammatory thickening of the tendon sheaths (as in rheumatoid arthritis), osteoarthritis of the wrist, thickening after fracture of the lower end of the radius, and myxoedema. In many cases no primary cause can be discovered.

Pathology. The median nerve lies beneath the flexor retinaculum in company with the flexor tendons of the hand. If the available space within this strong-walled tunnel is reduced the nerve is compressed against the flexor retinaculum. When the retinaculum is divided in such a case the nerve may be found constricted where it lay behind it. The ulnar nerve does not pass behind the flexor retinaculum; so it is not liable to compression in this way.

Clinical features. The condition is commonest in women in or beyond middle life. The symptoms are sensory and motor. There is tingling, numbness, or discomfort in the radial three and a half digits (that is, in the median distribution), and there is a feeling of clumsiness in carrying out fine movements such as those concerned in sewing. Distressing tingling is often prominent during the night: the patient may have to work the fingers or shake the hand to gain relief.

On examination the findings vary with the degree and duration of the compression. At first there are no objective findings. Later there may be blunting of sensibility in the median distribution. In a severe case there may eventually be evident wasting and weakness of the median-innervated small muscles of the hand.

Investigations. Electrical tests may show decreased conduction velocity in the affected part of the median nerve.

Diagnosis. Care must be taken to exclude other causes of neurological disturbance in the hand, especially those arising in the neck from interference with the brachial plexus, and lesions of the median nerve elsewhere in its course.

Treatment. A trial may be made of conservative treatment by supporting the wrist for three weeks with a simple splint. When the symptoms arise in pregnancy, relief that lasts until after delivery (when the symptoms usually subside spontaneously) may be gained by the injection of hydrocortisone alongside the nerve at wrist level. This may be tried also in other cases. If it is unsuccessful full relief is assured by dividing the flexor retinaculum to decompress the nerve, an operation that may be done either through an open incision or (with slightly greater risk to the median nerve) by an endoscopic technique.

GANGLION
(Simple ganglion)

A ganglion is the commonest cystic swelling at the back of the wrist.

Pathology. Conflicting views have been put forward on the origin of ganglia. Some believe that they represent a degenerative process. Others claim that they are benign tumours of tendon sheath or joint capsule. The cyst wall is of fibrous tissue and there is no true endothelial lining. It is connected at some point with a joint capsule or tendon sheath, but there is no communication between the joint cavity or tendon sheath and the interior of the cyst. The cyst is usually unilocular. The contained fluid is clear and viscous.

Clinical features. Ganglia are commonest at the back of the wrist, where they are often seen in adults of any age (Fig. 232). They also occur, less commonly, at the front of the wrist, or in the palm or fingers. Ordinarily there are no symptoms other than the swelling itself and, sometimes, discomfort or slight pain. *On examination* the swelling may be soft and obviously cystic, but more often it is tense. It is often mistaken for a bony prominence—but careful tests will show that it is fluctuant.

Fig. 232
A simple ganglion at the back of the wrist. This is the commonest site.

Complications. A ganglion arising deeply in the wrist or palm may interfere mechanically with the ulnar or the median nerve or their branches. There will be motor and usually sensory impairment in the distribution of the particular branch affected.

Treatment. A ganglion is harmless and in the absence of pain or complications it may safely be left alone. Sometimes the ganglion can be dispersed subcutaneously by firm local pressure. This rather dramatic treatment is harmless and temporarily effective, but the ganglion may slowly reappear. An alternative method of providing temporary relief is to aspirate the cyst with a wide-bore needle. Lasting cure can be ensured only by complete excision of the ganglion—not always an easy task because the thin-walled sac often tracks deeply between the tendons, where it may be torn and a fragment left behind. In children there is a tendency to spontaneous resolution; so the question of excision may be deferred.

A ganglion that is interfering with a peripheral nerve demands operative excision without delay.

DUPUYTREN'S CONTRACTURE
(Contracture of the palmar aponeurosis; Dupuytren's disease)

This is an easily recognised condition characterised in the established phase by flexion contracture of one or more of the fingers from thickening and shortening of the palmar aponeurosis.

Cause. This is unknown. There is a hereditary predisposition. In a predisposed person injury possibly plays a part but its exact significance is uncertain. There is an increased incidence of the disorder among epileptics,

Fig. 233

Early Dupuytren's contracture. There is a nodule of thickened aponeurosis in the palm, opposite the base of the ring finger, with slight puckering of the skin; but so far there is no flexion contracture of the fingers.

Fig. 234

A typical example of Dupuytren's contracture of the palmar aponeurosis in which the ring finger has been drawn down into flexion. Note the tight band of thickened aponeurosis immediately under the skin. The band has sometimes been mistaken for a contracted flexor tendon.

but this is possibly related to the use of anticonvulsant drugs rather than to the underlying disease.

Pathology. The palmar aponeurosis (palmar fascia) is normally a thin but tough membrane whose fibres radiate from the termination of the palmaris longus tendon at the front of the wrist to gain insertion into the proximal and middle phalanges of the fingers. It lies immediately beneath the skin. In Dupuytren's contracture the aponeurosis, or part of it, becomes greatly thickened (often to half a centimetre or more), and it slowly contracts, drawing the fingers into flexion at the metacarpo-phalangeal and proximal interphalangeal joints. The medial half of the aponeurosis is affected most, and serious flexion deformity is usually confined to the ring and little fingers, with only moderate deformity of the middle finger (Figs 233 and 234). The joints themselves are unaffected at first, but in long-established cases secondary capsular contractures occur.

Fig. 235
Typical nodule in the sole of the foot in Dupuytren's disease.

The plantar aponeurosis in the foot is occasionally affected, but in the foot the lesion usually takes the form of a firm nodule under the instep rather than of a contracture involving the toes (Fig. 235). Other parts that may be affected include the penis. Thus although the hands are primarily affected, the condition is sometimes much more widespread (Dupuytren's disease).

Clinical features. The affection is much more common in men than in women. Often both hands are affected. The earliest sign is a small thickened nodule in the mid-palm opposite the base of the ring finger (Fig. 233). The area of thickening gradually spreads from this point, giving rise eventually to firm cord-like bands that extend into the ring or little finger, or both, and prevent full extension of the metacarpo-phalangeal and proximal inter-phalangeal joint (Fig. 234). The skin is closely adherent to the fascial bands, and is often puckered. The flexion deformity becomes progressively worse in the course of months or years.

In some cases these changes in the palm are accompanied by thickening over the dorsum of the interphalangeal joints (knuckle pads). The feet may also show nodules in the sole (Fig. 235). Occasionally the penis is distorted by thickened bands.

Diagnosis. The thickened bands of palmar aponeurosis must not be mistaken for contracted flexor tendons. It is easily confirmed that the bands are distinct from tendons because they do not move when the fingers are flexed and extended.

Treatment. The only effective treatment is by operation. That does not imply, however, that operation is necessary in every case: a contracture that is not progressing rapidly is often better left alone, especially in an elderly patient. Operation entails excision of the thickened part of the palmar aponeurosis by painstaking dissection. Simple division of the taut contracted bands is unsatisfactory because the contracture tends to recur. Even after competent excision there is a group of patients—often relatively young—who show a strong tendency to recurrence.

RUPTURE OR SEVERANCE OF TENDONS IN THE HAND

Most tendon divisions in the hand are caused by cuts with sharp objects such as glass or knives. Certain tendons are prone to rupture: thus the extensor tendon of a finger is easily torn from its insertion into the distal phalanx by sudden forced flexion of the finger; and the extensor pollicis longus tendon is liable to rupture spontaneously after fractures of the lower end of the radius in consequence of its becoming frayed where it crosses the roughened bone. In rheumatoid arthritis, also, spontaneous rupture—especially of an extensor tendon—is common.

Clinical features and diagnosis. Loss of function of a tendon is obvious clinically. When the findings are correlated with the history the diagnosis is usually clear.

Treatment. This varies according to the tendon affected and the site of severance or rupture (see below and Figs 236 and 237). Sometimes treatment is unnecessary or undesirable, but more often operative reconstruction is to be advised: the tendon is either sutured directly or replaced by a free tendon graft or by a tendon transfer, according to circumstances.

SPECIAL FEATURES OF INDIVIDUAL LESIONS
INJURIES OF FLEXOR TENDONS

DIVISION WITHIN A FIBROUS FLEXOR SHEATH OF A FINGER. Severance at this site presents the most difficult problem of all tendon injuries. The prognosis is uncertain after operative repair or reconstruction because of the proclivity of the tendon to adhere to the sheath.

Treatment. If a flexor superficialis tendon alone is divided and the flexor profundus is intact treatment is not required, for there is virtually no disability.

If a flexor profundus tendon alone is divided, the flexor superficialis being intact, the loss of active flexion at the distal interphalangeal joint can often be accepted. Attempted repair of the tendon is usually better avoided because of its uncertain results. Arthrodesis of the distal interphalangeal joint in slight flexion reduces the disability to a negligible level.

If both tendons are divided, operative repair or later reconstruction is advised. When the injury is recent (within one week) and the wound clean, and when good conditions and skilled staff are available, primary repair is often the method of choice. In all other cases only the skin should be sutured initially, and tendon reconstruction should be deferred until the wound is well healed and the joints are mobile.

Technique. Direct suture of the severed ends demands high technical skill and long experience. Both the superficialis tendon and the profundus tendon should be repaired, usually with sutures of fine stainless steel wire.

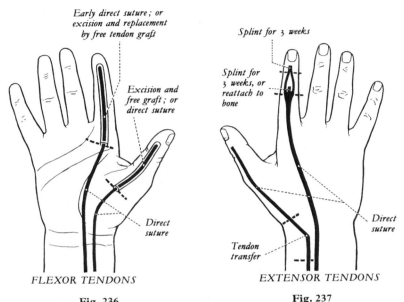

FLEXOR TENDONS

EXTENSOR TENDONS

Fig. 236　　　　　　　　**Fig. 237**

Treatment of tendon injuries at various sites. Figure 236—Flexor tendons. Figure 237—Extensor tendons. For details, see text.

Late reconstruction, in cases unsuitable for primary direct suture, is also technically demanding. The standard method is to remove the flexor superficialis tendon entire (to make more room in the sheath) and to replace the whole of the digital part of the flexor profundus tendon by a free tendon graft (from the palmaris longus or from a toe extensor) sutured proximally to the profundus tendon in the palm or at wrist level, and inserted distally into a drill hole in the distal phalanx (Fig. 238). This method eliminates the need for a tendon junction within the sheath.

In a recent two-stage modification of this technique a new synovial sheath is prepared in advance by laying in a flexible silicone-rubber rod for eight weeks before the tendon graft is inserted.

DIVISION OF FLEXOR POLLICIS LONGUS IN THE THUMB. The problem is less difficult than that presented by division of both flexor tendons in a finger. Repair may be made by direct suture, by advancement of the tendon, or by replacement of the digital part of the tendon by a free graft as described for the fingers.

DIVISION OF FLEXOR TENDONS IN THE PALM OR WRIST. Direct suture is advised. It may be done primarily if the wound is clean. The prognosis is good if a single tendon is affected but it is uncertain in cases of multiple tendon divisions at the front of the wrist, especially if the nerves are also injured.

INJURIES OF EXTENSOR TENDONS

SEVERANCE OF EXTENSOR TENDONS AT THE BACK OF THE HAND. This injury has a good prognosis. There is a tendency to spontaneous union with recovery of normal function. *Treatment*: Primary suture should be undertaken if the injury is recent. If there has been delay, freshening and direct suture of the divided ends is advised. Repair of a spontaneously ruptured extensor tendon in rheumatoid arthritis has a less satisfactory prognosis because the tendon is of impaired quality. Operative repair should usually be attempted.

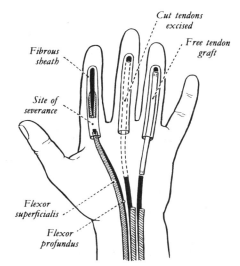

Fig. 238
Tendon graft for reconstruction of severed flexor tendons in the digital sheath. Successive stages of the operation are shown in the index, middle, and ring fingers. The use of a free graft eliminates the need for a tendon junction within the sheath.

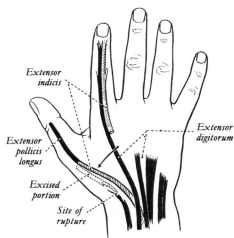

Fig. 239
Transfer of extensor indicis to replace a ruptured extensor pollicis longus. The tendon of extensor indicis is divided opposite the neck of the second metacarpal, re-routed towards the thumb, and sutured to the freshened distal stump of the extensor pollicis longus. This transfer is to be preferred to direct suture when the ends of the ruptured tendon are frayed.

RUPTURE OF EXTENSOR POLLICIS LONGUS TENDON may complicate fracture of the lower end of the radius. The tendon gives way after becoming frayed by repeated movement over the roughened lower end of the radius. Spontaneous rupture may also occur in drummers. The extensive fraying makes direct suture unsatisfactory. *Treatment*: A clean rupture should be sutured end-to-end. If the tendon is frayed, as is usually the case, a tendon transfer operation is to be preferred. The tendon of extensor indicis is divided at the level of the neck of the second metacarpal bone, re-routed towards the thumb, and sutured to the freshened distal stump of the extensor pollicis longus (Fig. 239).

RUPTURE OF MIDDLE SLIP OF EXTENSOR EXPANSION. This is caused by sudden forced flexion of the proximal interphalangeal joint, the middle slip of the extensor expansion being torn from its attachment to the middle phalanx. The patient is unable to extend the proximal interphalangeal joint fully. The distal joint becomes hyperextended. *Treatment*: The choice lies between immobilisation on a splint in the straight position for three weeks, or operative repair. In a fresh case simple splintage probably gives the better results, though restoration of full function is seldom achieved.

Fig. 240
Mallet finger (baseball finger). The extensor tendon is avulsed from its insertion. The terminal joint cannot be extended fully.

AVULSION OF EXTENSOR TENDON from distal phalanx of a finger. This is known as 'mallet' finger or 'baseball' finger. It is caused by sudden forced flexion of the distal interphalangeal joint—for instance, by a blow on the tip of the finger from a ball. In a few cases a small fragment of bone is avulsed with the tendon. The patient is unable fully to extend the distal interphalangeal joint (Fig. 240). *Treatment*: Immediate treatment is to splint the finger for three weeks with the distal interphalangeal joint fully extended. Splintage must be continuous and uninterrupted if a good result is to be achieved. The avulsed tendon always unites to the bone, but often with lengthening, in which case some deformity persists. However, the disability is usually insignificant and acceptable.

DE QUERVAIN'S TENOVAGINITIS
(Tenovaginitis of the abductor pollicis longus and extensor pollicis brevis)

This is a common and well recognised condition characterised by pain over the styloid process of the radius and a palpable nodule in the course of the abductor pollicis longus and extensor pollicis brevis tendons.

Cause. The precise cause is unknown. Excessive friction from over-use may be a factor, because the condition seems prone to follow oft-repeated actions such as wringing clothes.

Pathology. The fibrous sheaths of the abductor pollicis longus and extensor pollicis brevis tendons are thickened where they cross the tip of the radial styloid process. The tendons themselves appear normal. The condition is possibly analogous to that other common form of tenovaginitis, 'trigger' finger (see below).

Clinical features. The condition is commonest in middle-aged women. The main symptom is pain on using the hand, especially when movement tenses the abductor pollicis longus and extensor pollicis brevis tendons (as in lifting a saucepan or a teapot). *On examination* there is local tenderness at the point where the tendons cross the radial styloid process (Fig. 241); the thickened fibrous sheaths are usually palpable as a firm nodule. Passive adduction of the wrist or thumb causes the patient to wince with pain.

Treatment. There is a tendency to very slow natural recovery with rest, or after the local injection of hydrocortisone. But operation provides so

Fig. 241
Site of tenderness in de Quervain's tenovaginitis.

certain a cure that it should always be advised if the disability is severe. All that is necessary is to slit or 'de-roof' the offending tendon sheaths.

DIGITAL TENOVAGINITIS STENOSANS
('Trigger' finger; snapping finger)

In this rather common condition thickening and constriction of the mouth of a fibrous digital sheath interfere with the free gliding of the contained flexor tendons.

Cause. This is unknown.

Pathology. The proximal part of the fibrous flexor sheath at the base of a finger or thumb is thickened and the mouth of the sheath is constricted. The contained tendons become 'waisted' opposite the constriction, and swollen

Swelling of tendon

Thickened tendon sheath

Fig. 242
Mechanism of trigger finger. The swollen part of the tendon is reluctant to enter the constricted mouth of the fibrous sheath when an attempt is made to extend the finger. When sufficient force is exerted it enters with a snap. The thickening forms a palpable nodule at the base of the finger.

proximal to it. The swollen segment enters the mouth of the sheath only with difficulty when an attempt is made to straighten the finger from the flexed position (Fig. 242).

Clinical features. The condition occurs: 1) in the fingers of the middle-aged (especially women); and 2) in the thumb in infants or young children.

The adult type. There is complaint of tenderness at the base of the affected finger and of locking of the finger in full flexion (Figs 243 and 244). The locking can be overcome either by a strong effort or by extending the finger passively with the other hand, when the flexion is released with a distinct snap. *On examination* there is a palpable nodule, usually slightly tender, at the base of the affected finger or thumb—that is, over the mouth of the fibrous flexor sheath. The snapping cannot be reproduced on passive movements; it can be demonstrated only when the patient flexes the finger fully with its own muscles.

Fig. 243   **Fig. 244**

Trigger finger. The fingers can be flexed without difficulty (Fig. 243), but when the patient attempts to straighten them the affected finger sticks in the position shown (Fig. 244).

The infantile type (contracted thumb of infants). The infant is unable to straighten the thumb, which is locked in flexion. *On examination* it may be possible to extend the thumb passively with a snap, but in many cases the flexed position of the joint cannot be corrected even by moderate force. A palpable nodule is present at the base of the thumb in the position of the mouth of the fibrous flexor sheath—that is, at the level of the head of the metacarpal bone. It should be noted that because the deformity is often resistant to correction this condition in infants is often mistaken for a dislocated thumb or for a congenital deformity.

Treatment. Both the adult and the infantile type can be cured by the simple operation of incising the mouth of the fibrous flexor sheath longitudinally.

EXTRINSIC DISORDERS SIMULATING DISEASE OF THE FOREARM OR HAND

DISORDERS OF THE NECK

Certain disorders of the neck interfere with the brachial plexus or its roots, and thereby produce their predominant symptoms—or even their only symptoms—in the lower arm or hand. By far the commonest of such disorders are osteoarthritis of the cervical spine (cervical spondylosis) and prolapse of a cervical intervertebral disc. Less common as causes of peripheral symptoms are cervical rib, tumours of the spinal column or of the spinal cord, and soft-tissue tumours involving nerves. All these conditions were described in Chapter 9.

Rarely, neck disorders affect the lower arm or hand by interfering with the subclavian artery. Examples are occasionally seen in cases of cervical rib, or when the artery is obstructed by a tumour or aneurysm.

TUMOUR AT THE THORACIC INLET

A mass at the thoracic inlet is an occasional cause of peripheral symptoms in the upper limb. The commonest cause is an apical tumour of the lung (Pancoast tumour) involving the nerves of the brachial plexus.

DISORDERS OF THE UPPER ARM

Rarely, a disorder of the upper arm may produce its chief effects in the lower arm or hand, usually through the medium of the major nerve trunks. A well known example is crutch palsy, in which there is weakness or paralysis of the extensor muscles of the wrist, fingers and thumb from repeated pressure of a crutch upon the radial nerve in the axilla. Occasionally the axillary artery has been injured in the same way, with consequent ischaemic manifestations in the digits. These complications are avoided if elbow crutches can be used instead of axillary crutches.

DISORDERS OF THE ELBOW

Affections of the elbow may be associated with vague referred pain in the forearm. This is especially true of tennis elbow, in which the pain extends along the extensor aspect of the forearm, often to the hand. Almost always, however, the local symptoms in the elbow overshadow the referred symptoms; so mistakes in diagnosis are unlikely.

In the condition of friction neuritis of the ulnar nerve, the symptoms and signs are predominantly in the hand, and one might suspect a local disorder of the hand itself if the possibility of a lesion at the elbow were not considered and investigated.

References and bibliography, page 403.

14. The hip region

The hip presents some of the most fascinating problems in the whole field of orthopaedic surgery. Practically and economically, its injuries and diseases are important because they so often cause prolonged suffering and serious disablement—even total incapacity. Academically, the region is of interest for several reasons: the mechanics of the joint are complex; it is one of the most difficult joints to examine with accuracy; and—of special significance to students—cases of hip disease are often presented as tests of clinical acumen in the examinations in surgery. Time spent on learning how to examine the hip correctly will usually be well rewarded.

Table IX
Usual age incidence of common hip disorders at time of diagnosis

Age at time of diagnosis (years)	Disease
0–2	Congenital dislocation
2–5	Tuberculous arthritis; transient synovitis
5–10	Perthes' disease; transient synovitis
10–20	Slipped upper femoral epiphysis
20–50	Osteoarthritis (secondary to previous injury or disease)
50–100	Osteoarthritis (primary)

SPECIAL POINTS IN THE INVESTIGATION OF HIP COMPLAINTS

History
The characteristics of hip pain. Pain in the region of the hip is notoriously misleading, for often it is referred from the spine or pelvis and has no connection with the hip joint itself. Therefore one must always be cautious in attributing such pain to a hip lesion without first investigating the possibility of an extrinsic cause.

Pain arising in the hip is felt mainly in the groin and in the front or inner side of the thigh. Pain is often referred also to the knee; indeed pain in the knee is sometimes the predominant feature. In contrast, the 'hip' pain that is referred from the spine is felt mainly in the gluteal region, whence it often radiates down the back or outer side of the thigh.

True hip pain is made worse by walking, whereas gluteal pain referred from the spine is aggravated by activities such as stooping and lifting, and it is often eased by walking.

Age incidence of hip disorders. Many of the important disorders of the hip occur in childhood, and often at a particular period of childhood. So true is this with some disorders that the age of the patient at the onset of symptoms affords some indication of the likely nature of the trouble, as shown in Table IX. (For ease of memorising, round figures have been given in the table but some latitude must be allowed.)

Table X
Routine clinical examination in suspected disorders
of the hip

1. LOCAL EXAMINATION OF THE HIP REGION

(Patient supine)
Position of pelvis
Determine the lie of the pelvis and set it square with the limbs if possible

Inspection
Bone contours and alignment
Soft-tissue contours
Colour and texture of skin
Scars or sinuses

Palpation
Skin temperature
Bone contours
Soft-tissue contours
Local tenderness

Measurement of limb length
Real or true length:
Measure from anterior superior iliac spine to medial malleolus. (Angle between pelvis and limbs to be equal on each side)
If discrepancy found, determine site of shortening:
(a) Above trochanter (Bryant's triangle; Nelaton's line; Schoemaker's line)
(b) Below trochanter (measure each bone)
'Apparent' or false discrepancy:
Measure from xiphisternum to medial malleolus. (Limbs to be parallel and in line with trunk)

Examination for fixed deformity
Including Thomas's manoeuvre for detection and measurement of fixed flexion deformity

Movements (active and passive)
Flexion
Abduction; abduction in flexion
Adduction
Medial (internal) rotation
Lateral (external) rotation

Power (tested against resistance of examiner)
Estimate strength of each muscle group: flexors, extensors, abductors, adductors, rotators

Examination for abnormal mobility
Test for longitudinal (telescopic) movement
Click test (in new-born)

(Patient standing)
Examination for postural stability
Trendelenburg's test

Gait

2. EXAMINATION OF POTENTIAL EXTRINSIC SOURCES OF HIP SYMPTOMS

This is important if a satisfactory explanation for the symptoms is not found on local examination. The investigation should include: 1) the spine and sacro-iliac joints; 2) the abdomen and pelvis; 3) the knee; and 4) the major blood vessels (arterial circulation).

3. GENERAL EXAMINATION

General survey of other parts of the body. The local symptoms may be only one manifestation of a widespread of generalised disease.

Exposure
For the proper examination of the hip the patient should be stripped except for a pelvic slip or underpants and, in women, a brassière. The first part of the examination is conducted with the patient lying supine; afterwards the patient is examined standing and walking.

Steps in clinical examination
A suggested routine for clinical examination of the hip is summarised in Table X.

Setting the pelvis square
This is an important preliminary step. Determine from the position of the anterior superior iliac spines whether or not the pelvis is lying square with the limbs (Fig. 245). If it is not, an attempt is made to set it square. If this is impossible it means that there is incorrectable

Fig. 245
First step in the clinical examination of the hip: determining the lie of the pelvis.

adduction or abduction at one or other hip (or, rarely, a severe and rigid curvature of the spine): in that event the fact that the pelvis is tilted should be noted and borne in mind during the subsequent steps of the examination.

Figs 246 and 247
'Apparent' or false discrepancy in limb length is caused entirely by incorrect- able lateral tilting of the pelvis, which effectively abducts one hip and adducts the other hip (Fig. 246). If the pelvis is square with the limbs there can be no 'apparent' discrepancy in limb length (Fig. 247).

Fig. 246

Fig. 247

Measuring the length of the limbs
Methods of measuring the lower limbs are often confusing to the uninitiated, but it is important that they should be properly understood. Accuracy in measurement is of more than academic significance; it is of practical importance when corrective operations or adjustments to the shoes are contemplated. Limb length can be measured clinically within an error of one centimetre. If greater accuracy is needed, radiographic measurement (scanography) is recommended.

It is necessary to measure, first, the real or *true length* of each limb. Secondly, it is necessary to determine whether there is any '*apparent*' or *false discrepancy* in the length of the limbs from fixed pelvic tilt (Figs 246 and 247). Whereas it is always necessary to measure the true length, it is necessary to measure 'apparent' discrepancy only when there is an incorrectable pelvic tilt.

Measurement of true length. Ideally it would be desirable to measure from the normal axis of hip movement—that is, the centre of the femoral head—but since there is no surface landmark at that point it is impracticable to do so clinically. The measurement is therefore taken from the nearest convenient landmark—namely, the anterior superior spine of the ilium. Distally, measurement is usually made to the medial malleolus.

Fixed
adduction
deformity

Sound limb
adducted
through
equal angle

Fig. 248   **Fig. 249**

Figure 248—Since the anterior superior spine is lateral to the hip joint abduction approximates the foot to it and adduction carries the foot away from it. For this reason measurements of true length, taken from the anterior superior spine, are inaccurate if the angle of abduction or adduction is not equal on the two sides. Figure 249—Correct way of measuring the true length when there is a fixed adduction deformity of one hip. The other hip must be adducted through an equal angle. (Position of tape measure shown by interrupted lines.)

It should be noted that the anterior superior spine is well lateral to the axis of hip movement. This is of no consequence if the angle between limb and pelvis is the same on each side. But it will render the measurements fallacious if the angle between limb and pelvis is not the same on each side. This will be understood best by reference to Figure 248. It will be seen that abduction of a limb brings the medial malleolus nearer to the corresponding anterior superior spine, whereas adduction of the limb carries the medial malleolus away from the anterior superior spine. Thus if measurements are made while the patient lies with one hip adducted and the other abducted (a common posture in cases of hip disease) inaccurate readings will be obtained: the length will be exaggerated on the adducted side and belittled on the abducted side.

The rule is, therefore, that *to obtain an accurate comparison of their true length by surface measurement the two limbs must be placed in comparable positions relative to the pelvis.* Thus if one limb is adducted and cannot be brought out to the neutral position the other limb must be adducted through a corresponding angle by crossing it over the first limb before the measurements are taken (Fig. 249). Similarly, if one hip is in fixed abduction the other must be abducted through the same angle before the measurements of true length are made.

Fixing the tape measure at the anterior superior spine. A flat metal end (as found on the ordinary tailor's measure) is essential. The metal end is placed immediately *distal* to the anterior superior spine and is pushed up against it. The thumb is then pressed firmly backwards against the bone and the tape end together (Fig. 250). This gives rigid fixation of the tape measure against the bone.

Fig. 250
Fixing the tape measure at the
anterior superior spine.

Taking the reading at the medial malleolus. The tip of the index finger is placed immediately distal to the medial malleolus and pushed up against it. The thumb nail is brought down against the tip of the index finger so that the tape measure is pinched between them (Fig. 251). The point of measurement is indicated by the thumb nail.

Fig. 251
Taking the measurement at the
medial malleolus.

Determining the site of true shortening. If measurements reveal real shortening of a limb it is necessary to determine whether the shortening is above the trochanteric level (suggesting an affection in or near the hip), or below the trochanteric level (suggesting an affection of the limb bones).

Shortening above the greater trochanter.[1] Tests for shortening above the trochanteric level are: 1) the measurement of Bryant's triangle; 2) the construction of Nelaton's line; and 3) the construction of Schoemaker's line.

Bryant's triangle. In principle, this is nothing more than a method of comparing the distance between the greater trochanter and the wing of the ilium on the two sides. With the patient lying supine a perpendicular is dropped from the anterior superior spine of the ilium towards the couch. A second line is projected upwards from the tip of the greater trochanter to meet the first line at a right angle. This is the important line of the triangle: it is measured and compared on the two sides. (The third side of the triangle is unimportant. It joins the anterior superior spine to the tip of the greater trochanter.)

---

[1]The measurements described under this heading are seldom if ever carried out in practice because the information that they give is more easily obtained from radiographs. Nevertheless the student is still expected sometimes to know the principles of the tests for examination purposes.

Measurement of Bryant's triangle gives a comparison between the pelvis-to-trochanter distance on each side.[1] Relative shortening on one side indicates that the femur is displaced upwards in consequence of a lesion in or near the hip. But if there is a possibility that both sides are abnormal measurement of Bryant's triangle is not helpful.

Nelaton's line. With the patient lying on the sound side, a tape measure or string is stretched on the affected side from the tuberosity of the ischium to the anterior superior spine of the ilium. Normally the greater trochanter lies on or below that line. If the trochanter lies above the line the femur has been displaced upwards.

Schoemaker's line. This is a similar test. A line is projected on each side of the body from the greater trochanter through and beyond the anterior superior spine. Normally the two lines meet in the midline above the umbilicus. If one femur is displaced upwards owing to shortening above the greater trochanter the lines will meet away from the midline on the opposite side. If both femora are displaced upwards the lines will meet at or near the midline but below the umbilicus.

Shortening distal to the trochanter. True shortening is sometimes caused by an abnormality below the trochanteric level, such as a congenital defect of development, impaired epiphysial growth, or a previous fracture with overlapping of the fragments. To investigate this possibility individual measurements should be made of the femur (tip of greater trochanter to line of knee joint) and of the tibia (line of knee joint to medial malleolus) on each side.

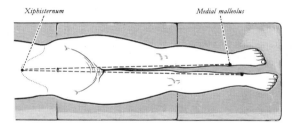

Xiphisternum   *Medial malleolus*

Fig. 252

For correct measurement of 'apparent' discrepancy in limb length the limbs must be parallel and in line with the trunk. (Position of tape-measure shown by interrupted lines.)

Measurement of 'apparent' discrepancy in limb length. 'Apparent' or false discrepancy in limb length is due entirely to incorrectable sideways tilting of the pelvis (Fig. 246). The usual cause is a fixed adduction deformity at one hip, giving an appearance of shortening on that side, or a fixed abduction deformity, giving an appearance of lengthening. Exceptionally, fixed pelvic obliquity is caused by severe lumbar scoliosis.

To measure apparent discrepancy the limbs must be placed parallel to one another and in line with the trunk. Measurement is made from any fixed point in the midline of the trunk (for example, the xiphisternum) to each medial malleolus (Fig. 252).

If there is a discrepancy of true length it must be allowed for when 'apparent' discrepancy is determined.

Examination for fixed deformity

Contracture of the joint capsule or of muscles may cause fixed deformity at the hip, preventing its being placed in a neutral position. Fixed flexion, fixed adduction, and fixed lateral rotation are common in some forms of arthritis.

Fixed adduction deformity. This is detected by judging the relationship between pelvis and limbs. It will already have been noted at an earlier stage of the examination. If fixed adduction is present the transverse axis of the pelvis (as indicated by a line joining the two anterior superior spines) cannot be set at right angles to the affected limb, but lies at an acute angle with it.

---

[1] A simpler and equally informative method is to measure, on each side, the distance between the tip of the greater trochanter and the highest point of the iliac crest.

Fixed abduction deformity. The angle between the transverse axis of the pelvis and the limb is greater than 90 degrees.

Fixed flexion deformity. This is determined by a manoeuvre known as Thomas's test.

Principle of Thomas's test. If a patient has a fixed flexion deformity at the hip he compensates for it, when lying on his back, by arching the spine and pelvis into exaggerated lordosis, as shown in Figure 253. This allows the affected limb to lie flat on the couch. To measure the angle of fixed flexion deformity it is necessary to correct the lumbo-pelvic lordosis. This is done by flexing the pelvis (and with it the lumbar spine) by means of the fully flexed sound limb (Fig. 254).

Fig. 253

Fig. 254

Thomas's test for fixed flexion deformity. Figure 253—Flexion deformity masked by arching of spine and pelvis. Figure 254—Deformity revealed by flexing the sound hip and, by continuing the flexion force, correcting the arching of spine and pelvis.

Technique of the manoeuvre. One hand is placed behind the lumbar spine (between it and the couch) to assess the degree of lumbar lordosis. If there is no lordosis when the affected limb lies flat on the couch there can be no fixed flexion deformity and there is no need to proceed with the test. If there is excessive lordosis, as indicated by arching of the back, it is corrected in the following way: The *sound* hip is flexed to the limit of its range. The limb is then pushed further into flexion, thereby rotating the pelvis on a horizontal transverse axis until the arching of the spine is obliterated. During this manoeuvre the thigh of the disordered limb, if in fixed flexion, is automatically raised from the couch as the lumbar lordosis is reduced (Fig. 254). The angle through which the thigh is raised from the couch is the angle of fixed flexion deformity.

Fixed rotation deformity. The most reliable index of the rotational position of the thigh is the patella, which normally points forwards when the hip is in the neutral position. If there is fixed lateral rotation or fixed medial rotation the limb cannot be rotated to the neutral position. The angle by which it falls short of the neutral when rotated as far as possible is the angle of fixed rotation deformity.

Movements

The accurate determination of hip movements demands much care, because restriction of hip movement is easily masked by movement of the pelvis It is therefore essential to place one hand upon the pelvis to detect any movement there, while the other guides and supports the limb.

Flexion. The range of hip flexion is best demonstrated by flexing the hip and knee together; not by lifting the leg with the knee straight. Movement of the pelvis is best detected by grasping the crest of the ilium (Fig. 255). Only in this way is it possible to distinguish between true hip movement and the false flexion imparted by rotation of the pelvis. The normal range of true hip flexion is about 120 degrees, but it varies according to the build of the patient.

Fig. 255
Testing hip flexion. The right hand supports the limb while the left hand grips the ilium to detect incipient rotation of the pelvis. Hip and knee are flexed together.

Fig. 256
Testing abduction of the hip. The right hand supports the limb while the left, bridging the two anterior superior spines, is ready to detect tilting of the pelvis. Adduction is tested in the same way.

Abduction. The limb to be tested is supported by one hand while the other hand bridges the pelvis from anterior superior spine to anterior superior spine (Fig. 256). In this way true abduction at the hip can be differentiated from the false abduction that is imparted by tilting of the pelvis. The normal range of true abduction at the hip is 30 to 35 degrees (more in children).

Abduction in flexion. This is often the first movement to suffer restriction in arthritis of the hip. The patient flexes his hips and knees by drawing the heels towards the buttocks. He then allows the knees to fall away from one another towards the couch (see Fig. 260). The normal range is about 70 degrees (90 degrees in young children).

Adduction. The limb to be examined is crossed over the other limb. Again care must be taken to differentiate between true adduction and the false movement imparted by tilting of the pelvis. The normal range of adduction is about 25–30 degrees.

Lateral rotation and medial rotation. Judge the range by an imaginary pointer thrust axially into the patella, not by the position of the foot. The normal range both of medial and of lateral rotation is about 40 degrees.

Extension. Contrary to what has often been written, the range of extension at the hip is nil. Extension of the hip joint beyond the neutral position is prevented by the strong anterior capsule and reinforcing Y-shaped ligament. Seeming backward movement of the thigh is in fact contributed entirely by rotation of the pelvis and extension of the spine, not by extension at the hip joint proper.

Examination for abnormal mobility

In cases of marked instability of the hip longitudinal movement or 'telescoping' can sometimes be demonstrated—especially in children with congenital dislocation of the hip. To carry out the test the limb is grasped firmly in one hand and alternately pushed and pulled in its long axis, the trunk being steadied by the examiner's other hand upon the iliac crest.

In infants it is important to examine for dislocation by the click test of Ortolani and others. This is described on page 295.

Examination for postural stability: the Trendelenburg test

The Trendelenburg manoeuvre is a test of the stability of the hip, and particularly of the ability of the hip abductors (gluteus medius and gluteus minimus) to stabilise the pelvis upon the femur when the subject is standing.

Principle of the test. Normally, when one leg is raised from the ground the pelvis tilts upwards on that side, through the action of the hip abductors of the standing limb (Fig. 257). (This automatic mechanism allows the lifted leg to clear the ground in walking.) If the abductors are inefficient they are unable to sustain the pelvis against the body weight and it tilts downwards instead of rising on the side of the lifted leg (Fig. 258).

Technique. Stand behind the patient. Instruct him first to stand upon the sound limb and to raise the other from the ground. Having thus got the idea of what he is required to do, he should now stand on the affected limb and lift the sound leg from the ground. By inspection, or by palpation with a hand upon the iliac crest, observe whether the pelvis rises or falls on the lifted side. Remember that the limb upon which the patient stands is the one under test. If the pelvis rises on the opposite side (normal) the test is negative (Fig. 257). If it falls, the test is positive (Fig. 258); in other words the abductor muscles are incapable of stabilising the pelvis upon the femur.

Fig. 257

Negative Trendelenburg test. The hip abductors are acting normally, tilting the pelvis upwards when the opposite leg is raised from the ground.

Fig. 257

Fig. 258

Positive Trendelenburg test. The hip abductors are unable to control the dropping of the pelvis when the opposite leg is raised.

Fig. 258

Causes of positive Trendelenburg test. There are three fundamental causes: 1) paralysis of the abductor muscles (example—poliomyelitis); 2) marked approximation of the insertion of the muscles to their origin by upward displacement of the greater trochanter, so that the muscles are slack (examples—severe coxa vara; congenital dislocation of the hip); 3) absence of a stable fulcrum (example—ununited fracture of the femoral neck). Sometimes two of these factors may operate together: for instance, in a case of upward dislocation of the hip there may be an unstable fulcrum as well as approximation of the origin of the abductor muscles to their insertion.

Gait

Watch how the patient stands and observe his gait on walking. Note that a patient with an unstable or painful hip prefers to use a stick in the *opposite* hand, and tends to shorten the period of weight-bearing on the affected limb. Characteristic gait patterns that are recognised include: 1) antalgic gait (weight-bearing minimised to reduce pain); 2) short-leg gait; and 3) Trendelenburg gait (patient leans towards the affected side to lift the sound leg clear of the ground).

Extrinsic causes of pain in the hip region

If examination of the hip itself fails to reveal abnormalities sufficient to account for the patient's symptoms, possible causes outside the hip must be investigated. Attention should be directed particularly to the spine and sacro-iliac joints (including a neurological survey of the lower limbs), to the abdomen and pelvis (including rectal or bimanual examination if necessary), and to the vascular system (state of the peripheral pulses).

Imaging

Radiographic examination. *Plain radiographs* should include an antero-posterior projection showing the whole pelvis with both hips, and lateral films of each hip separately. It is recommended that the lateral films be obtained by slightly abducting the affected hip and directing the x-ray beam horizontally beneath the opposite flexed thigh. In special cases there is a place for *tomography* and for *arthrography* (that is, radiography after the intra-articular injection of radio-opaque fluid). When there is a possibility that the symptoms may be referred from the back radiographs of the spine and sacro-iliac joints must be obtained.

Radioisotope bone scanning. This is of value especially in the diagnosis of inflammatory lesions in or about the hip. It may also be helpful in the early detection of metastatic neoplastic deposits in the pelvis or upper end of the femur.

Computerised tomography (CT scanning) provides clear cross-sectional images of the pelvis or thigh and is useful in special circumstances. For instance, it can show accurately the orientation (degree of anteversion) of the acetabulum or of the neck of the femur. Or it may be used to outline bony or soft-tissue tumours in or about the pelvis or hip (see Fig. 10 p. 17).

Magnetic resonance imaging (MRI) may also be useful, especially in showing the extent of soft-tissue changes—for instance in the case of an invasive tumour.

CLASSIFICATION OF DISORDERS IN THE HIP REGION

ARTICULAR DISORDERS OF THE HIP

Congenital deformities
Congenital dislocation of the hip
(Developmental dysplasia of the hip)

Arthritis
Transient synovitis of children
Pyogenic arthritis
Rheumatoid arthritis
Tuberculous arthritis
Osteoarthritis

Osteochondritis
Perthes' disease

Mechanical disorders
Slipped upper femoral
epiphysis

EXTRA-ARTICULAR DISORDERS IN THE REGION OF THE HIP

Deformities
Coxa vara

Infections
Tuberculosis of the trochanteric bursa

Mechanical disorders
Snapping hip

ARTICULAR DISORDERS OF THE HIP

DEVELOPMENTAL DYSPLASIA OF THE HIP

The term *developmental dysplasia* of the hip includes congenital dislocation of the hip, nearly always diagnosed either within a few days of birth or within the first two years of life; and dysplasia of the hip in adults, characterised by shallow configuration of the acetabulum, defective congruity between the femoral head and the socket, and a predisposition to osteoarthritis in middle or later life. Despite a trend towards re-naming congenital dislocation of the hip as developmental dysplasia of the hip, the title 'congenital dislocation' of the hip is so well established that it seems unnecessary to discard it. That title is therefore retained here for dislocation diagnosed in infancy.

CONGENITAL DISLOCATION OF THE HIP

This is a spontaneous dislocation of the hip occurring either before or during birth or shortly afterwards. In Western races it is one of the commonest of the congenital skeletal deformities: it is also of special importance because neglect or inefficient treatment incurs the penalty to the patient of lifelong crippling.

Cause. Much remains to be learnt, but it now seems to be clear that a number of factors are concerned in the causation—some genetic and some environmental. One such abnormality acting alone may not always be sufficient in itself to bring about dislocation, and it may well be that a combination of factors is often at work.

1) *Genetically determined joint laxity.* Generalised ligamentous laxity is found in a proportion of the patients, and may also be present in a parent or relatives. It leads to lack of stability at the hip, so that dislocation may easily occur in certain positions of the joint.

2) *Hormonal joint laxity.* It is possible that in females a ligament-relaxing hormone ('relaxin') may be secreted by the foetal uterus in response to oestrone and progesterone reaching the foetal circulation. This may cause instability in the same way as does genetically determined joint laxity. It is possible, also, that laxity of the hip ligaments from this cause might help to explain the greater incidence of dislocation in girls (the relaxing agent is not produced in boys). This factor requires further investigation.

3) *Genetically determined dysplasia of the hip.* There is little doubt that defective development of the acetabulum, and probably also of the femoral head, can be inherited as a distinct entity. The defect appears always to be bilateral, and is probably as common in boys as in girls. It predisposes to dislocation, which indeed may often occur before birth. If dislocation does not occur, the defect may show itself in adult life in the form of unduly shallow acetabula, with a tendency to subluxation and later osteoarthritis (acetabular dysplasia: see p. 301).

4) *Breech malposition.* The incidence of hip dislocation is slightly greater when the infant is delivered by the breech than with normal delivery. It is possible that the act of extending the hips during delivery may precipitate dislocation when there is already a predisposition to it from ligamentous laxity or acetabular dysplasia.

The relative importance of these various factors is not fully understood. Present evidence suggests, however, that there may be two distinct types of congenital dislocation of the hip. The first type is caused predominantly by ligamentous laxity—whether genetically determined or hormonal—in which dislocation occurs as it were accidentally when some precipitating movement such as extension of the hips during delivery is the adjuvant cause, the dislocation in this type often being unilateral and readily correctable. The second type is due predominantly to genetically determined dysplasia of the acetabulum, which is always bilateral and often much more difficult to treat.

Pathology. *The femoral head*: In a case of persistent dislocation the bony nucleus appears late and its development is retarded. The femoral head is dislocated upwards and laterally from the acetabulum. *The femoral neck*: In most cases the neck is anteverted (directed forwards) beyond the normal angle for infants of 25 degrees. *The acetabulum:* The ossific centre for the roof of the acetabulum, like that for the femoral head, is late in developing. The bone slopes upwards at a steep angle instead of forming a nearly horizontal roof for the acetabulum. The cartilaginous part of the roof is often well formed at first, but if the dislocation is allowed to persist development does not proceed normally, and the socket assumes a shallow contour with steeply sloping roof. *The fibrocartilaginous labrum*: The labrum or 'limbus' is often folded into the cavity of the acetabulum and may impede complete reduction of the dislocation (Somerville 1978). *The capsule*: This is gradually elongated as the femoral head is displaced upwards.

Clinical features. Girls are affected six times as often as boys. In one-third of all cases both hips are affected. Unless it is specially looked for in infancy—as it always should be—abnormality may not be noticed until the child begins to walk. Walking is often delayed, and there is a limp or a waddling gait.

On examination at that time, the main features in unilateral cases are asymmetry (notably of the buttock folds), shortening of the affected limb (Fig. 259), and restricted abduction in flexion. In bilateral cases the striking features are widening of the perineum and marked lumbar lordosis. The range of joint movements is full except for abduction in flexion, which is characteristically slightly restricted (Fig. 260). In most cases the affected limb is abnormally mobile in its long axis (telescopic movement).

Imaging. *Plain radiographs* show three important features (Fig. 261): 1) The ossific centre for the head of the femur is late in appearing and its development is retarded; 2) the bony acetabular roof has a pronounced upward slope; and 3) the femoral head (as judged from the position of the

Fig. 260

Congenital dislocation of the right hip. Figure 259—The right lower limb was slightly shorter than the left, as suggested here by the typical extra skin folds in the thigh. Figure 260 shows the reduced range of abduction of the affected hip—another typical and important diagnostic feature.

Fig. 259

Fig. 261

Congenital dislocation of the right hip in a child of 2. The three points to note are the retarded development of the capital epiphysis, the steeply sloping acetabular roof, and the lateral and upward displacement of the upper end of the femur.

ossific centre) is displaced upwards and laterally from its normal position in the centre of the acetabulum. These changes are not always shown conclusively before the age of 4 months.

Arthrography (radiography after injection of opaque fluid into the joint) is useful in showing the outline of the cartilaginous elements of the joint.

Ultrasound scanning allows the position of the femoral head to be determined in the new-born, when radiographic examination tends to be inconclusive.

Diagnosis. *In the new-born*: Nearly always—though there are a few exceptions—dislocation or instability of the hip may be detected in the first few days of life by a diagnostic manoeuvre (Barlow 1962) similar to that described by Ortolani in 1937. In this test the surgeon faces the child's perineum and grasps the upper part of each thigh between fingers behind and thumb in front, the child's knees being fully flexed and the hips flexed to a right angle (Fig. 262). While each thigh in turn is steadily abducted

Fig. 262
Examining the hips of a new-born infant for instability. While the hip is abducted through the full range forward pressure is applied by the middle finger behind the greater trochanter. For details, see text.

towards the couch the middle finger applies forward pressure behind the greater trochanter and alternately the thumb placed anteriorly applies backward pressure. One of two abnormal states may be detected: 1) a dislocated femoral head snaps back into the acetabulum with a palpable and audible jerk or jolt; or 2) backward pressure with the thumb dislocates a joint that is unstable.

The Barlow manoeuvre must be combined with assessment of the range of abduction in flexion at each hip (Fig. 260). If abduction is restricted it may indicate persistent or irreducible dislocation, and in such a case the absence of the characteristic jerk or jolt may mislead the observer into believing that all is well. In such a case, if unilateral, shortening may be observed when the knees are placed together, with the hips flexed.

In newborn infants radiography may be inconclusive because the high proportion of radiolucent cartilage in the femoral head and acetabulum makes interpretation difficult. It becomes diagnostic after the age of about four months. As the necessary skill in examination is more widely acquired, ultrasound scanning will become increasingly important in diagnosis in early infancy.

In older children. Delay in beginning to walk or abnormality of gait in early childhood should always arouse suspicion. The most important clinical sign in children one or two years old is a restricted range of abduction when the hip is flexed (Fig. 260). If for any reason suspicion arises that all is not well with the hips, radiographic examination must be insisted upon. In these older children radiography is always conclusive.

Course and prognosis. The earlier the dislocation is reduced the better the prognosis. Even under the best conditions only about half or two-thirds of the patients treated after the first year of life can be expected to remain permanently free from trouble. Gradual redislocation or subluxation is all too frequent, and pain from secondary degenerative changes often develops in middle adult life.

It is therefore important that, through careful examination of every newborn infant, congenital dislocation be detected within the first week of life, when simple treatment can nearly always assure normal development of the hip.

Treatment. This varies according to the age of the patient when advice is sought. Four groups will be discussed: 1) neonatal cases (instability or dislocation); 2) age 6 months–6 years; 3) age 7–10 years; 4) adolescents and adults.

Neonatal cases (within six months of birth)

These are the cases in which instability or dislocation is found on neonatal screening, either by the Ortolani-Barlow test or by ultrasound examination. In most of these cases the hip becomes stable spontaneously within three weeks. Accordingly, there is much to be said for delaying a decision on definitive treatment until the time of reassessment three weeks after birth, when it will be found that a large proportion of the infants do not need treatment. In the interval between the first examination and the reassessment at three weeks the limbs are left free, though it seems sensible to advise the use of bulky double nappies to encourage abduction of the hips.

If at three weeks the hip is found to be stable, treatment is unnecessary, and the parents may be tentatively reassured. Nevertheless it is important that the child should be reviewed at the age of 5 or 6 months, when radiography gives conclusive findings, and again at one year of age.

If on the other hand the hip is still unstable at three weeks, splinting in the reduced position in moderate (not extreme) abduction for three months is recommended. Splintage may be by plaster of Paris or by one of the many types of abduction harness that are made for the purpose.

Age 6 months–6 years

This still forms a substantial group, but with more regular diagnosis in early infancy the proportion of patients treated as late as this should progressively decrease. There are three essential principles of treatment: 1) to secure concentric reduction; 2) to provide conditions favourable to continued stability; and 3) to observe the hips regularly in order to detect any failure of normal development of the acetabulum and to apply appropriate treatment when necessary.

Reduction of dislocation. It is desirable whenever possible to obtain reduction by non-operative means, operation being used only when con-servative methods fail. In practice, it is found that closed reduction is often possible in babies up to eighteen months of age, but that thereafter the proportion that require operation progressively increases, so that operative reduction becomes almost routine after the age of 3 years.

Closed reduction. The standard practice is to apply weight traction to the limbs with the child either on a frame or in gallows (Bryant's) suspension, and while traction is maintained, gradually to abduct the hips, a little more each day, until 80 degrees of abduction is reached after three to four weeks. Cross traction by slings round the upper thighs may then be applied. In many cases reduction is obtained by this method alone. If however the hip is

Fig. 263
A method of holding the hips in moderate abduction and medial rotation. Extreme positions of abduction or rotation are nowadays avoided because of the risk of damaging the blood supply to the capital epiphysis of the femur.

not reduced at four weeks an attempt is made to complete the reduction by gentle manipulation under anaesthesia. It is essential that reduction be complete, so that the femoral head fits the socket concentrically. If neces-sary, arthrography, CT scanning or magnetic resonance imaging may be employed to establish whether reduction is complete or whether interposed soft tissue is blocking it.

If full reduction is secured, the limbs are immobilised for an initial period in plaster of Paris, usually in a position of moderate medial rotation and moderate abduction (Fig. 263): extreme positions must not be used. This has superseded the 'frog' position of right-angled flexion and abduction, formerly widely used, which has been found to prejudice the blood supply of the capital epiphysis of the femur, with risk of necrotic changes resembling those of Perthes' disease.

Operative reduction. If reduction is not obtained by traction and abduction, with or without manipulation, operation should be undertaken without delay. At operation, it will usually be found that full engagement of the femoral head in the acetabulum is prevented by inturning of the acetabular labrum (limbus), or occasionally by a voluminous ligament of the femoral head or a tight psoas tendon. Any such obstruction is removed or released to allow the femoral head to be fully engaged. While the femoral head is exposed to view, note should be made of the angle of anteversion of the femoral neck. This will often be found to be increased beyond the normal angle of 25 degrees. At the completion of the operation the limbs are immobilised in plaster in the same way as after closed reduction.

Maintenance of stability. A major hazard to continued stability in a child whose hip dislocation has been concentrically reduced comes from excessive anteversion of the femoral neck, which is a common if not a constant feature in children beyond eighteen months of age. Excessive anteversion has its main adverse effect when the child assumes the erect posture for walking: with the hips extended excessive anteversion brings the femoral head anteriorly, and radiographs may show it to lie eccentrically in the acetabulum. If uncorrected, this initial subluxation may progress eventually to redislocation.

The diagnosis of excessive anteversion is simple if operative reduction has been undertaken, for with the hip exposed the angle of anteversion can be measured under direct vision. When reduction has been by closed methods, however, diagnosis presents some difficulty—indeed to some extent it may be a matter of guesswork. Methods of radiographic measurement are available (Dunn 1952; Harris 1965) but they are not always easy to apply successfully in a small child and have been largely superseded. A more empirical method is often used: antero-posterior radiographs are taken with the hip first in the neutral position and then medially rotated. A more central position of the capital epiphysis in the acetabulum when the hip is medially rotated suggests that excessive anteversion is prejudicing stability. Definitive information on the angle of anteversion can best be gained from computerised tomography (CT scanning) or magnetic resonance imaging.

There are two methods of correcting excessive anteversion: 1) non-operative; and 2) operative (rotation osteotomy).

Non-operative management of anteversion. Long-continued harnessing of the hips in flexion and moderate abduction, a limited amount of walking being allowed, has been found to favour spontaneous correction of anteversion. Correction may, however, take a year or more.

Rotation osteotomy. Excessive anteversion is easily corrected by rotating the femur through an osteotomy at its upper end. The femur is divided a little below the trochanteric level to allow the shaft fragment to be rotated laterally in relation to the upper end of the femur. The fragments are then fixed with a plate and screws. After operation immobilisation in plaster is maintained until union occurs—usually a matter of about six weeks. Thereafter all splintage is discarded.

Counteracting defective development of the acetabulum. In a proportion of cases—greater when treatment has been started late than when it has been begun in the first year of life—the acetabulum fails to develop normally from the stimulus of the femoral head within it, and remains unduly shallow. The femoral head is not well contained within it, being partly uncovered by the acetabular roof. If this deficiency is not corrected the femoral head may become slowly displaced upwards, so that the joint is subluxated, the head no longer articulating congruously with the socket. The treatment of such acetabular deficiency is operative, and it should be carried out as soon as it is observed that this adverse situation has arisen. Mention will be made of four of the several operations that are available for improving the acetabulum: 1) osteotomy of the hip (innominate) bone (Salter's pelvic osteotomy); 2) pericapsular osteotomy of the ilium (Pemberton's pelvic osteotomy); 3) shelf acetabuloplasty (Wainwright's shelf operation); and 4) Chiari's displacement osteotomy of the ilium.

Bone graft
Roof levered down

Fig. 264   Fig. 265

Fig. 266   Fig. 267

Four methods of improving a poorly developed acetabulum to provide better cover for the femoral head. Figure 264—Salter's osteotomy of the ilium. Figure 265—Pemberton's pericapsular osteotomy of the ilium. Figure 266—Wainwright's shelf acetabuloplasty. Figure 267—Chiari's pelvic displacement osteotomy. For details see text.

Osteotomy of hip (innominate) bone (Salter 1961; 1969). The iliac bone is divided completely just above the acetabulum, the cut emerging at the greater sciatic notch. The whole of the lower half of the bone, bearing the intact acetabulum, is then sprung outwards and forwards, hinging at the symphysis pubis (Fig. 264). The effect is that the femoral head is more fully covered by the roof of the acetabulum, and stability of the hip is correspondingly increased. This operation is most suitable for young children.

Pericapsular osteotomy of ilium (Pemberton 1964; 1965; 1974). This operation has a similar aim of providing increased cover for the femoral head by the roof of the acetabulum. A curved osteotomy is made part-way across the thickness of the pelvic wall from the outer aspect of the ilium a few millimetres proximal to the attachment of the capsule to the upper margin of the acetabulum. The osteotomy extends to the triradiate cartilage, which forms a flexible hinge about which the roof of the acetabulum is deflected downwards over the femoral head. The triangular osteotomy gap is held open by bone obtained locally from the ilium (Fig. 265). This operation is most suitable for young children.

Cortical turn-down acetabuloplasty (Wainwright 1976). This so-called shelf operation also has the aim of increasing the surface area of the acetabular roof. A sizeable area of the outer table of the ilium is turned down as a flap into contact with the upper and outer aspect of the capsule of the hip joint (Fig. 266). The flap, thus reflected, is held in place by strut grafts. This operation is suitable mainly for adolescents and young adults.

Chiari's pelvic displacement osteotomy. The iliac bone is divided almost transversely immediately above the acetabulum, and the lower fragment (bearing the acetabulum) is displaced medially (Fig. 267). The cut surface of the upper fragment thus forms an extension of the acetabular roof, with capsule and newly formed fibrous tissue intervening. The operation is suitable mainly for adolescents and young adults.

Age 7–10 years

In these older children with untreated dislocations, the first point to be decided is whether or not treatment should be undertaken at all. In some of these children with well developed false acetabula symmetrically placed on both sides, functional disability is slight, and appearance and gait may be acceptable. Accordingly it may often be wise to advise against attempted reduction of the dislocation. In contrast there are others with high-lying femoral heads and poorly developed false sockets who can benefit greatly from operative reduction up to the age of 10 years or sometimes even later. This applies particularly when the dislocation is unilateral. Treatment in such cases entails open reduction of the dislocation, to accomplish which the femur may have to be shortened in the subtrochanteric region. Any

False joint

Site of osteotomy

Fig. 268
Low abduction femoral osteotomy (Schanz), used in selected cases of painful unreduced congenital dislocation of both hips in adults. The osteotomy is at the level of the ischial tuberosity.

excessive anteversion of the femoral neck is corrected at the same time by rotation at the site of bone resection. Either at the same time or later, one of the operations mentioned above for deepening the acetabulum may be carried out. An obvious advantage of reducing the dislocation in these older children is that conditions are made suitable for replacement arthroplasty should the need for it arise in later life.

Age 11 years onwards

After the age of 10 years, and often in younger children, treatment of freshly diagnosed congenital dislocation of the hip is not advised unless secondary degenerative changes lead to severe pain. If increasing pain justifies operative treatment, the choice of method depends largely upon whether the dislocation affects one or both hips. If only one hip is affected total replacement arthroplasty may sometimes be practicable once adult life is reached; but if not, consideration should be given to the advisability of arthrodesis, which can offer a satisfactory solution. If both hips are affected abduction osteotomy at the level of the ischial tuberosity (Schanz) may be appropriate (Fig. 268), though when it is practicable replacement arthroplasty is usually to be preferred.

The Schanz operation. This operation helps to stabilise the hip by preventing adduction of the pelvis on the femur, thereby eliminating the Trendelenburg 'dip' on walking. At the same time the adducted upper fragment of the femur, lying close to the side wall of the pelvis, affords it greater support, and stability is further improved by the medial shift of the femoral shaft.

DYSPLASIA OF THE HIP IN ADULTS

The gene that is responsible for many cases of congenital dislocation of the hip may also cause dysplasia, or failure of normal development, of the joint that may not become apparent in childhood.

Hip dysplasia in adults may become symptomatic at any time from early adult life up till middle age, or later. The common presenting symptom is

Fig. 269
Congenital dysplasia of the hip in a woman aged 42. Note that the acetabulum is very shallow. The femoral head is ill-formed and higher than normal. The cartilage space is greatly narrowed, indicating degenerative arthritis.

pain, usually in one hip, but often occurring later in the opposite hip as well. Examination shows good mobility of the hip, but often with complaint of pain at the extremes of the range, especially of flexion and abduction. On radiological examination the affected acetabulum is seen to be shallow, often with a steeply sloping roof (Fig. 269). The femoral head does not fit concentrically in the acetabulum: it may be shown to be displaced slightly upwards and outwards, so that Shenton's line, the normally smooth arch formed by the medial/inferior border of the femoral neck prolonged into the inferior border of the pubic ramus, is broken.

Dysplasia of the hip is important not only because it may cause pain and instability in its own right, but because it predisposes to the later development of degenerative arthritis, usually in middle life, with slowly increasing pain and difficulty in walking.

Treatment. Operative treatment is often appropriate, but it should be deferred until the disability becomes severe enough to demand it. The choice of operation is usually between osteotomy of the upper end of the femur to displace the femoral head and neck into more varus (Fig. 285); and pelvic osteotomy above the acetabulum to increase the coverage of the femoral head and improve stability of the hip (Fig. 264). In patients with advanced arthritic changes total replacement arthroplasty of the hip may have to be recommended.

TRANSIENT SYNOVITIS OF THE HIP

(Traumatic synovitis; transient arthritis; observation hip; irritable hip)

The so-called transient arthritis or synovitis of childhood is a short-lived affection of the hip of uncertain pathology, characterised clinically by pain, limp, and limitation of hip movements.

Cause. This is unknown. Injury is possibly a factor but the evidence in support of it is slender.

Pathology. This is unknown. Possibly there is a mild inflammation of the synovial membrane, initiated by minor injury; or perhaps a viral infection.

Clinical features. The condition is virtually confined to children under 10, especially boys. The child complains of pain in the groin and thigh and he is noticed to limp. *On examination* the only physical sign is limitation of hip movements. *Radiographs* do not show any alteration from the normal.

Diagnosis. Transient arthritis of the hip is important only because it resembles clinically the earliest stages of tuberculous arthritis or of Perthes' disease, before the characteristic radiographic features have become apparent. Transient arthritis should be diagnosed only after the hip has recovered—never while the symptoms and signs are present. While the symptoms and signs last, the case should be regarded as one of suspected tuberculous arthritis or Perthes' disease and the child placed under observation in bed; full recovery within a few weeks excludes tuberculous arthritis and justifies a retrospective diagnosis of transient synovitis.

Course. Full recovery, with return of a normal range of hip movements, invariably occurs within three to six weeks.

Treatment. Rest in bed until the pain has settled and full movements have been restored is the only treatment required.

PYOGENIC ARTHRITIS OF THE HIP

(General description of pyogenic arthritis, p. 109)

Pyogenic arthritis of the hip is uncommon. It occurs mostly in children, in whom it is often secondary to osteomyelitis of the upper end of the femur. Its features resemble those of pyogenic arthritis elsewhere (p. 109); but in infants there are particular characteristics that require special description.

Pathology. Organisms (usually staphylococci or streptococci) may reach the joint directly through the blood stream, or the infection may spread from an adjacent focus of osteomyelitis. Rarely a penetrating wound is responsible. In new-born babies the infection may enter through the umbilicus. There is an acute inflammatory reaction in the joint tissues, with an effusion of turbid fluid or pus. In favourable cases healing with restoration to normal can occur, but often the joint is permanently destroyed or damaged, and in older children and adults bony ankylosis may occur.

In infants bony ankylosis does not occur because the femoral head and the acetabulum are composed almost entirely of cartilage rather than of bone, but there may be total destruction of the developing femoral head with secondary dislocation of the hip (pathological dislocation) (Tom Smith's disease). The femur may remain short, from destruction of the upper femoral growth cartilage. Additional shortening will occur if the dislocation is allowed to persist and the femur to slide upwards on the ilium; so the discrepancy in length may be marked by the time adolescence is reached.

Clinical features. The clinical features differ so much in infants and in older patients that separate descriptions are required.

Pyogenic arthritis of infants. The onset is within the first year of life. Often there has been a known septic lesion somewhere on the body (for example, umbilical sepsis), but it may have caused little anxiety. Then the child becomes unwell and pyrexial.

On examination it is not always apparent at first that the hip is the seat of the trouble. But careful examination will show thickening in the hip area, and movements of the joint are restricted. Sometimes an abscess points at the skin surface in the buttock or thigh.

Radiographic features. In the early stages there is no alteration of the bone shadows, but the soft-tissue shadows may suggest swelling about the hip. If the infection progresses to the stage of destroying the capital epiphysis of the femur the ossific nucleus fails to appear as it should before the age of one year. In such a case subsequent radiographs may show gradual dislocation of the hip. This 'pathological' dislocation is distinguished from congenital dislocation by the facts that the acetabular roof is of normal shape and that the capital epiphysis is permanently absent (Fig. 270). Radioisotope scanning reveals increased uptake in the region of the hip.

Fig. 270

Old pyogenic arthritis of left hip in an infant (Tom Smith's disease). The epiphysis of the head of the femur has been destroyed and the hip is dislocated. Note the almost normal appearance of the acetabular roof, which helps to distinguish this from a congenital dislocation. The normal hip is shown for comparison.

Investigations. Ultrasound scanning may show the hip joint to be distended with fluid. Aspiration of the hip yields pus from which the causative organism may be identified.

Pyogenic arthritis in older children and adults. The onset is acute or subacute, with pain in the hip made worse by attempted weight-bearing, and severe limp. There is constitutional illness with pyrexia. *On examination* there may be some fullness about the hip region from swelling of the joint. All movements of the hip are markedly restricted, and painful if forced.

Radiographic features. There may be no change in the early stages, but sometimes the space between the acetabulum and the femoral head is widened on account of distension of the joint with pus. There may be evidence of osteomyelitis in the upper metaphysis of the femur. Later, if the infection persists, the bone is rarefied and the cartilage space is narrowed. Finally, there may be bony ankylosis of the joint (Fig. 271).

Fig. 271
Bony ankylosis of the hip caused by pyogenic arthritis. The infection spread to the hip from a focus of osteomyelitis in the upper metaphysis of the femur. This is a common outcome of pyogenic arthritis in older children and adults.

Radioisotope bone scanning shows increased uptake in the region of the hip.

Investigations. The erythrocyte sedimentation rate is raised. There is a polymorphonuclear leucocytosis. Aspiration of the joint yields pus from which the causative organism may be identified.

Treatment. *Constitutional treatment* is by rest and appropriate antibiotic therapy—for instance by flucloxacillin and fusidic acid, depending upon the nature of the infecting organism.

Local treatment. Rest for the joint and relief of muscle spasm are best ensured by weight traction through adhesive skin strapping applied to the leg. The joint is aspirated daily until pus ceases to re-form; after each aspiration a solution of the appropriate antibiotic is injected into the joint. In severe cases more effective drainage may be obtained by incision into the joint. When the infection has been overcome active movements are encouraged.

Pathological dislocation complicating pyogenic arthritis of infants, with total destruction of the upper femoral epiphysis (Tom Smith's disease). Definitive treatment of this rare but crippling condition must await adolescence. In childhood the aim of treatment is to prevent progressive upward displacement of the femur and thereby to minimise shortening. Provided the infection has settled, operation should be undertaken to deepen the acetabulum, to place the upper end of the femur within it and, if necessary, to lever down a 'shelf' of ilium over it. In adolescence, when the bones are nearing full development, arthrodesis may be recommended if the hip is painful. If the hip has fused spontaneously (Fig. 271) the situation is best accepted, provided that fusion has occurred in a good functional position.

RHEUMATOID ARTHRITIS OF THE HIP
(General description of rheumatoid arthritis, p. 111)

The hip joints often escape in cases of rheumatoid arthritis; but when they are affected the consequent disability is serious. The main features of the disease are like those of rheumatoid arthritis in general, as described on page 111.

Clinical features. The changes may affect one or both hips, in common with several other joints. The main symptoms are pain and limitation of movement, aggravated by activity.

On examination swelling is not obvious because the joint is so deeply situated; for the same reason the temperature of the overlying skin is not increased as it is in rheumatoid affection of the more superficial joints. The range of all hip movements is impaired and movement is painful if forced. Fixed flexion deformity or adduction deformity may develop. The gluteal and thigh muscles are wasted.

Fig. 272
Left—Long-established rheumatoid arthritis of the hip, with destruction of the cartilage space. The marginal osteophytes indicate that osteoarthritis is becoming superimposed upon the old rheumatoid disease. *Right*—The left hip of another patient, showing marked encroachment of the femoral head into the softened acetabulum (protrusio acetabuli).

Imaging. *Radiographic features.* In the early stages there are no radiographic changes. Later, there is diffuse rarefaction in the area of the joint. Later still, destruction of articular cartilage leads to narrowing of the cartilage space between femur and acetabulum, often with inward protrusion of the softened medial wall of the acetabulum (Fig. 272). *Radioisotope bone scanning* shows increased uptake in the region of the hip from an early stage.

Investigations. The erythrocyte sedimentation rate is increased during the active stage. The latex fixation test and the Rose-Waaler test may be positive.

Course. The disease becomes inactive after months or years, but the hip is seldom restored to normal. In long-established cases degenerative changes are superimposed upon the original inflammatory condition, giving rise to secondary osteoarthritis (Fig. 272).

Treatment. Constitutional treatment is the same as that for rheumatoid arthritis in general (p. 115). Local treatment for the hip joints depends upon the activity and severity of the inflammatory reaction. In most cases rest in bed is required, but when the reaction is moderate or mild, exercises and active use within the limits of pain are encouraged. Intra-articular injections of hydrocortisone have sometimes given relief, but they cannot safely be repeated. Various physiotherapeutic methods may be given a trial in attempts to reduce discomfort and hasten resolution.

Operative treatment. When pain is severe and walking is limited to a few yards operation is justified. Replacement arthroplasty (Figs 278 and 280) is the method of choice.

TUBERCULOUS ARTHRITIS OF THE HIP
(General description of tuberculous arthritis, p. 117)

The hip is one of the joints most frequently affected by tuberculosis. In Western countries, however, its incidence has declined so sharply that it is now seldom seen, and it is mainly confined to poorer countries or to immigrants from such countries.

Fig. 273
Early stage of tuberculous arthritis of the right hip. The bone is rarefied but the cartilage space is not reduced. The joint might be saved.

Clinical features. The patient is usually a child—often 2 to 5 years old—or a young adult. There is often a history of contact with a person with active pulmonary tuberculosis. The symptoms are pain and limp. The general health is usually impaired. *On examination* a thickening is often palpable in the region of the hip. All movements of the hip are limited, often markedly, and attempts to force movement provoke pain and muscle spasm. The gluteal and thigh muscles are wasted. A 'cold' abscess is sometimes palpable in the upper thigh or buttock. A tuberculous lesion may be apparent elsewhere in the body.

Imaging. *Radiographic features.* The earliest sign is diffuse rarefaction in the area of the hip. This is detected most easily when the bones are compared with those of the sound side, taken on the same film (Fig. 273). At first the changes are slight, but it must be emphasised that even slight rarefaction is significant. In the more fully developed stage the rarefaction is obvious; and later there are fuzziness of the joint margins and narrowing of the cartilage space, indicating erosion of the articular cartilage (Fig. 274). Later still, bone may also be eroded; but in a favourable case the disease is arrested before these later changes occur. *Radioisotope bone scanning* shows increased uptake in the region of the hip.

Fig. 274
Tuberculous arthritis of right hip in a more advanced stage. The cartilage has been destroyed and the articular surfaces of the acetabulum and femoral head have lost their sharp definition. The joint is permanently destroyed.

Diagnosis. This is mainly from transient synovitis, Perthes' disease (osteochondritis), low-grade pyogenic arthritis, and rheumatoid arthritis. Important features supporting a diagnosis of tuberculosis are: a history of contact with tuberculosis (often parental); the presence of a tuberculous lesion elsewhere; a positive Mantoux reaction in children; a 'cold' abscess; the characteristic radiographic changes; a high sedimentation rate; and the typical histological appearance on biopsy of the synovial membrane.

Course and prognosis. In a reasonable proportion of cases, especially in children, the lesion is aborted by treatment and a sound joint is preserved, provided there has been no destruction of cartilage or bone when treatment is begun. If cartilage or bone are eroded the joint is permanently damaged and often totally destroyed, with eventual fibrous ankylosis. Unless this is converted by operation to bony fusion there is some risk that the disease may become active again later.

Treatment. Essentially, treatment is the same as that for other tuberculous joints. The mainstay of treatment is a prolonged course of antibacterial agents, as described on page 120.

Local treatment is initially by rest for the hip, usually in plaster, for a first period of three months. The subsequent treatment depends upon the progress made. If radiographs show no destruction of cartilage or bone, if the general health is good, and if the erythrocyte sedimentation rate has shown steady improvement, the hip is left free for a clinical trial. Joint movements are practised in bed for a further month, and if there is no evidence of deterioration full activity is gradually resumed.

On the other hand, if at the end of three or six months' treatment radiographs show marked destruction of cartilage or bone (Fig. 274), there is no possibility of preserving the joint intact. The choice then lies between total replacement arthroplasty, which must await full quiescence of the infection, and arthrodesis (see Fig. 16, p. 29). In children these operations should be deferred until adolescence.

OSTEOARTHRITIS OF THE HIP
(General description of osteoarthritis, p. 120)

Osteoarthritis of the hip is a common cause of severe disablement, especially in the elderly. It is not uncommon even in younger patients, when it is usually secondary to previous injury or disease. Indeed operations for the relief of osteoarthritis of the hip now make up a considerable part of the work of an orthopaedic department.

Cause. It is sometimes regarded as a wear-and-tear process; but in fact it reflects an inability of articular cartilage fully to repair itself. Any injury or disease that damages the joint surfaces initiates or accelerates the process of degeneration. Common examples of such predisposing causes are fracture of the acetabulum, Perthes' osteochondritis, slipped upper femoral epiphysis, and ischaemic necrosis of part of the femoral head from any cause. In another group the joint degeneration is secondary to a developmental imperfection (dysplasia) or congenital subluxation. In many cases there is no evidence of an underlying cause, and for want of any other explanation such cases are regarded as primary or idiopathic.

Pathology. The articular cartilage is worn away, especially where weight is transmitted. The underlying bone becomes hard and eburnated. Hypertrophy of bone at the joint margins leads to the formation of osteophytes.

Fig. 275
Osteoarthritis of the hip. The characteristic features are narrowing of the cartilage space, sclerosis of the subchondral bone and osteophytes at the joint margins.

Clinical features. The patient is usually elderly; but when osteoarthritis is secondary to previous hip disease or to injury it often arises in middle life. There is pain in the groin and front of the thigh; often also in the knee. The pain is made worse by walking and eased by rest. Later, there may be complaint of stiffness, which manifests itself in everyday life by inability to reach the foot to tie the shoe laces or cut the toe nails. The symptoms tend to increase progressively month by month and year by year until they eventually cause severe painful limp and incapacity for normal activities.

On examination all hip movements are impaired. Limitation of abduction, adduction and rotation is marked, but a good range of flexion is often preserved. Forced movements are painful. Fixed deformity (flexion, adduction or lateral rotation, or a combination of these) is common (Fig. 276).

Radiographic features. The changes are characteristic. There is diminution of the cartilage space, with a tendency to sclerosis of the subchondral bone (Figs 275 and 276). Hypertrophic spurring of bone (osteophyte formation) is usually seen at the joint margins.

Fig. 276
Advanced osteoarthritis of right hip. Note the adduction deformity—a common feature that causes apparent shortening of the limb from tilting of the pelvis. As in Figure 275, the characteristic features are narrowing of the joint space, subchondral bone sclerosis, and marginal osteophytes.

Treatment. The treatment required depends upon the severity of the disability. Mild osteoarthritis is best left untreated; in cases of moderate severity conservative treatment suffices; in severe cases operation is often advisable.

Conservative treatment. Clearly no form of conservative treatment can possibly influence the distorted anatomy of the joint. At best such treatment is only palliative; it may alleviate but cannot abolish the pain. Four methods will be mentioned. 1) *'Relative' rest.* By this is meant a modification of the patient's mode of life by change of occupation or adjustment of duties so that the work thrown upon the hip is reduced. The use of a stick (cane) and the correction of shortening by a shoe raise also come into this category, and they often afford considerable relief. 2) *Drugs:* Mild analgesic medication is often helpful, especially when the

pain disturbs sleep. 3) *Physiotherapy:* Local deep heat by short-wave diathermy, with exercises to strengthen the muscles and to preserve mobility,
often provides temporary relief. 4) *Injections into the joint:* The injection into
the joint of hydrocortisone, with or without a local anaesthetic solution, has
been tried, and in a few cases temporary relief has been claimed. Repeated
injections may do harm and are not to be recommended.

Fig. 277
Displacement osteotomy of the femur
(McMurray). The femur is divided between
the greater and the lesser trochanters, and the
shaft fragment is displaced medially through
a distance equal to about a quarter of its
diameter. The fragments have been fixed
with a nail-plate.

Operative treatment. Operation may be required if pain is severe—
especially if it hinders sleep and interferes seriously with the patient's
capacity for walking or work. Three types of operation must be considered:
1) upper femoral osteotomy (Fig. 277); 2) arthroplasty (Figs 278 and 279);
and 3) arthrodesis.

Fig. 278   **Fig. 279**
Methods of arthroplasty of the hip. Figure 278—Total
replacement arthroplasty. The femoral head is of metal,
the socket of plastic. Figure 279—Excision arthroplasty
(Girdlestone pseudarthrosis). Head and neck of femur
removed; muscle interposed.

Upper femoral osteotomy (McMurray displacement osteotomy). This operation is now little used. The femur is divided between the greater and the
lesser trochanter, and the lower (shaft) fragment is displaced medially

through about a quarter of its diameter (Fig. 277). Internal fixation of the fragments by nail-plate and screws is usually employed. Relief of pain is often satisfactory and some joint movement is retained. The question of why an upper femoral osteotomy should relieve the pain of an osteoarthritic hip has not been answered satisfactorily. It is possible that in some way the remodelling of bone trabeculae necessitated by the displacement stimulates repair processes in the damaged articular cartilage: certainly in a favourable case the cartilage thickens appreciably in the first two or three years after operation, as shown radiologically.

Fig. 280
Total replacement arthroplasty of hip. The hemispherical socket, of polyethylene, is not seen, but its mouth is indicated by the wire marker.

Arthroplasty. The method commonly used in primary management is total replacement arthroplasty (Figs 278 and 280). Excision arthroplasty is also used, but almost entirely as a salvage operation after other methods of treatment have failed.

In *replacement arthroplasty* the femoral head is excised and replaced by a metal prosthesis which is designed to remain permanently fixed in the femoral shaft, being usually embedded in an acrylic filling compound or 'cement'. At the same time the acetabulum is deepened to receive a hemispherical socket, usually of high density polyethylene, which is likewise usually secured by acrylic cement. This two-component substitution is illustrated in principle in Figure 278 and in a radiograph in Figure 280.

In *excision arthroplasty* (Girdlestone pseudarthrosis) a false joint is created by excising the head and neck of the femur and the upper half of the wall of the acetabulum, and suturing a mass of soft tissue (such as the gluteus medius muscle) in the gap thus created, to act as a cushion between the bones (Fig. 279).

Arthrodesis. The joint is fused in a position of 15–20 degrees of flexion but without any abduction, adduction or rotation (Fig. 16, p. 29). There is complete relief of pain, and good function is possible so long as the other hip, the knees and the spine are normal.

Choice of method. The three operations that require consideration as primary treatment are displacement osteotomy, replacement arthroplasty and arthrodesis. A fourth operation, excision arthroplasty, is used mainly as a salvage procedure. In recent years total replacement arthroplasty (replacement of both the femoral head and the acetabulum) has achieved such spectacular success and acclaim that the other operations have been largely displaced. It is necessary therefore to emphasise that it is not a panacea, and that there is still a place for each of the other operations mentioned, even though the indications for them have considerably narrowed since total replacement arthroplasty was introduced.

Displacement osteotomy is suitable for relatively young patients (say under 55) with moderately early osteoarthritis, a reasonably spherical femoral head well centred in the acetabulum, and a fair range of movement still preserved. If these criteria are fulfilled it can give good and lasting relief of pain in over 70 per cent of patients. So long as displacement does not exceed about a quarter or at most a third of the diameter of the femoral shaft the operation does not prejudice the undertaking of total replacement arthroplasty later, should the result of the osteotomy prove disappointing.

Total replacement arthroplasty gives excellent results in a high proportion of cases, with full relief of pain and a reasonable range of movement. It also offers the advantage of rapid convalescence. It is by far the most satisfactory solution to the problem of osteoarthritis in the elderly patient, no matter whether it be unilateral or bilateral. It is still necessary, however, to exercise caution in recommending it for younger patients, because it is not yet known to what extent a good result is lasting, and what are the risks of loosening or breakdown of the prosthesis in the long term. The risk of complications has also to be borne in mind—particularly of infection, a catastrophe that virtually destroys any chance of success from replacement arthroplasty. In these younger patients, therefore, it is necessary to weigh the likely advantages and possible hazards of the operation against the degree of disability that is imposed by the diseased hip.

Arthrodesis has a very limited application. It may be appropriate as an alternative to other methods in young patients (under 40) with severe, strictly unilateral osteoarthritis, especially when the anatomy is much distorted and hip movement already greatly restricted. Arthrodesis is accepted very reluctantly in countries where squatting is the normal habit; and in general it is not favoured in North America. It has the advantage, however, of ensuring permanent relief of pain.

Excision arthroplasty (Girdlestone pseudarthrosis) is best regarded as a salvage operation, to be resorted to only if other methods are inappropriate or have failed. It is the only operation available in the event of irretrievable failure of a total replacement arthroplasty. It can give a painless hip with reasonable movement, but at the cost of appreciable shortening and instability, usually necessitating the permanent use of a stick (cane) and a shoe raise.

PERTHES' DISEASE
(Legg-Perthes' disease; coxa plana; pseudocoxalgia; osteochondritis of the femoral capital epiphysis)

Perthes' disease is osteochondritis of the epiphysis of the femoral head. The general features of osteochondritis were described in Chapter 5 (p. 96). Like most examples of osteochondritis, Perthes' disease is an affection of childhood. The femoral head is temporarily softened and may become deformed. The main importance of the condition is that it may lead to the development of osteoarthritis of the hip in later life.

Cause. A temporary, and possibly repeated, local disturbance of blood supply is believed to be the major factor, but the precise cause of the vascular disturbance is unknown.

Pathology. The bony nucleus of the epiphysis of the femoral head undergoes necrosis either in whole or in part, presumably from ischaemia. This sets up a sequence of changes which occupies two to three years. The

Fig. 281
Perthes' disease of the left hip. Note the shrunken appearance of the bony nucleus of the femoral epiphysis, the corresponding increase in depth of the cartilage space, the patchy changes of density, and the suggestion of fragmentation.

Fig. 282	**Fig. 283**
Same patient as above, two years after the onset of symptoms. The shape of the head is virtually normal, and the femoral neck is of normal length. There is little risk of osteoarthritis.	In this patient, despite prolonged relief from weight-bearing, the femoral head is markedly flattened and the femoral neck is short. The deformity of the femoral head predisposes to osteoarthritis in later life.

first stage is that of ingrowth of new blood vessels and removal of dead bone by osteoclasts. In the second stage, which is not distinct but overlaps the first stage so that both processes are going on together, new bone is laid down on the dead trabeculae, gradually reconstituting the bony nucleus. The third stage is that of remodelling: this may continue for several years. This sequence of necrosis and replacement of bone is patchy rather than uniform, so that the nucleus has an appearance of fragmentation as seen radiographically. During this period structural rigidity is lost, and deformation of the epiphysis may occur from pressure across the joint.

In the early phases of the cycle of changes growth of the bony element of the epiphysis is temporarily arrested, but the cartilage surrounding the bony nucleus, which forms a considerable proportion of the femoral head, continues to grow and so is disproportionately thick (Fig. 281). Nevertheless it may sometimes follow the bone in suffering deformation, so that the femoral head as a whole may become much flattened (Fig. 283). At the same time there is often some enlargement of the femoral head. As the acetabulum grows, it tends to follow the contours of the femoral head, so that it may end up abnormally large and shallow (Fig. 284).

Fig. 284
Old untreated Perthes' disease. The femoral head is markedly flattened and the femoral neck is short. There is already some narrowing of the cartilage space, suggesting early osteoarthritis.

In consequence of interrupted growth at the epiphysial plate the femoral neck—and the limb as a whole—may be shorter than on the normal side, though the discrepancy is not great.

Clinical features. The disease occurs mainly in children of 5 to 10 years. It usually affects only one hip. The child complains of pain in the groin or thigh, and is noticed to limp. There is no disturbance of general health. *On examination* the only striking sign is moderate limitation of all hip movements, with pain and spasm if movement is forced.

Imaging. *Radiographic features.* The earliest radiographic changes are usually, though not always, present by the time advice is sought. There is a slight decrease in the depth of the ossific nucleus of the femoral head, whereas the clear cartilage space is often increased in depth: in other words the bony nucleus seems to have shrunk within its surrounding bed of cartilage (Fig. 281). The nucleus becomes denser than that of the normal side, though the density is patchy rather than uniform, so that there is an appearance of fragmentation. In severe cases the nucleus becomes progressively more flattened. Eventually the texture of the bone returns to normal (Fig. 282), but if flattening has occurred the femoral head is permanently deformed (Figs 283 and 284). *Radioisotope scanning* shows failure of uptake of the isotope in the region corresponding to the bony nucleus of the femoral head. Since this 'void' is seen at an early stage of the disease the examination may prove to be important in early diagnosis (Sutherland *et al.* 1980).

Diagnosis. Perthes' disease is distinguished from tuberculous arthritis, which it may resemble clinically, mainly by the radiographs. A normal erythrocyte sedimentation rate and blood count, and good general health, are other distinguishing features.

Prognosis. The disease has no direct adverse effect upon the general health. The main risk is to the future function of the affected hip joint, because if the femoral head suffers permanent deformity there is a risk of secondary osteoarthritis in later life, often in the fifth or sixth decade (Fig. 284).

The outcome depends largely upon whether the whole of the epiphysis is affected or whether part of it escapes, as it often does. In the latter case the prognosis is favourable (Fig. 282), whereas if the whole epiphysis is affected marked flattening of the femoral head may occur despite the most careful treatment (Fig. 283). The state of the cartilaginous part of the head, as determined from arthrography or from comparison of the measured 'head height' on radiographs of both hips, is also important in prognosis. If head height is well preserved, the outlook is favourable, whereas if there has been early collapse of cartilage permanent deformation of the head is to be expected. In general, the outlook is more favourable in younger children than in older children.

Treatment. It has to be admitted that the treatment of Perthes' disease is often disappointing: no universally satisfactory method has yet been evolved. Indeed it has sometimes been questioned whether treatment has any effect on the final state of the hip.

The former method of preventing weight-bearing pressure upon the softened femoral head by prolonged recumbency (often for two years or more) has been abandoned because the results were not commensurate with the severe disruption of home life that this treatment entailed. Other methods of trying to prevent pressure upon the head while still allowing the child to be up and about, such as slings or ischial-bearing calipers, have also fallen into disfavour because they are seldom effective and because they may embarrass the child psychologically.

The present trend is to grade the cases according to the likely outcome, so far as the shape of the femoral head is concerned, as judged from the radiographic features in the early stages (Catterall 1972), and to regulate the treatment accordingly. In the 'favourable' category are placed those with only half the head affected (as seen in the lateral radiographs) and with no sign of lateral extrusion of part of the femoral head from under the roof of the acetabulum. In the 'unfavourable' grade are placed those with the whole head affected or with some lateral extrusion of the head beyond the roof of the acetabulum. In general, patients with a favourable prognosis do not require treatment other than by rest for a few weeks to allow the pain to subside—though it is essential that they attend periodically for radiological review. In contrast, those with an unfavourable prognosis, with the femoral head in danger of becoming badly deformed, are advised to have treatment to try to prevent this.

Fig. 285

Diagrams to show how adduction (varus) osteotomy of the femur improves the containment of the femoral head in the acetabulum. *Left*—Site of bone wedge to be removed. *Right*—Gap closed after removal of wedge, so that femoral neck is turned down into varus. The osteotomy has the effect that the upper part (head and neck) of the femur is abducted in the socket, while the femoral shaft remains in the neutral position.

Present thought is that treatment, when needed, should be by 'containment' of the femoral head within the acetabulum. This means that the femoral head must be centered within the acetabulum so that the two are co-axial, and thus the whole circumference of the femoral head is embraced by the socket. The socket then acts as a mould, to keep the head hemispherical while it is in the softened state.

In practice, ensuring maximal containment of the femoral head demands that the femoral head and neck (or the whole limb) must be abducted in relation to the acetabulum, to make them co-axial (Fig. 285). This has sometimes been achieved by splinting the limbs in 20 or 30 degrees of abduction, but the child is thus greatly handicapped in walking. Most surgeons therefore prefer to realign the femoral head and neck by dividing the femur below the greater trochanter and deflecting the neck downwards to coincide with the central axis of the acetabulum (Fig. 285). Alternatively, the acetabulum itself may be redirected after osteotomy of the innominate bone (Fig. 264, p. 299).

Comment

These current thoughts on the management of Perthes' disease have not yet been fully tested by analysis of sufficient numbers of cases, and further experience must be gained before it can be established whether or not treatment by containment is consistently effective.

SLIPPED UPPER FEMORAL EPIPHYSIS
(Adolescent coxa vara; epiphysial coxa vara)

This is an affection of late childhood in which the upper femoral epiphysis is displaced from its normal position upon the femoral neck. The displacement occurs at the growth plate (epiphysial line).

Cause. This is unknown. The condition is often associated with overweight from endocrine dysfunction, but in other cases the patient is of normal build.

Pathology. The junction between the capital epiphysis and the neck of the femur loosens. With the downward pressure of weight-bearing and the upward pull of muscles on the femur the epiphysis is displaced from its normal position. Displacement is always backwards and downwards, so that the epiphysis comes to lie at the back of the femoral neck (Figs 286 and 287).

Upper end of child's femur seen from the side. Figure 286—Normal position of epiphysis. Figure 287—Slipped epiphysis. The displacement is always backwards and downwards.[1]   **Fig. 286**   **Fig. 287**

The displacement usually occurs gradually, but occasionally a sudden displacement is caused by injury, such as a fall. Left undisturbed, the epiphysis fuses to the femoral neck in the abnormal position. The consequent deformity of the articular surface then predisposes to the later development of secondary osteoarthritis.

Clinical features. The patient is between 10 and 20 years of age. In about half the cases there is evidence of an endocrine disturbance leading to marked overweight. In a little less than half the cases both hips are affected, though seldom simultaneously. Typically, there is a gradual onset of pain in the hip, with limp. Sometimes the pain is felt mainly in the knee, which may confuse the diagnosis. Rarely, these symptoms develop acutely after an injury, such as a fall.

On examination the physical signs are characteristic, for there is selective limitation of certain hip movements, the other movements being full or even increased. The movements that are restricted are flexion, abduction, and medial rotation. Lateral rotation and adduction are often increased, and the limb tends to lie in lateral rotation. Forcing movement in the restricted range exacerbates the pain.

Fig. 288
This radiograph shows how a slipped epiphysis may easily be overlooked if antero-posterior films alone are examined. The only indications that the right femoral epiphysis is displaced are a slight reduction of its vertical depth and slight rounding of the upper corner of the femoral neck. Now see the lateral radiograph in Figure 289.

Fig. 289
Lateral radiograph of the right hip shown in Figure 288. Slight backward slipping of the epiphysis is clearly revealed.

Fig. 290
Another patient. Slipped epiphysis of severe degree.

Fig. 289   **Fig. 290**

Radiographic examination. Even a slight displacement of the epiphysis is recognisable, provided good *lateral* radiographs are obtained. It must be stressed that a slight displacement is easily overlooked if antero-posterior films alone are examined (Fig 288). Lateral radiographs are essential. In the lateral film the epiphysis is seen to be tilted over towards the back of the femoral neck,[1] the posterior 'horn' being lower than the anterior, whereas in the normal hip they are level (Figs 287–290).

Diagnosis. Slipped upper femoral epiphysis should be suspected in every patient of 10–20 years of age who complains of pain in the hip or knee. The characteristic clinical features, together with the radiographic evidence of epiphysial displacement, are conclusive. The condition is nevertheless often missed, partly because pain may be predominantly in the knee, the hip therefore being not examined; or because lateral radiographs are not obtained (Fig. 288).

Fig. 291
Osteoarthritis developing twenty years after uncorrected slipped epiphysis.

Complications. These include avascular necrosis of the epiphysis of the femoral head, cartilage necrosis, and late osteoarthritis.

Avascular necrosis and consequent collapse of the epiphysis may occur if its blood supply is damaged. This complication is usually a consequence of attempted reduction of the slip by manipulation or of operation, but it may occur spontaneously, especially after a sudden acute slip.

Cartilage necrosis is a rare and unexplained thinning of the articular cartilage, with marked restriction of joint movement. It is commonest after operative treatment and may possibly represent an auto-immune reaction.

If severe displacement is allowed to remain uncorrected *osteoarthritis* is likely to develop in later life (Fig. 291).

A careful watch must be kept for slipping of the opposite femoral epiphysis.

Treatment. The treatment depends upon the degree of displacement. This may be graded as *slight* or *severe*.

---

[1]Students often have difficulty in determining in lateral radiographs of the upper end of the femur which is the back and which is the front of the bone. The key is the bony projection formed by the trochanters: this is always posterior.

Slight displacement. When displacement is slight (less than 40 degrees as measured on the lateral radiograph) (Fig. 289) the position may be accepted and all that is necessary is to prevent further displacement. This is

Fig. 292
Slipped epiphysis with only slight displacement. Threaded wires have been inserted to prevent further slipping.

achieved by driving threaded wires or slender screws[1] along the neck of the femur into the epiphysis (Fig. 292). It should be remembered that even though the position that has been accepted may be imperfect, improvement can occur spontaneously in the succeeding years, through a process of remodelling.

Severe displacement. When displacement is severe (Fig. 290) the position cannot easily be accepted because of the virtual certainty that painful osteoarthritis will develop in adult life. The position should therefore be improved. Three methods are available: manipulation, operative replacement of the epiphysis at the site of slipping, and compensatory osteotomy at a lower level.

Manipulation, with or without preliminary weight traction, is seldom successful; it is worth trying only in the rare cases of recent sudden displacement, especially if caused by injury. Manipulation—predominantly by medial rotation—should be carried out very gently lest the blood supply to the epiphysis be damaged. After successful manipulative reduction further slipping should be prevented by inserting threaded wires or screws.

Operative replacement of the epiphysis, with fixation by wires or a screw, has sometimes been practised when symptoms have been present for less than three months, provided the growth plate is still open. At its best it can restore the hip virtually to normal (Dunn and Angel 1978). Nevertheless the operation has the serious hazard that it may destroy the blood supply to the femoral head, leading to avascular necrosis of the femoral head and precipitating the onset of disabling osteoarthritis. In the opinion of many surgeons this major hazard negates any indication for the operation.

---

[1] A three-flanged nail, formerly sometimes used for fixation instead of threaded wires, is not recommended because it does not easily penetrate the hard epiphysis and may damage its blood supply.

Compensatory osteotomy is an alternative method that is preferred by most surgeons. The osteotomy is done just below the trochanteric level (Fig. 293). An anteriorly-based wedge of bone is removed so that the shaft of the femur is angled into flexion relative to the upper fragment. The operation thus compensates for the backward tilting of the epiphysis; correction should be sufficient to bring the epiphysis once more into the weight-transmitting segment of the acetabulum. The operation entails no risk of damage to the blood supply of the femoral head, so there is no risk of disastrous avascular necrosis; but it leaves the articular surface of the upper end of the femur deformed, and therefore does not altogether remove the risk of secondary osteoarthritis in later years.

Fig. 293
Subtrochanteric osteotomy for slipped femoral epiphysis of severe degree. By removal of an appropriate wedge of bone (shown outlined in the left-hand diagram), the epiphysis is restored to its proper relationship with the acetabulum. The operation has the advantage that the blood supply of the epiphysis is not endangered.

Comment
There is general agreement that when the displacement is slight it is best to accept the position and to prevent further slipping by inserting threaded wires.

Agreement is less complete in the matter of deciding which slips should be classed as 'slight' and treated by fixation with pins, and which are 'severe' and unsuitable for simple pinning. The experience of most surgeons suggests that it is wise to lean towards conservatism, and to resort to the more radical operation of corrective osteotomy only when displacement is extreme. In cases of severe displacement compensatory osteotomy is much to be preferred to operative replacement of the epiphysis at the site of slip. Because of the severe risk of avascular necrosis the latter operation is not to be recommended.

EXTRA-ARTICULAR DISORDERS IN THE REGION OF THE HIP

COXA VARA

The general term *coxa vara* includes any condition in which the neck-shaft angle of the femur is less than the normal of about 125 degrees (Figs 294 and 295). The angle is sometimes reduced to 90 degrees or less. The deformity is caused mechanically by the stress of body weight acting upon a femur that is defective or abnormally soft.

Causes. The most important causes of coxa vara are: 1) *Congenital*. Part of the femoral neck remains as unossified cartilage, which gradually bends during childhood (congenital coxa vara; infantile coxa vara). This type is uncommon. 2) *Slipped upper femoral epiphysis* (epiphysial coxa vara). This was described on page 317. 3) *Fracture*. Coxa vara is common after fractures in the trochanteric region with mal-union, and in ununited fractures of the neck of the femur. 4) *Softening of bone*, in general affections such as rickets, osteomalacia, or Paget's disease.

Effects. Coxa vara leads to true shortening of the limb. Approximation of the greater trochanter to the ilium impairs the efficiency of the hip abductors, leading in severe cases to a Trendelenburg 'dip', with consequent limp (p. 289).

Fig. 294   **Fig. 295**
Figure 294—Normal neck-shaft angle. Figure 295—Coxa vara: the neck-shaft angle is reduced.

Treatment. The treatment is mainly that of the underlying condition. Often a mild deformity is best accepted. In appropriate cases the neck-shaft angle can be corrected by osteotomy just below the greater trochanter.

TUBERCULOSIS OF THE TROCHANTERIC BURSA

The extensive bursa between the greater trochanter and the gluteal aponeurosis is occasionally the site of tuberculous infection. This type of bursitis has now become rare in Britain and other Western countries.

Pathology. Tubercle bacilli presumably reach the bursa through the blood stream from a focus elsewhere. There is a chronic inflammatory reaction in the walls of the bursa, usually with the formation of a tuberculous abscess. The abscess may burst through the skin to form a chronic discharging sinus. Later, the surface of the greater trochanter is sometimes eroded, with loss of the normal smooth surface.

Clinical features. The patient, often a young adult, complains of a swelling in the trochanteric region, with local discomfort and sometimes a persistent discharge of pus. *On examination* the trochanteric area is thickened, warmer than normal, and perhaps reddened. Often there is a palpable abscess or a discharging sinus. Movements of the hip are not impaired. *Radiographs* typically do not show any abnormality, but in long-standing cases there is sometimes superficial roughening or erosion of the lateral aspect of the greater trochanter. *Investigations*: The erythrocyte sedimentation rate is increased. Biopsy of the walls of the bursa shows the typical histological features of tuberculosis.

Treatment. After a preliminary one-month period of rest and antituberculous drugs, with aspiration as required, the bursa should be excised entire.

SNAPPING HIP

Snapping hip is a harmless condition in which a distinct snap is heard and felt on certain movements of the joint. It does not denote any underlying injury or disease and it is seldom of practical significance. The snap is attributed to slipping of a tendinous thickening in the aponeurosis of the gluteus maximus over the bony prominence of the greater trochanter. It is heard easily when the patient flexes the hip actively, but it is not reproduced by passive movement with the muscles relaxed. Treatment is required only exceptionally, when disability is severe. The offending ridge of aponeurosis is simply divided transversely from its under surface.

EXTRINSIC DISORDERS SIMULATING DISEASE OF THE HIP

As has already been mentioned, it frequently happens that a patient complains of symptoms in the region of the hip or thigh when in fact they arise at a distance. The conditions that may confuse the diagnosis in this way fall into three main groups: 1) disorders of the spine or sacro-iliac joints; 2) disorders of the abdomen or pelvis; and 3) occlusive vascular disease.

DISORDERS OF THE SPINE AND SACRO-ILIAC JOINTS

PROLAPSED INTERVERTEBRAL DISC

The pain of a prolapsed lumbar intervertebral disc or strained ligament is often referred to the gluteal region or lateral aspect of the thigh: indeed this is the commonest clinical feature in cases of intervertebral disc injury of slight or moderate degree. The patient himself, and often his doctor, may ascribe the symptoms to a lesion of the hip. But the history is unlike that of a hip affection. On examination other evidence of a spinal disorder will usually be found, whereas the hip itself is normal clinically and radiographically.

SACRO-ILIAC ARTHRITIS

The pain caused by arthritis of a sacro-iliac joint—whether it be tuberculous, pyogenic, or the early stages of ankylosing spondylitis—spreads diffusely over the gluteal area and may simulate an affection of the hip. Mistakes should be prevented by careful clinical examination and by routine radiography of the whole pelvis in cases of alleged hip complaints.

DISORDERS OF THE ABDOMEN AND PELVIS

PELVIC OR LOWER ABDOMINAL INFLAMMATION

Inflammation involving the side wall of the pelvis may mimic a hip lesion very closely; indeed even experienced surgeons have been deceived. The condition responsible is usually a subacute suppurative lesion such as a deep peri-appendicular abscess or a pyosalpinx. The hip symptoms arise partly from irritation of the obturator nerve, causing referred pain in the thigh, and partly from irritative spasm of the hip muscles that have their origin within the abdomen or pelvis—namely the psoas, iliacus, pyriformis, and obturator internus. The muscle spasm may cause marked restriction of hip movements, with pain if movement is forced. Differentiation from an intrinsic lesion of the hip depends upon a careful history and a complete physical examination including an investigation of the abdomen and pelvis. It is always important to bear in mind the possibility of abdominal or pelvic inflammation when the nature of an alleged hip complaint remains in doubt after clinical and radiographic examination of the joint.

OCCLUSIVE VASCULAR DISEASE

THROMBOSIS OF LOWER AORTA OR MAIN BRANCHES

Ischaemic pain in the muscles of the buttock or thigh, from occlusion of the lower abdominal aorta or its main branches, may occasionally simulate disease of the hip. Distinction should not be difficult: in occlusive vascular disease the pain is brought on by activity and is quickly relieved by rest; the femoral pulses will be weak or absent even though the pulses in the foot may be strong; and the hip will show a full range of painless movement.

References and bibliography, page 403.

15. The thigh and knee

The knee depends for its stability upon its four main ligaments and upon the quadriceps muscle. The importance of the quadriceps cannot be over-emphasised. So efficiently can a powerful quadriceps control the knee that it can maintain stability despite considerable laxity of the ligaments. In many injuries and diseases of the knee the quadriceps wastes strikingly, and to some extent the condition of the muscle is an index of the state of the knee: if it is wasted it is probable that there is an abnormality within the joint.

Apart from its vulnerability to injury, the knee is also particularly prone to almost every kind of arthritis. Moreover, it is the joint most commonly affected by osteochondritis dissecans and intra-articular loose body formation.

The region of the knee is the zone of most active bone growth in the lower limb (contrast the upper limb, where most growth occurs towards the shoulder and the wrist). Perhaps partly for this reason the metaphyses near the knee are common sites of osteomyelitis and of primary malignant bone tumours.

The knee is, in fact, a region where nearly every kind of orthopaedic disorder may be represented.

In the diagnosis of knee complaints arthroscopy has secured for itself such an important place that it has become almost a routine investigation for any suspected intra-articular lesion. Arthroscopic techniques of surgery have also become routine for such common disorders as meniscal tears and intra-articular loose bodies. Arthroscopic surgery has the advantages that formal opening of the knee is avoided and that recovery and convalescence are greatly accelerated. Stay in hospital is reduced, often markedly. Because of these benefits, arthroscopic surgery is demanded increasingly for straight-forward procedures within the knee.

An important landmark in knee surgery in recent years has been the successful development of total replacement arthroplasty for the relief of disabling arthritis, whether rheumatoid or degenerative.

SPECIAL POINTS IN THE INVESTIGATION OF THIGH AND KNEE COMPLAINTS

History

The history is of particular importance in the diagnosis of disorders of the knee. In a case of torn meniscus, for instance, the history is often the most important factor in the clinical diagnosis. When there has been a previous injury to the knee, the exact sequence of events at the time of the injury and afterwards must be ascertained. Inquiry is made into the mechanism of the injury; what the patient was doing at the time; whether he was able to carry on afterwards. Was he able to finish the game? If not, was he carried from the field or was he able to walk? How soon after the injury did the knee swell? Was he able to straighten the knee fully? If not, how did he eventually get it straight? Was he able to bend it? These and many other details must be elicited by careful questioning because they are so important in building up a picture of what exactly happened to the knee. Caution is necessary in accepting the patient's story of 'locking' at its face value. Many patients speak of 'locking' when the knee simply feels stiff and painful, or when it causes momentary jabs of pain on movement. Locking from a torn meniscus means simply that the knee cannot be straightened fully; it can usually be flexed freely. In locking from a loose body within the joint the knee may be jammed so that it will neither flex nor extend, but this is rather uncommon and the knee usually unlocks itself after an interval.

Table XI
Routine clinical examination in suspected disorders of the thigh and knee

1. LOCAL EXAMINATION OF THE THIGH AND KNEE

Inspection
Bone contours and alignment
Soft-tissue contours
Colour and texture of skin
Scars or sinuses

Palpation
Skin temperature
Bone contours
Soft-tissue contours
Local tenderness

Measurement of thigh girth
Comparative measurements at precisely the same level in each limb. (Note particularly the bulk of the quadriceps muscle)

Movements (active and passive, against normal knee for comparison)
Flexion

Extension
? Pain on movement
? Crepitation on movement

Power (tested against resistance of examiner)
Flexion
Extension

Stability
Medial ligament
Lateral ligament
Anterior cruciate ligament: anterior draw test; Lachman test; pivot shift test
Posterior cruciate ligament

Rotation tests (McMurray)
(Of value mainly when a torn meniscus is suspected)

Stance and gait

2. EXAMINATION OF POTENTIAL EXTRINSIC SOURCES OF THIGH OR KNEE SYMPTOMS

This is important if a satisfactory explanation for the symptoms is not found on local examination. The investigation should include especially: 1) the spine; and 2) the hip.

3. GENERAL EXAMINATION

General survey of other parts of the body. The local symptoms may be only one manifestation of a widespread disease.

Exposure

For proper examination the whole length of the limb must be uncovered. Trousers (and long underwear) must be removed. It is impossible to examine a knee adequately when the thigh is half covered by tightly rolled trousers or underpants. The sound knee must also be exposed for comparison. For proper examination of the knee the patient must always be recumbent upon a couch.

Steps in clinical examination

A suggested routine for clinical examination of the thigh and knee is summarised in Table XI.

Determining the cause of a diffuse joint swelling

The knee exemplifies better than any other joint the different types of diffuse articular swelling. That the joint is in fact swollen should be obvious from inspection: comparison of the two knees will show that the concavities present at each side of the patella have been filled out on the affected side.

A diffuse swelling of the knee can arise only from three fundamental causes: 1) thickening of bone; 2) fluid within the joint; and 3) thickening of the synovial membrane (in practice it is found that this is the only soft tissue about the knee that swells appreciably). Determination of the particular cause or combination of causes in a given case depends entirely on careful palpation, as follows:

Thickening of bone. Thickening of bone is detected without difficulty by deep palpation if the affected side is compared with the normal. There may be a general enlargement, caused perhaps by a bone infection or by an expanding tumour or cyst; or there may be simply a local prominence, caused usually by osteophytes at the joint margin or by an exostosis.

Fluid within the joint. A fluid effusion is best detected by the fluctuation test. The palm of one hand is placed upon the thigh immediately above the patella—that is, over the suprapatellar pouch. The other hand is placed over the front of the joint, with the thumb and index finger just beyond the margins of the patella (Fig. 296). Pressure of the upper hand

Fig. 296
Fluctuation test for fluid in the knee joint. Fluctuation is elicited between the two hands. One hand compresses the suprapatellar pouch, while the thumb and fingers of the other hand receive the impulse at either side of the patella.

upon the suprapatellar pouch drives fluid from the pouch into the main joint cavity, where it bulges the capsule at each side of the patella and imparts an easily detectable hydraulic impulse to the finger and thumb of the lower hand. Conversely, by pressure of this finger and thumb the fluid can be driven back into the suprapatellar pouch, the hydraulic impulse being clearly received by the upper hand. In this way an unmistakable sense of fluctuation can be elicited between the two hands. With practice it is easy to detect even a small effusion in this way. The 'patellar tap' test, in which the patella is tapped backwards sharply so that it strikes the femur and rebounds, though sometimes still used, is not recommended because it is unreliable. The test is negative in the presence of fluid in two circumstances: first, when there is insufficient fluid to raise the patella away from the femur; and secondly, when there is a tense effusion. If used at all, the 'patellar tap' test should be used only as a supplementary method.

Distinction between effusions of blood, serous fluid, and pus is made partly from the history, partly from the clinical examination. An effusion of blood (haemarthrosis) appears within an hour or two of an injury and rapidly becomes tense and therefore painful. An effusion of clear fluid develops slowly (twelve to twenty-four hours) and is never as tense as a blood effusion. An effusion of pus is associated with general illness and pyrexia.

Thickening of synovial membrane. A thickened synovial membrane is always a prominent feature of chronic inflammatory arthritis. The thickening is often most obvious above the patella, where the reduplicated membrane forms the suprapatellar pouch. It has a characteristic boggy feel on palpation, rather as if a sheet of warm sponge-rubber had been placed between the skin and the underlying bone. It is worth emphasising that since it is highly vascular a thickened synovial membrane is always associated with increased warmth of the overlying skin.

Movements

Accurate assessment of the range of movement is particularly important in the knee, because even a slight impairment of movement is significant. It is important to note also whether movement is painful and whether it is accompanied by crepitation.

Flexion. The normal range varies with the build of the patient. Thin patients can flex more than fat patients—usually enough to bring the heel in contact with the buttock. The range of the sound knee must be taken as the normal for the individual.

Extension. There is a fairly wide variation in the normal range of extension: it is wrong to accept 0 degrees as the starting-point of movement.[1] Many normal women can hyperextend their knees whereas some normal men cannot extend quite to the straight position. It is important to detect even a slight impairment of knee extension: therefore the range on the sound side must be taken as the yardstick of normal extension and a very careful comparison must be made between the two sides.

Tests for stability

The integrity of each of the four major ligaments is tested in turn.

Testing the medial and lateral ligaments. For this test the joint must be in a position just short of full extension, so that the posterior part of the joint capsule is relaxed: with the knee fully extended even marked laxity of the collateral ligaments can be masked by the intact posterior capsule, held taut. It must be remembered, however, that with the knee slightly flexed the medial and lateral ligaments are normally somewhat slack and allow a little side-to-side wobble. *Technique:* Support the limb by a hand gripping the ankle region and by the other hand behind the knee, flexing it slightly. Instruct the patient to relax the muscles. Using the more proximal hand as a fulcrum on the appropriate side of the knee, apply first an abduction force to test the medial ligament (Fig. 297) and then an adduction force to test the lateral ligament. If the ligament is torn, the joint will open out more than in the normal knee when stress is applied.

Fig. 297   **Fig. 298**

Figure 297—Testing the medial ligament. The knee is held slightly flexed (see text). Figure 298—Testing the cruciate ligaments. The patient's foot is steadied by sitting upon it. Pulling the tibia forwards tenses the anterior ligament; pushing it backwards tenses the posterior ligament.

Testing the anterior and posterior cruciate ligaments. The *anterior* cruciate ligament prevents *anterior* glide of the tibia on the femur; the *posterior* cruciate ligament prevents *posterior* glide. First the ligaments are tested with the knee flexed 90 degrees. *Technique:* The patient's knee being flexed to a right angle and the foot placed firmly on the couch, sit lightly on the foot to prevent it from sliding (Fig. 298). With the interlocked fingers of the two

---

[1] 0 degrees = the anatomical position, with the knee straight.

hands form a sling behind the upper end of the tibia, and clasp the sides of the leg between the thenar eminences. Place the tips of the thumbs one upon each femoral condyle. Ensure that the patient has relaxed the thigh muscles. Alternately pull and push the upper end of the tibia to determine the amount of antero-posterior movement. Normally there is an antero-posterior glide of up to half a centimetre; but since the normal is variable it is wise to use the patient's sound limb for comparison. Excessive glide in one or other direction indicates damage to the corresponding cruciate ligament.

Fig. 299
In the Lachman test the amount of anterior or posterior glide of the tibia upon the femur is assessed with the knee flexed only about 20 degrees.

In a second test the ligaments are examined with the knee flexed only 15 or 20 degrees (Lachman test). One hand supports the thigh just above the knee, gripping the femoral condyles, while the other hand grasps the upper end of the tibia (Fig. 299). While the patient relaxes the muscles the extent of any anterior or posterior glide of the tibial condyles upon the femur is determined by push-and-pull movements of the tibia.

Lateral pivot shift. The test for lateral pivot shift is supplementary to the tests described above for deficiency of the anterior cruciate ligament: it may be positive when the foregoing test is equivocal. The test depends on the fact that when the anterior cruciate ligament and the lateral ligament are deficient or lax the pivot between the lateral femoral condyle and the lateral tibial condyle may be unstable. In that event the lateral tibial condylar surface may be displaced forwards in relation to the femoral condyle when the tibia is rotated medially with the knee straight. When the knee is then flexed the subluxation is spontaneously reduced with a visible or palpable 'jerk'. The test is thus an indication of antero-lateral instability.

Fig. 300
Test for lateral pivot shift. The test depends upon first rotating the tibia medially to provoke subluxa-tion of the lateral condyle of the tibia upon the lateral femoral condyle, and then correcting the subluxation by flexing the knee (see text).

Technique. The foot on the affected side is lifted by the examiner's corresponding hand (the right foot is lifted by the right hand; the left foot by the left hand) so that the knee drops into full extension with the muscles relaxed. With the other hand the examiner then presses against the outer aspect of the limb just below the knee, imparting a valgus strain (Fig. 300). At the same time the tibia is rotated medially upon the femur. The knee is now flexed slowly from the straight position. If the test is positive the lateral tibial condyle becomes spontane-ously relocated on the femoral condyle when the knee reaches 30 or 35 degrees of flexion. The relocation is evidenced by a visible or palpable jerk (hence the term 'jerk test' sometimes used for the manoeuvre).

Rotation test for pedunculated tag of meniscus

The object of this test, often known as McMurray's test and used only for suspected tears of the menisci, is to demonstrate a pedunculated tag of meniscus by causing it to be momentarily jammed between the joint surfaces: when the knee is then straightened a loud click may be heard and felt as the tag is disengaged.

The manoeuvre is carried out by repeatedly: 1) flexing the knee, first fully but in succeeding tests progressively less fully; then 2) rotating the tibia upon the femur, first laterally but in further tests medially; and finally 3) extending the knee while the rotation of the tibia is still maintained. A loud click, distinct from the normal patellar click and usually associated with pain, suggests a tag tear (not a 'bucket-handle' tear) of a meniscus. *Caution:* Loud clicks can often be produced in normal knees. Most of them arise from movements of the patella, and they are not accompanied by pain. Discretion must be used in interpreting a click as an abnormal finding.

Extrinsic causes of pain in the thigh and knee

In most cases symptoms felt in the knee have their origin locally in or near the joint; but there are exceptions that may trap the unwary. Most importantly, pain in the knee may be the predominant feature of a lesion of the hip, such as arthritis or slipped upper femoral epiphysis. Less commonly sciatic pain, perhaps from a prolapsed intervertebral disc, has its greatest intensity at the level of the knee. In the investigation of pain in the knee we must therefore recognise the possibility that it may be referred from the spine or hip, and extend the examination to those regions if a satisfactory explanation for the trouble is not found on local examination.

Imaging

Radiographic examination. In a straightforward case antero-posterior and lateral films are sufficient. They should always include a reasonable length of the femur and of the tibia and fibula. Tangential projections of the femoral condyles with the knee flexed are sometimes helpful, especially when osteochondritis dissecans is suspected. Tangential ('sky-line') views of the patella may also be required. *Arthrography* (p. 15) may be helpful in certain cases of internal derangement.

When it is suspected that the knee symptoms might be referred from a lesion of the hip or spine appropriate radiographs of those regions should be obtained.

Radioisotope bone scanning. This may be useful in the diagnosis of inflammatory or neoplastic lesions.

Magnetic resonance imaging. When adequate information cannot be obtained from plain radiography or arthrography, magnetic resonance imaging may be helpful.

Fig. 301
Arthroscopic photograph showing normal appearance of medial meniscus. The medial femoral condyle is seen above, and the upper surface of the tibia is at lower right. The concave edge of the meniscus is seen clearly lying upon the tibia.

Arthroscopy

Arthroscopy has become an important adjunct to clinical and radiographic examination in the diagnosis of knee complaints. Indeed it has become almost mandatory if an intra-articular disorder is suspected (Fig. 301).

In diagnostic arthroscopy, usually carried out with the patient anaesthetised, the joint cavity is filled with saline through a hollow needle, and a cannula and telescope are entered at the appropriate site—usually antero-laterally or antero-medially, depending upon whether the surgeon is concerned to inspect mainly the medial or the lateral compartment. By correctly manoeuvring and rotating the arthroscope, and if necessary by the use of alternative sites of entry, almost the whole extent of the interior of the joint can be brought into view with the possible exception of the postero-lateral recess. The information gained can be enhanced by probing the menisci and other intra-articular structures with an instrument introduced at a site away from the arthroscope.

CLASSIFICATION OF DISORDERS OF THE THIGH AND KNEE

DISORDERS OF THE THIGH

Infections
Acute osteomyelitis
Chronic osteomyelitis
Syphilitic infection

Tumours
Benign bone tumours
Malignant bone tumours

ARTICULAR DISORDERS OF THE KNEE

Arthritis
Pyogenic arthritis
Rheumatoid arthritis
Tuberculous arthritis
Osteoarthritis
Haemophilic arthritis
Neuropathic arthritis
Anterior knee pain

Mechanical disorders
Tears of the menisci
Cysts of the menisci
Discoid lateral meniscus
Osteochondritis dissecans
Intra-articular loose bodies
Recurrent dislocation of the patella
Habitual dislocation of the patella

EXTRA-ARTICULAR DISORDERS IN THE REGION OF THE KNEE

Deformities
Genu varum
Genu valgum

Cystic swellings
Prepatellar bursitis
Popliteal cysts

Injuries
Rupture of the quadriceps
apparatus
Apophysitis of the tibial
tubercle (Osgood-Schlatter's
disease)

Post-traumatic ossification
Pellegrini-Stieda's disease of the
medial femoral condyle

DISORDERS OF THE THIGH

ACUTE OSTEOMYELITIS
(General description of acute osteomyelitis, p. 69)

The femur is one of the bones most commonly affected by pyogenic osteomyelitis. The infection is carried to the femur either through the blood stream (haematogenous osteomyelitis), when it usually affects the lower metaphysis; or it is introduced through an external wound, especially in cases of compound fracture. The clinical features and treatment are the same as those of osteomyelitis elsewhere (p. 69).

CHRONIC OSTEOMYELITIS
(General description of chronic osteomyelitis, p. 74)

Chronic pyogenic osteomyelitis is nearly always a sequel to acute infection that has been neglected or has responded poorly to treatment. As with the acute disease, the lower end of the femur is affected more often than the upper; but in many cases the infection spreads to involve a large part of the femoral shaft. Clinical features and treatment are like those of chronic osteomyelitis elsewhere (p. 74).

SYPHILITIC INFECTION
It is well to be aware that an unusual thickening of the femoral shaft may be due to syphilitic gumma or to diffuse syphilitic osteo-periostitis (see p. 78). These affections are now so uncommon in Western countries that they tend to be forgotten.

BONE TUMOURS IN THE THIGH
The femur is one of the commonest sites of the important bone tumours.

BENIGN TUMOURS
(General description of benign bone tumours, p. 80)

Of the four main types of benign bone tumour—osteoma, chondroma, osteochondroma, and giant-cell tumour—only the giant-cell tumour requires further consideration here.

GIANT-CELL TUMOUR (Osteoclastoma)
The lower end of the femur is a particularly frequent site for this uncommon tumour. The upper end of the femur is affected much less often. The tumour usually arises in young adults. It begins in what was the metaphysial region, but since the epiphysis is fused there is no obstacle to its spread to the articular end of the bone (see Fig. 71, p. 83). The bone is gradually expanded, the cortex becoming very thin. Pathological fracture may occur.

Though classed with the benign tumours, a giant-cell tumour tends to recur after inadequate removal and in some cases it has the character of a sarcoma, metastasising through the blood stream.

Treatment. Thorough curettage of the tumour and filling of the resultant cavity with bone grafts has been widely used but it is attended by a high incidence of recurrence. It may still be appropriate for small tumours but careful monitoring afterwards is essential so that any recurrence may be detected early. If the tumour is large most surgeons now prefer to excise the tumour-bearing lower end of femur entire, and to fuse the knee by means of bone grafts, stability being maintained in the meantime by a long intramedullary nail driven down the femur and across the gap into the tibia. An alternative method of reconstruction after radical excision of the tumour-bearing area is to fit a custom-made metal prosthesis to replace the lower end of the femur.

MALIGNANT TUMOURS
(General description of malignant bone tumours, p. 84)

The femur is a common site for all of the four main types of malignant bone tumour. Metastatic tumours are much more common than any of the primary malignant tumours, of which three require mention—namely osteosarcoma, Ewing's sarcoma and multiple myeloma.

OSTEOSARCOMA (Osteogenic sarcoma)
This is usually a tumour of childhood or early adult life: when it occurs in patients beyond middle age it is usually a complication of Paget's disease. Typically it arises in the metaphysis of a long bone, and the lower metaphysis of the femur is the favourite site. The tumour is highly malignant, with a mortality still in the region of 50 per cent or more despite recent advances in treatment. Treatment is discussed on page 89.

EWING'S TUMOUR
This also occurs mainly in children or adolescents. Unlike most bone tumours, it affects the shaft of the bone, which it expands in a fusiform manner. Over it, layer upon layer of new bone is laid down, giving a typical 'onion-peel' appearance as seen in the radiographs. Although the tumour responds dramatically to chemotherapy, usually in combination with radiotherapy or surgical excision, the prognosis remains poor, with a mortality in the region of 50 per cent from blood-borne metastases. Treatment is discussed on page 92.

MULTIPLE MYELOMA (Myelomatosis)
This is a tumour of later life. There are multiple tumour foci scattered through several bones, especially those containing abundant red marrow. The upper half of the femur is a favourite site (see Fig. 75, p. 86). The tumour responds temporarily to radiotherapy and chemotherapy (see p. 94) but it is eventually fatal.

Fig. 302
Metastatic tumour in the femur—a common site. Pathological fracture has occurred. The later radiograph at right shows the bone after internal fixation of the fragments by an intramedullary device.
The primary tumour was in the lung.

METASTATIC (SECONDARY) TUMOURS
The femur is commonly invaded by metastatic tumours, especially in its proximal half (Fig. 302).

Pathology. The tumours that metastasise most readily to bone are carcinomas of the lung, breast, prostate, kidney, and thyroid. The bone structure is destroyed by the tumour (except in the occasional osteoblastic or bone-forming metastasis from the prostate). Pathological fracture is common (Fig. 302).

Clinical features. Pain is the predominant symptom, but sometimes the tumour causes little disturbance until a pathological fracture occurs.

Treatment. The principles of treatment of metastatic tumours in bone were described on page 95. Most pathological fractures of the femur lend themselves well to internal fixation with a long modified intramedullary nail (Fig. 302). This facilitates nursing and greatly increases the patient's comfort because external splints can be dispensed with.

ARTICULAR DISORDERS OF THE KNEE

PYOGENIC ARTHRITIS OF THE KNEE
(General description of pyogenic arthritis, p. 109)

Pyogenic arthritis is commoner in the knee than in most other joints, partly because the knee is so exposed to injury and partly because of the close relationship of the joint cavity to the lower metaphysis of the femur, which is one of the commonest sites of acute osteomyelitis. The onset is acute or subacute, with pain, swelling, and loss of function. *Radiographs* do not show any abnormality in the early stages.

Treatment. Appropriate antibiotic therapy must be started immediately (see p. 110). *Local treatment:* The joint is rested in a plaster splint in a position of 20 degrees of flexion. The purulent effusion is removed daily by aspiration so long as it re-forms, and a solution of the appropriate antibiotic drug is injected into the joint. Rest is continued until the infection has been overcome; thereafter active movements are encouraged.

RHEUMATOID ARTHRITIS OF THE KNEE
(General description of rheumatoid arthritis, p. 111)

The knees are among the joints most frequently affected by rheumatoid arthritis, and they often suffer severe permanent disability. Both knees are often affected simultaneously with several other joints.

The knees are painful, swollen from synovial thickening, and warm to the touch. Bow-leg, knock-knee or flexion deformity may occur. Movement is impaired, and painful if forced.

Imaging. *Radiographs* do not show any abnormality at first. Later there is diffuse rarefaction in the area of the joint. In long-established cases destruction of articular cartilage leads to narrowing of the cartilage space (Fig. 303), and there may be clear-cut erosions of bone characteristically at the articular margins. *Radioisotope bone scanning* shows increased uptake of isotope in the region of the joint.

Course and prognosis. The inflammation dies down after months or years, but the knee is seldom restored to normal. The joint surfaces are usually damaged and wear out sooner than those of a normal joint. Thus in the late stages osteoarthritis is liable to be superimposed upon the original rheumatoid condition.

Fig. 303
Long-established rheumatoid arthritis of the knee. The bone is rarefied and the cartilage space is narrowed.

Treatment. In the active stage the treatment is that for rheumatoid arthritis in general (p. 115). Local treatment for the knees depends upon the severity of the inflammatory reaction. If it is severe, rest in bed or even temporary immobilisation in plaster is advisable. When it is moderate or slight, activity within the limits of pain is encouraged. Physical treatment is worth a trial. The most effective methods are exercises to preserve muscle power and joint movement, and local heat in the form of short-wave diathermy. Injections of hydrocortisone into the joint have sometimes given relief, but oft-repeated injections are inadvisable because they may accelerate the destructive process.

Operative treatment. Three types of operation are employed in suitable cases: 1) synovectomy; 2) replacement arthroplasty; and 3) arthrodesis. In deciding between them each case must be considered on its merits, and no hard-and-fast rules can be laid down.

Synovectomy. When there is persistent boggy thickening of the synovial membrane but when the articular cartilage is well preserved, the operation of synovectomy (excision of the synovial membrane) is worth considering. Comfort may be much improved and the advance of the disease is possibly slowed. This operation alone has no place in the later stages of the disease.

Replacement arthroplasty. Replacement arthroplasty of the knee has not reached quite the state of development that has been achieved at the hip. Nevertheless excellent and durable results are now being achieved in a high proportion of patients. In a favourable case pain is well relieved and good function is restored, with perhaps 90 degrees or more of flexion movement. Even at the best, however, the knee is unlikely to stand up indefinitely to vigorous activity. Replacement arthroplasty of the knee is therefore generally reserved for patients with severe disorganisation of the joint, and especially for elderly patients with involvement of several other joints.

Fig. 304   Fig. 305
Replacement arthroplasty of knee. Figure 304—Replacement of gliding surfaces; the femoral component of metal, the tibial component of plastic. Figure 305—Hinged prosthesis; both components of metal.

Several techniques of knee arthroplasty are available: all of them rely upon replacement of the articular surfaces by a metal or plastic (polyethylene) prosthesis. Most of the earlier devices took the form of a hinge, the upper and lower arms of which are cemented into the shafts of the femur and tibia respectively (Fig. 305). Such devices are still in use, though only

Fig. 306
Total replacement arthroplasty of knee. The femoral component is of metal. The tibial component (radiolucent and therefore not seen) is of high-density polyethylene.

on a small scale. The present trend is to provide gliding articular surfaces rather than a pivoted hinge. Thus the femoral condyles may be replaced by metal caps cemented in place, and the tibial condyles by a matching polyethylene prosthesis (total condylar replacement, Figs 304 and 306). The medial or the lateral femoral condyle may be replaced alone (in unicompartmental arthritis); but in most cases bicondylar replacement is preferred (Fig. 306).

Arthrodesis. This is a reliable operation for the disorganised rheumatoid knee, for it ensures total abolition of pain and good stability. But it is appropriate only if the other joints of the lower limbs are healthy—a condition that is seldom met in rheumatoid disease. The joint is usually fused in about 20 or 25 degrees of flexion, a position that is more convenient than the fully straight position. A stiff knee is, of course, an awkward handicap, but it is a price that is often acceptable to a patient who has been incapacitated by relentless pain over a long period.

TUBERCULOUS ARTHRITIS OF THE KNEE

(General description of tuberculous arthritis, p. 117)

After the hip, the knee is the limb joint most often affected by tuberculosis, usually in children or young adults. It is now an uncommon disease in Britain and other Western countries, though seen more often in developing countries. The knee is painful, diffusely swollen from thickening of the synovial membrane, and warm. Movements are restricted, the thigh muscles are wasted, and an abscess or sinus is sometimes apparent.

Fig. 307

Tuberculous arthritis of right knee in a child. The normal left knee is shown for comparison. Note the rarefaction, the diminution of cartilage space, and the small area of erosion near the lateral margin of the tibial joint surface. Destruction is only moderate, and a reasonably good result may be achieved with conservative treatment.

Radiographic features. The earliest change is diffuse rarefaction throughout the area of the knee (Fig. 307). Later, unless the disease is arrested, there is narrowing of the cartilage space and erosion of the underlying bone.

Treatment. *Constitutional treatment,* by antituberculous drugs, is the same as that for other tuberculous joints (p. 120). *Local treatment* is at first by rest in a splint or plaster, generally for two to three months in the first instance, depending on severity and progress.

Subsequent management depends upon the response to treatment and the state of the joint at the end of this period of immobilisation. If the articular cartilage and bone are still intact, if the general health is good and the local signs have subsided, and if the erythrocyte sedimentation rate has steadily improved, it is likely that the disease has been aborted. In that event active joint movements are encouraged and walking is gradually resumed.

On the other hand, if the review at the end of the initial period of immobilisation shows that the disease is still active and that articular cartilage or bone has been destroyed, sound bony fusion should usually be the ultimate aim, though arthroplasty may sometimes be considered. Immobilisation is therefore continued until the disease becomes quiescent. Arthrodesis may then be undertaken, provided the growth epiphyses have closed. In children still growing it is better to defer arthrodesis lest growth be disturbed, and in the meantime to protect the knee in a walking caliper or splint.

OSTEOARTHRITIS OF THE KNEE
(General description of osteoarthritis, p. 120)

The knee is affected by osteoarthritis more often than any other joint. The condition is particularly common in elderly, fat women.

Cause. It is caused by wear and tear; but nearly always some factor is present that has caused the joint to wear out sooner than usual. Overweight is the commonest factor: for some reason it seems to impose a harmful stress upon the knee whereas it does not adversely affect the hip or ankle. Other important predisposing factors are: previous fracture causing irregularity of the joint surfaces; previous disease with damage to articular cartilage (especially old rheumatoid arthritis or infective arthritis); previous intra-articular mechanical damage, as from a torn meniscus or from osteo-chondritis dissecans; and mal-alignment of the tibia on the femur (as in long-established bow-leg or knock-knee deformity from any cause).

Pathology. The articular cartilage is worn away and the underlying bone becomes eburnated. There is hypertrophy of bone at the joint margins, with the formation of osteophytes. The changes may affect predominantly the femoro-tibial joint or the patello-femoral joint; but usually the whole joint is affected.

Clinical features. The patient is commonly an elderly, heavy woman, in whom both knees may be affected. In another group, mostly in men, there is a history of previous mechanical derangement from a sports injury. There is slowly increasing aching pain in the joint, worse after unusual activity, and 'grating' may be felt or heard on movement. The symptoms are often exacerbated by a slight strain or twist. There is usually evidence of one of the predisposing factors mentioned above.

On examination the knee is slightly thickened from hypertrophy of bone at the joint margins, where a rim of osteophytes may be palpable. Effusion of fluid into the joint is unusual, except after much activity. Movement is moderately restricted and is accompanied by coarse crepitation. The quadriceps muscle is wasted. In severe cases there is a tendency to varus (bow-leg) deformity (less often a valgus (knock-knee) deformity), often with inability to straighten the knee fully.

Radiographic features. Narrowing of the cartilage space, which is the first sign of osteoarthritis in most joints, is often not discernible until a later stage in the case of the knee. The first clear sign of osteoarthritis in the knee is sharpening or 'spiking' of the joint margins, especially of the patella (Fig. 308) and tibia. Later, narrowing of the cartilage space is obvious,

Fig. 308
Spiking of the articular margins of the patella, as seen in the lateral radiograph, is an early sign of osteo-arthritis. The normal state (*right*) is shown for comparison.

osteophytes form at the joint margins, and the subchondral bone may become sclerotic (Fig. 309). Opacities that appear to be loose bodies are often seen; most are not in fact loose but are attached to the synovial membrane.

Fig. 309
Advanced osteoarthritis of the knee. Note the narrowing of the cartilage space, especially on the medial side and in the patello-femoral compartment. Note also the sclerosis of the subchondral bone, and osteophytes at the joint margins.

Treatment. In the usual case of moderate severity, conservative treatment is often successful in relieving the symptoms, although the structural changes in the joint are clearly irreversible. The most effective method is by physiotherapy. Intensive active exercises are carried out to strengthen the wasted quadriceps muscle. Local heat therapy is often also given, but it is less important than the exercises. The knee is largely dependent upon the quadriceps for its stability, and if a powerful muscle can be developed symptoms may remain in abeyance despite marked osteoarthritis.

Intra-articular injections of hydrocortisone have been tried, but the results are uncertain. Repeated injections are not recommended because they seem sometimes to accelerate the degenerative process.

Operative treatment. In the worst cases, with severe persistent pain, especially when associated with deformity, operation may be advisable. Its nature will depend upon the circumstances of each case. The following are the operations most used: 1) removal of loose bodies; 2) upper tibial osteotomy; 3) excision of patella; 4) arthroplasty; 5) arthrodesis.

    Removal of loose bodies. When loose bodies cause recurrent locking of the joint they should be removed. This is a simple operation, usually carried out by an arthroscopic technique, that gives good results. Any evident irregularities or excrescences of the articular surfaces may be trimmed at the same time.

| **Fig. 310** | **Fig. 311** |

Figure 310—Bow-leg deformity from uneven destruction of articular cartilage, that of the medial compartment being much thinner than that of the lateral. Body weight is now transmitted mainly through the diseased medial half of the joint. Interrupted line shows wedge of bone to be removed for correction of deformity. Figure 311—After corrective osteotomy and fixation with staples the line of weight transmission is shifted towards the more healthy lateral compartment.

    Upper tibial osteotomy. Tibial osteotomy aims to relieve pain and to correct deformity. It is especially valuable when wear of articular cartilage and bone has proceeded more in one half of the joint than in the other. For instance, if the medial half of the joint is markedly narrowed whereas the lateral compartment remains relatively healthy, there will be obvious bow-leg deformity and pain is likely to be prominent in the degenerate medial compartment, which is forced by the mal-alignment to take most of the weight (Fig. 310). Correction of the mal-alignment by removal of a wedge of bone based laterally (Fig. 311) transfers the weight-bearing thrust towards the more healthy lateral compartment and is often effective in relieving pain. Likewise if the lateral compartment is worn more than the medial, with consequent genu valgum, a medially based wedge may be excised. The osteotomy is done about 1.5 centimetres below the upper articular surface of the tibia, and to permit early walking the fragments are usually fixed together at operation by metal staples (Fig. 311).

Excision of patella. This is appropriate only when the arthritic process is largely confined to the patello-femoral joint, the femoro-tibial joint being relatively healthy.

Arthroplasty (Figs 304–306). This is undertaken less often for osteoarthritis than for rheumatoid arthritis, because the disability is seldom severe enough to justify an operation that is still unpredictable in its results and particularly in its durability. Methods of replacement arthroplasty were outlined on page 335.

Arthrodesis. This is now seldom undertaken, but is may be appropriate in a severe case, especially when other operations have failed and when the other knee and the hips are normal.

HAEMOPHILIC ARTHRITIS OF THE KNEE

(General description of haemophilic arthritis, p. 125)

Haemophilic arthritis affects the knee more often than any other joint.

Pathology. Initially there is simply a haemorrhage into the joint (haemarthrosis). With rest, this is slowly absorbed. But further bleeding usually occurs, and it leads eventually to degenerative changes in the articular cartilage and to fibrous thickening of the synovial membrane.

Clinical features. The findings on examination vary according to the phase and duration of the disease. After each fresh episode of bleeding the knee is swollen, partly from contained blood and partly from synovial thickening caused by interstitial extravasation of blood. The overlying skin is abnormally warm. Joint movements are restricted, and painful if forced.

In a quiescent phase between attacks of haemarthrosis there is some thickening of the joint from synovial fibrosis, movements are slightly impaired, and often there is moderate flexion deformity.

Investigations. The clotting time of the blood is increased.

Diagnosis. Because of the synovial thickening, increased warmth of the skin and restriction of knee movements, haemophilic arthritis is easily mistaken for chronic inflammatory arthritis. A history of previous bleeding incidents and the increased clotting time of the blood are the important distinguishing features. Biopsy should be avoided because it may cause further bleeding.

Treatment. In centres where the necessary haematological facilities are available the ideal treatment for acute haemarthrosis is to aspirate the knee under the temporary cover of antihaemophilic factor as if it were an ordinary traumatic haemarthrosis, and then to rest it in a plaster splint for two or three weeks. Such treatment may be expected to prevent or delay chronic joint changes. If antihaemophilic factor is not available the outlook for the future of the knee is much less favourable. Aspiration should usually be avoided. Instead, the knee should be bandaged and immobilised on a Thomas's splint or in plaster. After three to six weeks the residual blood is absorbed and cautious activity may be resumed.

The chronic degenerative arthritis that results from multiple repeated haemarthroses may have to be controlled by the permanent use of a polythene knee splint. Operative treatment—for instance arthrodesis—is practicable, but only under the cover of adequate doses of antihaemophilic factor.

NEUROPATHIC ARTHRITIS OF THE KNEE

(General description of neuropathic arthritis, p. 126)

Neuropathic arthritis (Charcot's osteoarthropathy) of the knee is now seen very seldom in Britain because of the rarity of tabes dorsalis, formerly the most prevalent underlying cause. Other occasional causes include denervation of the joint from a lesion of the cauda equina or from other neurological disease.

Pathology. The changes may be regarded as a much exaggerated form of osteoarthritis. The articular cartilage and parts of the underlying bone are worn away, but at the same time there is often considerable hypertrophy of bone at the joint margins. The ligaments become lax and the joint is unstable.

Clinical features. The knee is greatly thickened, mostly from irregular hypertrophy of the bone ends. There is slight or moderate restriction of movement, and there is marked lateral laxity, often allowing severe bow-leg deformity. Pain is slight or absent. Further examination will reveal evidence of the underlying neurological disease. *Radiographs* show marked destructive changes, usually with some new bone formation at the joint margins (Fig. 312).

Fig. 312
Neuropathic arthritis of the knee. Degenerative destruction is accompanied by massive new bone formation.

Treatment. In many cases function is adequate despite the marked disorganisation of the knee, and treatment is not required. In other cases marked deformity—usually lateral bowing—may demand some form of protective appliance (orthosis), such as a moulded plastic splint or a caliper. Arthrodesis is practicable but fusion is often slow. Because of this and the absence of severe pain operation should usually be avoided.

ANTERIOR KNEE PAIN
(Including chondromalacia of the patella)

Anterior knee pain is a generic term that almost certainly includes more than a single clinical entity. The non-specific nature of the label implies, correctly, that the pathogenesis of the pain is not always well understood. The clinical syndrome characteristically occurs in adolescents, especially girls. The description that follows relates to one well recognised type of lesion, namely chondromalacia of the patella. Similar symptoms may occur in the absence of demonstrable patellar changes, and their causation is often conjectural.

CHONDROMALACIA OF THE PATELLA
In chondromalacia of the patella the cartilage of the articular surface of the patella—particularly the medial facet—is roughened and fibrillated for reasons that are unknown. It is surmised that friction between the damaged area and the corresponding femoral condyle is responsible for the pain. The condition is distinct from osteoarthritis but osteoarthritis may be superimposed upon it in later years.

Clinical features. The patient is often a girl aged 15–18 years. There is aching pain deep in the knee, behind the patella. Pain is exacerbated by climbing or descending stairs. There is often effusion of fluid, and tenderness may be found on palpating the deep surface of the patella after displacing it to one side. There may also be a point of marked tenderness over the front of the medial femoral condyle. Movements may be accompanied by fine crepitation transmitted to the examiner's hand upon the patella, especially when the patient does a 'knees bend' exercise from the standing position.

Radiographs are normal. *Arthroscopy* will demonstrate the patellar lesions, if present.

Treatment. This should nearly always be expectant. A firm crepe bandage is applied and strenuous activities are curtailed. These precautions will usually reduce the symptoms to an acceptable level. Operative treatment should be avoided, for although a variety of procedures has been devised the results are almost universally disappointing.

TEARS OF THE MENISCI

Injuries of the menisci (semilunar cartilages) are common in men under the age of 45. A tear is usually caused by a twisting force with the knee semiflexed or flexed. It is usually a football injury, but it is also common among men who work in a squatting position. Thus it was common among coal miners excavating shallow seams, before the advent of full mechanisation. The medial meniscus is torn much more often than the lateral.

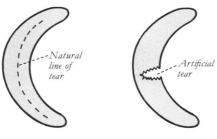

Fig. 313   **Fig. 314**

Figure 313—A tear of a meniscus nearly always takes the form of a longitudinal split, which may extend throughout the length of the meniscus or may emerge at the concave border. A transverse tear (Fig. 314) is nearly always an artefact, produced at the time of operation.

Pathology. In patients of athletic age there are three types of meniscus tear (Figs 315–317). All begin as a longitudinal split (Fig. 313). If this extends throughout the length of the meniscus it becomes a *bucket-handle tear*, in which the fragments remain attached at both ends (Fig. 315). This is much the commonest type. The 'bucket handle' (that is, the central fragment) is displaced towards the middle of the joint, so that the condyle of the femur rolls upon the tibia through the rent in the meniscus (Fig. 315). Since the femoral condyle is so shaped that it requires most space when the knee is straight, the chief effect of a displaced 'bucket-handle' fragment is that it limits full extension (= 'locking').

If the initial longitudinal tear emerges at the concave border of the meniscus a pedunculated tag is formed. In *posterior horn tear* the fragment remains attached at its posterior horn (Fig. 316); in *anterior horn tear* it remains attached at its anterior horn (Fig. 317). A transverse tear through the meniscus is nearly always an artefact, produced at the time of operation (Fig. 314).

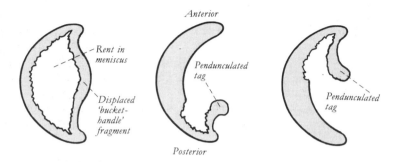

Fig. 315   Fig. 316   Fig. 317

The three types of meniscus tear. Figure 315—Bucket-handle tear, the commonest type. Figure 316—Posterior horn tear. Figure 317—Anterior horn tear.

The menisci are almost avascular; consequently when they are torn there is not an effusion of blood into the joint. But there is an effusion of synovial fluid, secreted in response to the injury. Major tears of the menisci do not heal spontaneously, probably because the torn surfaces are separated by fluid.

Clinical features of torn medial meniscus. The patient is 18–45 years old. The history is characteristic, especially with 'bucket-handle' tears. In consequence of a twisting injury the patient falls and has pain at the antero-medial aspect of the joint. He is unable to continue what he was doing, or does so only with difficulty. He is unable to straighten the knee fully. The next day he notices swelling of the whole knee. He rests the knee. After about two weeks the swelling lessens, the knee seems to go straight, and he resumes his activities. Within weeks or months the knee suddenly gives way again during a twisting movement; there are pain and subsequent swelling as before. Similar incidents occur repeatedly.

Locking. By 'locking' is meant inability to extend the knee fully. It is not a true jamming of the joint because there is a free range of flexion. Locking is a common feature of torn medial meniscus, but the limitation of extension is often so slight that it is not noticed by the patient. Persistent locking can occur only in 'bucket-handle' tears: tag tears cause momentary catching but not true locking in the accepted sense.

On examination in the recent stage the typical features are effusion of fluid, wasting of the quadriceps, local tenderness at the level of the joint antero-medially, and (characteristically in 'bucket-handle' tears) limitation of the *last few degrees* of extension by a springy resistance, with sharp antero-medial pain if passive extension is forced.

In the 'silent' phase between attacks there are often no signs other than wasting of the quadriceps.

Clinical features of torn lateral meniscus. The features are broadly similar, but the clinical picture is often less clearly defined. The history may be vague. Pain is at the lateral rather than the medial side of the joint, but it is often poorly localised.

Imaging. *Plain radiographs* are usually normal, whether the tear be of the medial or of the lateral meniscus. But in untreated cases of long duration signs of early degenerative arthritis may be noted in the affected compartment. *Arthrography* will often demonstrate the tear, but *magnetic resonance imaging* is even more reliable.

Arthroscopy. On arthroscopic examination a meniscal tear can be seen whatever its site, except sometimes at the posterior end of the lateral meniscus (Fig. 318).

Fig. 318
Arthroscopic photograph showing tear of medial meniscus.

Diagnosis. In the 'silent' phase clinical diagnosis often depends largely upon the history. The surgeon should be very cautious in diagnosing a torn meniscus unless there is a clear history of injury and unless there have been recurrent incidents, each followed by synovial effusion. If one is relying on clinical diagnosis alone a period of observation may be required before the diagnosis becomes reasonably certain. Arthroscopy, or a combination of arthroscopy with arthrography, should establish the nature of the lesion conclusively.

Late effects. Long-continued internal derangement from a torn meniscus predisposes to the later development of degenerative arthritis. Arthritis is also liable to develop years after a meniscus has been removed.

Treatment. Once the diagnosis is established the standard treatment is to excise either the whole meniscus or, more appropriately in most cases, the displaced 'bucket-handle' fragment alone. This operation is usually best carried out by the arthroscopic technique without formal opening of the joint—though of course the joint may be opened by incision if difficulty arises during the course of arthroscopic surgery. In selected cases of peripheral tear, repair by suture is sometimes undertaken.

Treatment of the locked knee. Manipulation under anaesthesia is a common practice when there is a marked block to extension. But it cannot be expected that manipulation will restore the displaced 'bucket handle' to its normal position: it merely extends the tear longitudinally and thus allows the 'bucket-handle' fragment to move further towards the middle of the joint—that is, to the intercondylar region. In this position the displaced fragment presents less impediment to joint movement, but completely full extension is seldom restored. Manipulation is therefore worthwhile only in so far as it increases the patient's comfort while he is awaiting admission for operation.

HORIZONTAL TEAR OF DEGENERATE MEDIAL MENISCUS

The meniscal tears described above are uncommon in patients over the age of 50, when the menisci begin to show degenerative changes. But a degenerate meniscus is liable to suffer a different type of lesion. The medial meniscus in particular may split horizontally at a point often near the middle of its convexity (Fig. 319). Such a split is usually of small dimensions, and since there is no separation of the fragments natural healing can occur.

Fig. 319
Horizontal tear of medial meniscus,
seen in plan and on section.

Clinically there is troublesome and persistent pain at the medial aspect of the knee at the joint level. The pain may be noticed after a minor injury, but often it seems to come on spontaneously, without any preceding incident. In the early stages there is usually a small effusion of fluid into the joint.

Treatment should be expectant at first, by bandaging and quadriceps exercises. In most cases the symptoms resolve in the course of several months. In the occasional case in which they fail to do so, excision of the meniscus should be advised.

CYSTS OF THE MENISCI

A cyst of a meniscus (semilunar cartilage) forms a tense, almost solid swelling at the level of the joint, usually on the lateral side.

Cause. Cysts arise spontaneously, but there is often a previous history of direct injury at the site of the cyst.

Pathology. The swelling is formed by a proliferation of fibrous tissue, which is honeycombed with small cystic cavities containing small quantities of clear gelatinous fluid.

Clinical features. The lateral meniscus is affected much more often than the medial. There is visible swelling, most obvious when the knee is held slightly flexed, at the level of the joint and usually anterior to the lateral (or medial) ligament (Fig. 320). The swelling tends to be painful at night and it is usually tender on firm pressure. The swelling is so tense that fluctuation can seldom be elicited—indeed it is sometimes mistaken for bone.

Fig. 320
Cyst of lateral meniscus.

Radiographic features. Radiographs may show an indentation of the side of the tibial condyle where the cyst has been in contact with it.

Treatment. If the disability justifies operation the cyst should be excised together with the meniscus from which it arises. Very occasionally, it may be practicable to excise the cyst while leaving the meniscus intact (Flynn and Kelly 1976).

DISCOID LATERAL MENISCUS

Rarely the lateral meniscus (semilunar cartilage) fails to assume its normal crescentic form during development, but persists in its embryonic form as a thick disc-like mass interposed between the lateral condyles of the femur and tibia.

A discoid meniscus may cause recurrent discomfort in the knee, with a tendency to giving way. Usually a loud 'clonk' can be demonstrated on flexion-extension movements. These symptoms often become prominent during childhood or adolescence. If the disability becomes troublesome the meniscus should be removed. There is a risk of the development of degenerative arthritis in later life.

OSTEOCHONDRITIS DISSECANS OF THE KNEE

(General description of osteochondritis dissecans, p. 130)

Osteochondritis dissecans is characterised by local ischaemic necrosis of a segment of the articular surface of a bone and of the overlying articular cartilage, with eventual separation of the fragment to form an intra-articular loose body. The knee is affected much more often than any other joint.

Cause. This is unknown. Impairment of the blood supply to the affected segment of bone by thrombosis of an end artery has been suggested. Injury is possibly a predisposing factor. There is also a constitutional predisposition to the disease, because it may affect several members of a family or several joints in the same patient.

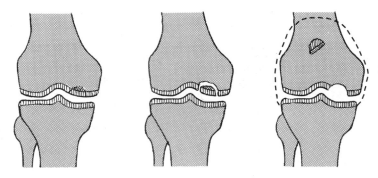

| Fig. 321 | Fig. 322 | Fig. 323 |

The evolution of osteochondritis dissecans. Figure 321—A segment of the articular surface dies. Figure 322—A line of demarcation forms around it. Figure 323—The fragment breaks away and lies loose in the joint, leaving a cavity in the femoral condyle.

| Fig. 324 | Fig. 325 |

Osteochondritis dissecans. Figure 324—Routine antero-posterior radiograph. Figure 325—Tangential postero-anterior projection with knee semiflexed—the so-called intercondylar view. This shows clearly the large crescentic cavity in the medial femoral condyle, with the separating fragment *in situ*. Inset shows the loose fragment after removal.

Pathology. The lesion nearly always affects the articular surface of the medial condyle of the femur (Figs 321–323). The size of the affected segment varies—it is often about 2 centimetres in diameter. Within the area of the lesion the subchondral bone is avascular and the overlying cartilage softens. A clear line of demarcation forms between the avascular segment and the surrounding normal bone and cartilage (Fig. 321). After many months the fragment separates as a loose body (sometimes two or three), leaving a shallow cavity in the articular surface which is ultimately filled with fibrocartilage (Figs 322 and 323). The damage to the joint surface predisposes to the later development of osteoarthritis, especially when the fragment is large.

Clinical features. The patient is an adolescent or a young adult, who complains of discomfort or pain in the knee after exercise, a feeling of insecurity, and intermittent swelling. When a loose body has already separated within the joint the predominant symptom is recurrent sudden locking. *On examination* there is a fluid effusion. The quadriceps muscle is wasted. Movements are not usually impaired.

Radiographic features. Radiographs show a clear-cut defect of the bone at the articular surface of the medial femoral condyle (Figs 324 and 325). At first the cavity is occupied by the separating fragment of bone; later the cavity may be empty, and a loose body will then be seen elsewhere in the joint. The lesion is shown best in tangential postero-anterior projections with the knee semiflexed (Fig. 325).

Arthroscopy. The osteochondritic lesion in the medial femoral condyle will be clearly evident in the later stages. Initially, however, the defect is concealed by articular cartilage that looks normal, though if it is probed an area of softening may be apparent.

Treatment. In the developing stage treatment should be expectant: the knee is supported with a crepe bandage and strenuous activities are curtailed. Sometimes in these early cases the lesion will heal spontaneously, especially in young adolescents.

When the lesion is 'ripe'—that is, when a clear line of demarcation has formed between the separating fragment and the surrounding normal bone—the loose piece should usually be removed, especially if it is small. This may be done arthroscopically when the necessary expertise is at hand. A shallow cavity is left in the femoral condyle, but this gradually fills with fibrocartilage and adequate function is usually restored.

Because of the risk of the later development of osteoarthritis if a large part of the femoral condyle has been excavated, some surgeons recommend that the loose fragment be replaced in position and fixed with a pin. It has been shown that the fragment may unite again with its bed, but it is by no means certain yet that the incidence of late osteoarthritis will be reduced by this method of treatment. Probably it should be reserved for cases in which the separated fragment is large.

LOOSE BODIES IN THE KNEE

The knee is the joint most commonly affected by the formation of loose bodies. There are four main causes: 1) osteochondritis dissecans (one to three loose bodies); 2) osteoarthritis (one to ten loose bodies); 3) chip fracture of a joint surface (one to three loose bodies); 4) synovial chondromatosis (five to five hundred loose bodies).

Pathology. *Osteochondritis dissecans* was described on page 347. The loose body or bodies are formed by spontaneous separation of a fragment of bone and cartilage from the articular surface of the medial femoral condyle. A shallow cavity remains in the condyle.

Osteoarthritis was described on page 338. Some of the loose bodies that may be found in osteoarthritis are probably formed by detachment of marginal osteophytes. Most separated osteophytes, however, retain a synovial attachment and cause no trouble: though they appear loose in radiographs they should not be regarded as such unless symptoms of locking indicate that they are moving freely within the joint. True loose bodies may possibly form from flakes of articular cartilage shed into the joint that gradually enlarge, nourished by synovial fluid.

Chip fracture of joint surface (osteochondral fracture) is an infrequent cause of intra-articular loose bodies. There is a clear history of the causative injury.

Synovial chondromatosis (osteochondromatosis) is a rare disease of the synovial membrane. It is characterised by the formation of numerous small villous processes, which become pedunculated. Later their bulbous extremities become cartilaginous and they are detached to lie free in the joint. Finally, some or all of the numerous loose bodies become calcified.

Whatever the cause of a loose body, its repeated jamming between the joint surfaces will predispose to osteoarthritis or will aggravate existing osteoarthritis.

Clinical features. The characteristic symptom of a loose body in the knee is recurrent locking of the joint from interposition of the loose piece between the joint surfaces. Suddenly, without warning, the knee becomes jammed during movement. Locking is accompanied by severe pain. After a variable interval the patient is usually able, by manoeuvring the limb, to disengage the loose body and free the joint. The next day the knee is found to be swollen with fluid. In many cases the patient is able to feel the mobile body through the soft tissues when it lies in a superficial part of the joint.

On examination the findings are often slight, for a patient is seldom seen when the knee is locked. If he is seen soon afterwards a fluid effusion is present. Between attacks there may be no objective signs other than perhaps slight wasting of the quadriceps. Sometimes the loose body can be palpated. The features of an underlying condition such as osteoarthritis may be present.

Fig. 326   **Fig. 327**

Figure 326—Loose body in the knee. As in this case, loose bodies often lie in the suprapatellar pouch. Figure 327—The fabella, a sesamoid bone in the lateral head of the gastrocnemius, present in many normal persons. It is sometimes mistaken for a loose body in the joint.

Radiographic features. With few exceptions, loose bodies are shown radiographically. They often lie in the suprapatellar pouch (Fig. 326). Care should be taken not to mistake the fabella (a sesamoid bone in the lateral head of the gastrocnemius) (Fig. 327) for a loose body. The position of the fabella is constant: it lies slightly above the level of the joint well behind the femur and towards the lateral side, and it is always oval in shape with its long axis vertical.

Treatment. In general the treatment for an intra-articular loose body is to remove it, when possible by an arthroscopic technique. Removal should always be advised if the loose body is causing recurrent locking. If there are no symptoms of locking operation is not essential. In such cases the fragment, though appearing loose in the radiographs, is often attached to the synovial membrane and is kept out of harm's way. This applies particularly to detached osteophytes in cases of osteoarthritis.

RECURRENT DISLOCATION OF THE PATELLA

The patello-femoral joint is one of the three joints that are most liable to recurrent displacement, the others being the shoulder and the ankle. In the case of the patello-femoral joint, unlike the other two, the instability is often caused by congenital factors rather than by an initial violent injury.

Pathological anatomy. In dislocations of the patella the displacement is always lateral, the patella slipping over the lateral condyle of the femur while the knee is flexed. Four factors predispose to recurrent dislocation: 1) general ligamentous laxity ('double-jointedness'), which may be an inherited defect; 2) under-development of the lateral femoral condyle, with a shallow intercondylar groove; 3) an abnormally high position of the patella, which consequently does not lie so deeply as usual in the intercondylar groove; and 4) genu valgum, which causes the line of pull of the quadriceps to lie too far to the lateral side; this last factor is seldom an important one.

Clinical features. Recurrent dislocation of the patella is more common in girls than in boys. Often both knees are affected. Trouble usually begins during adolescence. Dislocation occurs while the patient is engaged in some activity that entails flexing the knees—not necessarily a violent exertion. Suddenly, while the knee is flexed or semiflexed, there is severe pain in the front of the knee, and the patient is unable to straighten it. Often the displacement of the patella is recognised and reduced on the spot, either by the patient herself or by an onlooker.

On examination in the dislocated state the knee is swollen, and the patella is seen and felt upon the lateral side of the lateral femoral condyle. After reduction the main signs are an effusion (usually of blood-stained fluid), and tenderness over the medial part of the quadriceps expansion, which is usually strained or torn. One of the minor anatomical anomalies mentioned above may be observed. In particular, generalised ligamentous laxity is often found, as evidenced by the patient's ability to hyperextend the knee (genu recurvatum) or other joints such as the wrists or the joints of the fingers; this double-jointedness may be present also in parents or other relatives. The patella is often found to lie higher than normal, and it may be unduly small.

Radiographs are seldom obtained in the state of dislocation. After reduction the knee may appear normal radiographically, but commonly the patella is small and is seen at a slightly higher level than usual, often in both knees (patella alta).

Course. Dislocation of the patella does not always become recurrent: some patients have no further trouble after one or two dislocations. But in many cases dislocations recur with ever-increasing ease and frequency, so that the patient may become seriously handicapped. Moreover oft-repeated dislocations predispose to the later development of osteoarthritis.

Treatment. Treatment should be expectant at first. After a dislocation the patient should receive a course of physiotherapy designed to strengthen the quadriceps muscle, and especially the vastus medialis.

If the dislocations recur with such frequency that the patient is seriously disabled, operation should be advised. The method recommended is to detach the bony insertion of the patellar tendon and transpose it to a new bed in the tibia, medial and distal to the original insertion (Fig. 328). In this way the patella is drawn lower into the deeper part of the intercondylar groove of the femur, and the line of pull of the quadriceps mechanism is transferred more to the medial side.

Old insertion

New insertion

Fig. 328

Transposition of the insertion of the patellar tendon downwards and medially re-aligns the pull of the quadriceps and draws the patella down to lie in the intercondylar groove of the femur.

HABITUAL DISLOCATION

It is important to distinguish between recurrent dislocation of the patella and habitual dislocation. Whereas in recurrent dislocation the knee may seem normal for weeks or months between dislocations, in habitual dislocation the patella dislocates laterally each time the knee is flexed beyond a certain range. This condition becomes apparent at an earlier age than recurrent dislocation—usually in early childhood. The underlying pathology is also distinct: there is abnormality of the quadriceps muscle and in particular of the vastus lateralis, which may show a fibrous contracture; or there may be an abnormal fibrous band tethering the vastus lateralis to the ilio-tibial tract (Jeffreys 1963). It is this shortened vastus lateralis that pulls the patella laterally every time the knee is markedly flexed. In the absence of treatment the patella may eventually become permanently dislocated.

Treatment is by division of the tight muscle or band so far as is necessary to allow full flexion of the knee without displacement of the patella.

EXTRA-ARTICULAR DISORDERS IN THE REGION OF THE KNEE

GENU VARUM AND GENU VALGUM

Genu varum (bow leg) and genu valgum (knock knee) occur commonly in childhood. In the vast majority of instances there is no underlying disease, and the deformity need not cause anxiety because it is gradually corrected spontaneously.

Genu varum or valgum may also occur, either in children or in adults, in consequence of injury or disease. The commonest causes are: 1) fracture of the lower part of the femur or of the upper part of the tibia with mal-union (for example, depressed fracture of the lateral tibial condyle causing genu valgum); 2) rheumatoid arthritis or osteoarthritis; 3) rarefying diseases of the bones, such as rickets or osteomalacia; 4) other bone-softening diseases such as Paget's disease (osteitis deformans) (see Fig. 34, p. 51); 5) in children, uneven growth of the epiphysial plates, such as may occur after injury or osteomyelitis or in dyschondroplasia (p. 49).

In assessing a case of genu varum or genu valgum the surgeon must always be careful to exclude such underlying organic disorders by full clinical examination, and if necessary by radiography, before diagnosing the benign childhood affections described in the following sections.

BENIGN GENU VARUM OF TODDLERS

The knee and leg are bowed outwards (Fig. 329). A mild degree of this deformity is so common as to be almost normal in children aged 1 to 3 years. It does not require treatment unless it persists into later childhood. Care should be taken to exclude the possibility of rickets or other underlying disease.

Fig. 329   **Fig. 330**

Figure 329—Genu varum. Slight bowing is common in infants but it is usually corrected spontaneously as the child grows. Figure 330—Genu valgum. Deformity of this degree in young children is usually corrected spontaneously during growth.

BENIGN GENU VALGUM OF CHILDHOOD

The knee is angled inwards, the tibia being abducted in relation to the femur. With the knees straight, the medial malleoli cannot be brought into contact (Fig. 330). The deformity is common in children aged 3 to 5 years. In the absence of underlying bone disease it usually corrects itself spontaneously in the course of years.

Treatment. In early childhood treatment is unnecessary, but it is common practice (albeit of doubtful relevance) to fit a wedge, base medially and 3–5 millimetres deep, to the heel of the shoe to shift the line of weight-bearing medially (see Fig. 351, p. 382).

Severe genu valgum persisting after the age of 10 requires active treatment. In growing children two methods of correction are available. One is to retard the growth at the medial side of the epiphysial cartilage of femur or tibia by bridging the epiphysis to the diaphysis with metal staples (epiphysiodesis). The other and more certain method is by supracondylar osteotomy of the femur, or of the upper tibia if the fault lies there, with excision of a suitable wedge from the medial side. After the cessation of epiphysial growth genu valgum can be corrected only by osteotomy.

RUPTURE OF THE QUADRICEPS APPARATUS

The quadriceps muscle gains insertion into the tibia through the medium of the patella (enclosed within the quadriceps expansion) and the patellar tendon. Complete rupture may occur at three points (Fig. 331): 1) at the point of attachment of the quadriceps tendon to the upper pole of the

Fig. 331
The three points at which the quadriceps apparatus may rupture. 1. At insertion of quadriceps into patella. 2. Through the patella. 3. At insertion of patellar tendon into tibial tubercle.

patella; 2) through the patella and the surrounding quadriceps expansion (fractured patella); or 3) at the attachment of the patellar tendon to the tibial tubercle. In all cases the injury is caused by an unexpected flexion force, resisted automatically by a sudden contraction of the quadriceps.

AVULSION FROM PATELLA

Avulsion of the quadriceps tendon from the upper pole of the patella occurs mainly in elderly men, in whom the quadriceps tendon is often degenerate. It is not a common injury. The tendon should be re-attached to the bone by sutures of stainless steel wire.

DISRUPTION THROUGH PATELLA

This is the usual site of rupture, and it forms a common variety of fractured patella. The injury occurs mainly in adults of middle age. If the patella is cleanly broken into two pieces and the patient is under 40 the fragments should be fixed together by a screw. Otherwise the patellar fragments should be excised and the quadriceps expansion sutured.

This is the least common injury, occurring mainly in children or young adults. A fragment of bone may be pulled off with the tendon. The torn tendon should be re-attached by sutures.

APOPHYSITIS OF THE TIBIAL TUBERCLE
(Osgood-Schlatter's disease)

Apophysitis of the tibial tubercle is a childhood affection in which the tibial tubercle becomes enlarged and temporarily painful. Often known as Osgood-Schlatter's disease, it was formerly regarded as an example of osteochondritis juvenilis (p. 96), but it is now generally agreed that it is nothing more than a strain of the developing tibial tubercle, from the pull of the patellar tendon.

Fig. 332
Apophysitis of the tibial tubercle (Osgood-Schlatter's disease). The tibial tubercle appears enlarged and fragmented. The normal tubercle of the other tibia is shown for comparison.

Clinical and radiographic features. The patient is a child aged 10 to 14 years, usually a boy. The complaint is of pain in front of and below the knee, worse on strenuous activity. *On examination* the tibial tubercle is unduly prominent, and tender on palpation. Pain is increased when the quadriceps is tensed, as in straight leg raising against resistance. The symptoms and signs are confined to the region of the tibial tubercle, and the knee joint itself is normal.

Radiographs show enlargement and sometimes fragmentation of the tibial tubercle (Fig. 332).

Course. The disorder is self-limiting, and normal function is always restored.

Treatment. In most cases treatment is not required. If local pain and tenderness are severe the knee should be rested for two months in a plaster cylinder extending from groin to malleoli.

PREPATELLAR BURSITIS

The bursa that lies in front of the lower half of the patella and the upper part of the patellar tendon is prone to inflammation.

Types. There are two types of prepatellar bursitis: 1) irritative; and 2) infective or suppurative.

IRRITATIVE PREPATELLAR BURSITIS

This is caused by repeated friction; it occurs especially in those who do much kneeling. There is fibrous thickening of the wall of the bursa, which is distended with fluid.

Clinical features. There is a softly fluctuant swelling in front of the lower part of the patella ('housemaid's knee'). The swelling is clearly demarcated. It is manifestly confined to a plane in front of the joint, and the joint itself is unaffected.

Treatment. A trial may be made of aspiration under local anaesthesia, but the effusion tends to recur unless further friction can be avoided. The risk of recurrence may possibly be reduced if hydrocortisone is injected into the emptied sac. Operative excision of the bursa affords a more certain permanent cure.

SUPPURATIVE PREPATELLAR BURSITIS

This is caused by infection of the bursa with pyogenic organisms, which reach the bursa directly through a puncture wound, or through the lymphatics from an infected lesion on the leg. The wall of the bursa is acutely inflamed and the sac is distended with pus.

Clinical features. There are pain and swelling in front of the knee. There may be mild constitutional disturbance, with pyrexia. The swelling is confined to the site of the prepatellar bursa. It is acutely tender on palpation, and the overlying skin is hot and reddened. The inguinal lymphatic glands are often enlarged and tender. The knee joint itself is unaffected, but the patient is unwilling to bend it fully because flexion increases the pain by tensing the skin over the bursa.

Treatment. Appropriate antibiotic therapy should be instituted and the bursal abscess should be drained by incision.

POPLITEAL CYSTS

Cystic swellings are not infrequently found in the popliteal fossa. Most are examples of irritative bursitis, usually of the semimembranosus bursa. A few are caused by herniation of the synovial cavity of the knee (Baker's cyst).

Care must be taken to distinguish popliteal cysts from other, more serious swellings in this region, such as aneurysm of the popliteal artery and synovial sarcoma.

SEMIMEMBRANOSUS BURSITIS

The semimembranosus bursa lies between the medial head of the gastrocnemius and the semimembranosus. The bursa may become distended with fluid to form an elongated sac that bulges backwards between the muscle planes. *Clinically,* there is a soft cystic swelling at the back of the knee, close to the medial condyle of the femur.

Treatment is not always required. In children particularly, operation may usually be avoided because the cyst may disappear spontaneously. Nevertheless if the swelling becomes uncomfortably large the sac should be excised.

BAKER'S CYST

A Baker's cyst is simply a herniation of the synovial cavity of the knee, with the formation of a fluid-filled sac extending backwards and downwards (Fig. 333). It is not a primary condition but is always secondary to a disorder of the knee with persistent synovial effusion, such as rheumatoid arthritis or osteoarthritis. In long-standing cases the hernial sac is much elongated, and may extend a considerable distance down the calf.

Clinically there is a soft cystic bulge near the midline behind the knee or in the upper calf. The underlying abnormality of the knee, with synovial effusion, will usually be obvious.

Fig. 333
To show how a Baker's cyst is formed as a herniation of the synovial membrane.

Treatment. In most cases treatment should be directed towards the underlying condition of the knee rather than to the cyst itself. Nevertheless if the cyst is extensive it is sometimes advisable to excise it.

PELLEGRINI-STIEDA'S DISEASE

Pellegrini-Stieda's disease is the name sometimes used to describe ossification in the subligamentous haematoma after partial avulsion of the medial ligament from the medial condyle of the femur. *Clinically* there is persistent discomfort at the medial side of the knee after an injury to the medial ligament. There are thickening and slight tenderness over the site of attachment of the ligament to the medial femoral condyle. *Radiographs* show a thin plaque of new bone close to the medial condyle.

Treatment is by active mobilising and muscle-strengthening exercises.

CALCIFIED DEPOSIT IN MEDIAL LIGAMENT

It is probable that some supposed cases of Pellegrini-Stieda's disease are in fact examples of calcified deposit within the medial ligament. A similar deposit may occur in the lateral ligament. These lesions are homologous with the calcified deposit that occurs more commonly in the supraspinatus tendon (p. 223). If the symptoms are acute the calcified material should be removed by aspiration or by operation.

EXTRINSIC DISORDERS WITH REFERRED SYMPTOMS IN THE KNEE

From time to time patients are seen whose main complaint is of pain in the knee, but local examination reveals no satisfactory explanation for it. In such cases the possibility that the pain is referred from a disorder distant from the knee should always be considered. The commonest source of such referred pain is a disorder of the hip. Much less often a disorder of the spine is responsible.

DISORDERS OF THE HIP

The conditions of the hip in which the pain may be felt predominantly in the knee are the various types of arthritis, of which osteoarthritis is the most common. It is especially important to remember that pain in the knee may also be the main complaint, or even the only complaint, in cases of slipped upper femoral epiphysis: failure to bear this in mind has often led to the true diagnosis being missed. The pain is referred along the course of one of the nerves—especially the obturator nerve, which takes a large share in the innervation of the hip.

Differential diagnosis. There should be little difficulty in determining the true source of the pain if the possibility of a hip lesion is borne in mind. Whenever knee symptoms cannot be adequately explained after a local examination of the knee the hip should be investigated and, if necessary, radiographed.

DISORDERS OF THE SPINE

The only disorders of the spine that may cause symptoms predominantly in the region of the knee are those that cause pressure on the roots of the lumbar or sacral plexus, especially prolapsed intervertebral disc. It is only rarely that such referred symptoms are unassociated with other symptoms in the back, buttock or thigh.

References and bibliography, page 403.

16. The leg, ankle and foot

In the orthopaedic out-patient clinic disorders of the foot are second in frequency only to disorders of the back. Their prevalence may have several causes. *Hereditary factors*: The foot is probably in a state of relatively rapid evolution consequent upon man's assumption of the upright posture, and perhaps for that reason it is prone to variations in structure and form which may impair its efficiency. *Postural stresses*: Overweight throws an increased burden on the feet, and they may be unable to withstand the stress without ill-effect, especially if the intrinsic muscles are poorly developed. *Footwear*: The wearing of shoes is a potent cause of foot disorders. Many types of shoe interfere seriously with the mechanics of the foot, and the ladies' shoe with high heel and pointed toe is particularly to blame.

SPECIAL POINTS IN THE INVESTIGATION OF LEG, ANKLE AND FOOT COMPLAINTS

In nearly all cases symptoms in the leg, ankle or foot can be explained by a local abnormality. Only rarely are they referred from a distant lesion. In this respect the lower limb differs markedly from the upper, for in many cases symptoms in the hand have no local cause but are referred from a proximal lesion.

History

The precise distribution of pain should be ascertained. The occupation and habits of the patient, including sporting activities, may be significant, as may also be a history of previous injury. Specific enquiry should be made into the effect upon the symptoms of standing and walking.

Exposure

It is essential that socks or stockings be removed and that the whole leg be exposed up to the knee. Both limbs must always be examined so that the two may be compared. The first part of the examination is conducted with the patient lying upon a couch. Later, the foot is examined while the patient stands.

Steps in clinical examination

A suggested plan for the routine clinical examination of the leg, ankle and foot is summarised in Table XII.

Assessing the state of the peripheral circulation

An essential part of the examination of the foot that is often forgotten is to study the efficiency of the arterial circulation. A reasonably accurate assessment may be made on clinical

359

Table XII
Routine clinical examination in suspected disorders of the leg, ankle, and foot

1. LOCAL EXAMINATION OF THE LEG, ANKLE, AND FOOT

Inspection
Bone contours and alignment
Soft-tissue contours
Colour and texture of skin
Scars or sinuses

Palpation
Skin temperature
Bone contours
Soft-tissue contours
Local tenderness

State of peripheral circulation
Dorsalis pedis pulse
Posterior tibial pulse
Popliteal pulse
Femoral pulse
? Cyanosis of foot when dependent

Movements (active and passive,
compared with normal side)
At the ankle:
  Plantarflexion
  Extension (dorsiflexion)
At the subtalar joint:
  Inversion-adduction
  Eversion-abduction
At the midtarsal joint:
  Inversion-adduction
  Eversion-abduction

At the toes:
  Flexion
  Extension

Power (tested against resistance of
  examiner)
Each muscle group to be tested in turn.
  (Power of calf muscles is best tested
  with the patient recumbent and then
  standing)
(Compare with other side)

Stability
Integrity of ligaments—particularly the
  lateral ligament of the ankle

Appearance of foot on standing
Shape of longitudinal arch
Shape of forefoot
Efficiency of toes
Efficiency of calf muscles (? ability to
  raise heel from ground while standing
  on affected leg alone)

Gait

Condition of footwear
Sites of greatest wear. (Compare with
  other side)

2. GENERAL EXAMINATION

General survey of other parts of the body. The local symptoms may be only one
manifestation of a widespread disease.

evidence alone, but if surgical treatment is contemplated and vascular insufficiency is suspected it is necessary to have more precise information which can be provided only by certain special investigations.

Clinical assessment. This is based on a study of the texture of the skin and nails, colour changes, skin temperature, the arterial pulses, auscultation, and exercise tolerance. *Texture of skin and nails*: The skin of an ischaemic foot loses its hair and becomes thin and inelastic. The nails are coarse, thickened and irregular. Ulceration of the tips of the toes may be noted. *Colour changes*. A brick-red rubor or cyanosis occurring when the foot is made dependent after a period of elevation (Buerger's test) denotes serious impairment of the arterial circulation. *Temperature*: A foot with impaired arterial supply is colder than normal, but little reliance can be placed on this test as applied clinically at the bedside.

Arterial pulses: The pulses to be felt for are the dorsalis pedis, the posterior tibial, the popliteal and the femoral. The popliteal pulse is often difficult to feel even in normal individuals. Palpation should be made with the fingertips of both hands supporting the slightly flexed knee. Pulsation of the dorsalis pedis artery is best felt at the dorsum of the foot between the bases of the first and second metatarsals. The posterior tibial artery is felt about two centimetres behind and below the tip of the medial malleolus. Absence or impairment of arterial pulsation is an important sign of defective circulation. It should be remembered, however, that a normal pulse is easily masked by thickening or oedema of the soft tissues. *Capillary return*: In limb ischaemia capillary return is slowed after blanching of a digital pulp or nail by pressure. *Auscultation*: A bruit over one of the major limb vessels, caused by turbulence of blood flow, may denote partial obstruction or an arterio-venous communication.

Special investigations. These include ankle pressure recordings, Doppler ultrasound probe analysis, combined probe analysis and ultrasonography, pulse volume recording (plethysmography), and arteriography.

Ankle pressure recordings. The systolic blood pressure at ankle level is measured at rest and after walking at controlled speed on a treadmill, blood flow being monitored by an ultrasound probe utilising the Doppler principle. The brachial systolic pressure is also measured and the ratio of the two readings (leg/arm) is recorded. Normally this 'pressure index' is 1 or greater than 1. In arterial disease the ankle pressure is less than the brachial, and moreover it falls markedly on exercise and recovers slowly when exercise ceases, in proportion to the severity of the arterial narrowing.

Doppler ultrasound probe analysis has become increasingly sophisticated and informative. A number of different systems are in use. Bidirectional recording plots a wave form from blood flow and velocity in each direction. The wave form, displayed on a screen, provides information on the state of the artery proximally. Pulsed Doppler imaging is a development of this technique. *Duplex scanning* combines real-time ultrasonography of the vessel walls with Doppler probe analysis of the blood flow. These refined ultrasound techniques give accurate information and can often obviate the need for arteriography.

Pulse volume recording (segmental plethysmography) uses multiple cuffs round the thigh and leg, inflated to a pressure of about 65 mm Hg to obstruct the venous outflow. Small increases in the volume of the limb occurring with each arterial pulse are indicated by pressure changes in the cuffs. The rate of increase of limb volume can be related to the blood flow beneath each cuff.

Arteriography. The arterial tree is outlined by radiography after injection of opaque fluid into the main vessel. Any narrowing or occlusion of a vessel is clearly revealed.

Movements at the ankle and tarsal joints
Since the joints are close together, movement at the tarsal joints is easily mistaken for movement at the ankle, and vice versa. Careful examination is required to determine the range at each individual joint.

Fig. 334
Examining ankle movement. The examining hand grips the hindfoot rather than the forefoot, so that movements of the subtalar and midtarsal joints are eliminated.

Ankle movement. The ankle is strictly a hinge joint. The only movements are extension (dorsiflexion) and plantarflexion. The range should be judged from the excursion of the hindfoot rather than the forefoot, so that any contribution from the tarsal joints is disregarded. Similarly, in testing the passive range, the foot should be controlled from the heel (Fig. 334). The normal range of ankle movement varies in different subjects; so the normal ankle must be used as a control. An average range is about 25 degrees of extension (dorsiflexion) and 35 degrees of plantarflexion.

Subtalar and midtarsal movement. In normal use the subtalar and midtarsal joints work together as a single unit. The movements permitted are: 1) combined inversion and adduction (supination); and 2) combined eversion and abduction (pronation).

In clinical examination the range of movement contributed by each component can be determined separately. To test *subtalar movement* support the lower leg by a hand gripping

Fig. 335	**Fig. 336**
Examining subtalar movement. The calcaneus is gripped by the examining hand and moved upon the talus.	Examining midtarsal movement. The heel is gripped in the steadying hand to eliminate subtalar movement.

the ankle. With the other hand lightly grasp the calcaneus from below (Fig. 335). Instruct the patient alternately to invert and evert the foot, observing the range through which the heel rocks from side to side. Compare with the sound foot. The normal range is about 20 degrees on each side of the neutral position.

To test *midtarsal movement* grasp the calcaneus firmly so that subtalar movement is eliminated. With the other hand lightly grasp the midfoot near the bases of the metatarsals (Fig. 336). Instruct the patient alternately to twist the foot inwards and outwards into inversion and eversion, and compare the range with that on the sound side. The normal is a rotation of about 20 degrees on each side of the neutral position.

Toe movements. Determine the active and passive range at the metatarso-phalangeal and interphalangeal joints. It should be remembered that the normal range of dorsiflexion of the great toe at the metatarso-phalangeal joint is nearly 90 degrees (Fig. 337). Limitation to

Fig. 337
The normal range of dorsiflexion at the metatarso-phalangeal joint of the great toe is nearly 90 degrees.

less than 60 degrees of dorsiflexion is certainly abnormal. The range of downward flexion is about 15 degrees but it varies between individuals. Movement at the lesser toes is variable: there should be not less than 30 degrees of flexion at the metatarso-phalangeal joints and at the interphalangeal joints.

Examination of the feet under weight-bearing stress
Instruct the patient to stand evenly on both feet. Observe the general shape of the ankle, foot, and toes. Study the shape of the longitudinal arch. Is it of normal shape? Is it flattened so that the navicular region is in contact with the ground (pes planus or valgus)? Or is it higher than

normal (pes cavus)? It is important to view the heel from the back, so that any inward (varus) or outward (valgus) deviation may be noted. Next study the forefoot. Is it splayed and broader than normal? Assess the function of the toes. Normally they can be pressed upon the ground by the action of the intrinsic muscles so that the metatarsal heads are lifted up and relieved of weight-bearing pressure. Finally, examine the efficiency of the calf muscles. The crucial test is to ask the patient to stand on the affected leg and to raise the heel from the ground (see Fig. 338).

Examination of spine
Certain deformities of the foot—especially pes cavus with clawing of the toes—may be caused by a neurological abnormality in the thoraco-lumbar or lumbar region of the spine, associated with spina bifida or other developmental anomaly (see p. 138). Examination should therefore be made for a tell-tale dimple, pigmented area or tuft of hair on the overlying skin.

Gait
Look especially for abnormal posture of the feet such as turning in (intoeing) or turning out, or drop foot. Observe whether weight is borne correctly on the sole of the foot or whether it is taken too much on the medial or lateral border. Observe also whether the heel is raised normally from the ground at the beginning of each step.

For a more refined analysis of gait special force plates may be incorporated in a walkway to record the pressure beneath each component part of the foot in all phases of the step. It is thus possible objectively to compare the pattern of gait in a defective foot with the normal pattern; or to compare the gait pattern of a foot before and after operation.

Footwear
The examination of the foot is not complete until the patient's shoes have been inspected and compared on the two sides. Note the position of greatest wear. When the foot is normal the greatest wear in the sole occurs beneath the ball of the foot and slightly to the medial side. In the heel it is at the posterior border slightly to the lateral side. The state of the uppers is also important: excessive bulging on the medial side suggests a valgus foot and excessive bulging on the lateral side an inverted foot.

Radiographic examination

The ankle. Routine radiographs of the ankle comprise an antero-posterior and a lateral projection centred at the level of the joint. The films should include a reasonable length of the shafts of the tibia and fibula, and the whole of the talus.

When laxity of the lateral ligament is suspected a special inversion film is required. This is an antero-posterior projection taken while the heel is held in fullest inversion by an assistant. If the lateral ligament is torn or lax the talus will be shown tilted in the ankle mortise (see Fig. 340, p. 372).

In cases of suspected ligamentous injury antero-posterior stability should also be tested. Rupture of the anterior talofibular component of the lateral ligament allows anterior subluxation of the talus, as shown in a lateral radiograph taken while the foot is pushed forward upon the tibia.

The foot. Routine radiographs should comprise an antero-posterior (strictly a supero-inferior) projection and a lateral projection, preferably taken while weight is borne on the feet. An oblique projection (non-weight-bearing) is used to show the mid-foot. Special techniques are available to show the calcaneus (axial view).

CLASSIFICATION OF DISORDERS OF THE LEG, ANKLE AND FOOT

DISORDERS OF THE LEG

Injuries
Rupture of the calcaneal tendon

Infections
Acute osteomyelitis
Chronic osteomyelitis
Syphilitic infection

Tumours
Benign tumours of bone
Malignant tumours of bone

Circulatory disorders
Intermittent claudication

DISORDERS OF THE ANKLE

Arthritis
Pyogenic arthritis
Rheumatoid arthritis
Tuberculous arthritis
Osteoarthritis
Gouty arthritis

Haemophilic arthritis
Neuropathic arthritis

Post-traumatic mechanical derangements
Recurrent subluxation

DISORDERS OF THE FOOT

Deformities
Congenital club foot (talipes
  equino-varus)
Talipes calcaneo-valgus
Accessory bones in the foot
Pes cavus
Pes planus (flat foot)

Postural disorders
Foot strain

Arthritis
Osteoarthritis of the tarsal joints
Other forms of tarsal arthritis

Osteochondritis
Osteochondritis of the
  navicular bone (Kohler's
  disease)

Miscellaneous
Painful heel
Pain in the forefoot
Plantar wart
Callosities
Ganglion

DISORDERS OF THE TOES

Deformities
Hallux valgus
Hammer toe
Under-riding toe

Arthritis
Rheumatoid arthritis
Osteoarthritis
Gouty arthritis

Osteochondritis
Osteochondritis of a metatarsal
  head (Freiberg's disease)

Miscellaneous
Ingrowing toe nail
Subungual exostosis
Onychogryposis

DISORDERS OF THE LEG

RUPTURE OF THE CALCANEAL TENDON

Surprising as it may seem, a ruptured calcaneal tendon (tendo Achillis) is often overlooked, the symptoms being wrongly ascribed to a strain or to a ruptured plantaris tendon.

Pathology. The rupture is nearly always complete. It occurs about 5 centimetres above the insertion of the tendon. If it is left untreated the tendon unites spontaneously, but with lengthening.

Clinical features. While running or jumping the patient feels a sudden agonising pain at the back of the ankle. He may believe that something has struck him. He is able to walk, but with a limp. *On examination* there is tenderness at the site of rupture. There is general thickening from effusion of blood and from oedema of the paratenon, but a gap can usually be felt in the course of the tendon. The power of plantarflexion at the ankle is greatly weakened, though some power remains through the action of the tibialis posterior, the peronei, and the toe flexors. A useful test, to be carried out with the patient prone, is to squeeze the bulk of the calf muscles from side to side. Normally this causes a slight plantarflexion movement of the foot, but not if the tendon is ruptured.

Fig. 338
The crucial test of intact calf function is to raise the heel from the ground while standing only on the affected leg. Inability to do this after an injury to the calcaneal tendon is diagnostic of complete rupture.

Diagnosis. The retention of some power of plantarflexion may deflect the unwary from the correct diagnosis. The crucial test is to ask the patient to lift the heel from the ground while standing only upon the affected leg (Fig. 338). This is impossible if the tendon is ruptured. The gap in the tendon may be well demonstrated by ultrasound scanning.

Treatment. Non-operative treatment is usually by immobilisation in plaster for five weeks, with the foot in slight equinus to relax the tendon and thus to help to prevent lengthening.

Operative treatment entails repair of the tendon, preferably by non-absorbable sutures of synthetic material, tension on the suture line being relaxed by immobilising the limb with right-angled knee flexion and moderate ankle plantarflexion for two weeks. For the next four weeks a below-knee plaster with the ankle at 90 degrees is worn.

Whether treatment is by plaster alone or by operation, it must be completed after removal of the plaster by increasingly vigorous exercises for the calf muscles, practised until full strength is restored.

COMMENT
Whereas formerly a fresh rupture was regularly repaired by operation, more recently there has been a trend towards non-operative treatment in selected cases. There is certainly still a place for operation in athletic persons, to reduce the risk of lengthening of the tendon and consequent loss of 'spring-off'. If non-operative treatment is to be used it should be in more sedentary or elderly patients. If rupture has been overlooked or neglected for more than four weeks conservative treatment by graduated exercises is generally to be preferred.

ACUTE OSTEOMYELITIS
(General description of acute osteomyelitis, p. 69)

The tibia is one of the commonest sites of haematogenous osteomyelitis. Because of its liability to open (compound) fracture it is also the commonest site of osteomyelitis from direct contamination. The fibula is less often affected.

The pathological and clinical features and treatment conform to the general description on page 69.

CHRONIC OSTEOMYELITIS
(General description of chronic osteomyelitis, p. 74)

Chronic osteomyelitis in the lower leg, as elsewhere, is nearly always a sequel of acute osteomyelitis. It may follow either the haematogenous type of infection or an infected open fracture.

BRODIE'S ABSCESS
This rather uncommon lesion was described on page 76. It is a special form of chronic osteomyelitis which arises insidiously, without a recognised acute infection preceding it. The tibia is the commonest site (see Fig. 58, p. 76).

SYPHILITIC INFECTION OF THE TIBIA
(General description of syphilitic osteitis, p. 78)

Although skeletal syphilis is now rare in Western countries, when it does occur the tibia is often the bone affected. The infection may take the form of a localised gumma or of diffuse osteoperiostitis (see Figs 65 and 66, p. 80). There is a gradually enlarging swelling, with moderate pain. It is important to bear the possibility of syphilis in mind, because the swelling is easily mistaken for a tumour.

TUMOURS OF BONE

BENIGN TUMOURS
(General description of benign bone tumours, p. 80)

Of the four main types of benign tumours of bone—osteoma, chondroma, osteochondroma, and giant-cell tumour—only the chondroma and giant-cell tumour require further mention here.

CHONDROMA
In the tibia or fibula this is seldom found except in multiple form in the condition of dyschondroplasia (p. 49). The individual tumours in this condition resemble enchondromata. They arise from the growing epiphysial cartilage plate, and they interfere with the normal growth of the bone. An important effect is that the growth of the tibia and fibula may be unequal, with the consequence that the bones may become curved or the plane of the ankle joint may be tilted away from the horizontal (see Fig. 31, p. 50).

GIANT-CELL TUMOUR (Osteoclastoma)
The upper end of the tibia or fibula, like the lower end of the femur, is a favourite site for this tumour. It usually arises in a young adult, expanding the bone and extending to within a short distance of the articular surface.

Treatment. If the tumour is in the fibula the whole of the affected end of the bone should be excised together with an adequate margin of healthy bone. If the tumour is in the upper end of the tibia, the problem of treatment is much more difficult. The discussion relating to this tumour when it affects the lower end of the femur (p. 332) applies here also. As in the femur, to ensure full eradication of the tumour it is probably wise to excise the upper end of the tibia entire, to sacrifice the knee joint, to bridge the gap with bone grafts, and to provide stability by means of a long intramedullary nail. Alternatively, continuity may be restored after excision by the use of a custom-made prosthesis to replace the knee joint and the upper half of the tibia.

MALIGNANT TUMOURS
(General description of malignant bone tumours, p. 84)

The tibia, like the femur, is a common site for primary malignant bone tumours, especially osteosarcoma and Ewing's tumour.

OSTEOSARCOMA (Osteogenic sarcoma)
This tumour usually affects the upper metaphysis of the tibia: the lower end of the tibia and the fibula are affected much less often. The tumour metastasises rapidly through the blood stream, especially to the lungs. Treatment was described on p. 89.

EWING'S TUMOUR
This usually affects the shaft of a long bone, again in childhood or early adult life. The tibia is one of the commonest sites.
Treatment was described on page 91.

INTERMITTENT CLAUDICATION

Intermittent claudication is a symptom of arterial insufficiency in the lower limb. In its typical form it is characterised by cramp-like pain in the calf, induced by walking and relieved by rest.

Cause. The usual underlying cause is arteriosclerosis with consequent partial or total obstruction of the main limb vessel. Thrombo-angiitis obliterans and arterial embolism are less common causes. Tobacco smoking is a major contributory factor.

Pathology. The basic disturbance is ischaemia of muscle, in consequence of which metabolites cannot be removed speedily enough when the muscle is exercised. The accumulation of metabolites is believed to be responsible for the pain, which subsides within a few minutes when the muscle is rested. The muscles usually affected are those of the calf, but in some instances other muscle groups are involved, according to the site of the arterial obstruction. The vascular lesion is usually a complete occlusion of the femoral or the popliteal artery. In claudication affecting the buttock the aortic bifurcation or the iliac artery may be occluded.

Clinical features. Intermittent claudication is much more common in men than in women. In the usual arteriosclerotic type the patient is past middle life, but in cases due to thrombo-angiitis obliterans or embolism the symptoms may develop in early adult life. The patient is usually a regular smoker.

With gradual arterial occlusion the onset is insidious and the symptoms are slowly progressive; but in cases precipitated by thrombosis or embolism the onset may be sudden. In a typical case the patient complains that after walking a certain distance—perhaps a hundred metres or so—he is forced to stop by severe cramp-like pain in the calf, or occasionally in another muscle group, such as the buttock. After a few minutes' rest the pain disappears and he is able to walk on again for a similar distance.

On examination there is objective evidence of impaired arterial circulation in the lower limb (p. 359). The posterior tibial, dorsalis pedis, and popliteal pulses are absent. There may be ischaemic changes in the skin of the foot. Evidence of widespread arterial or cardiac disease is nearly always found on general examination.

Investigations. *Ankle pulse recordings* show a low arterial pressure compared to the arm pressure, and the pressure may fall markedly on exercise (see p. 361).

Doppler ultrasound probing and other tests may show reduced blood flow in the peripheral vessels.

Radiographic features. Plain radiographs often show patches of calcification in the walls of several arteries, from the aorta downwards. Arteriography will demonstrate the site and extent of the arterial occlusion.

Diagnosis. Intermittent claudication is frequently misdiagnosed. Unless a detailed history is obtained, the patient's complaint of pain in the calf may suggest to the unwary doctor the likelihood of foot strain or flat foot. Moreover, such a diagnosis may seem to be supported by the finding of flattened arches or deformed feet, common in the elderly. The clues to the correct diagnosis are the typical history and the impairment of the arterial pulses, and it may be confirmed by blood flow studies, including ankle pressure recordings, Doppler ultrasound examination and, if necessary, arteriography.

Intermittent claudication from vascular disease bears a resemblance to the symptoms of spinal stenosis (pseudoclaudication) (p. 200), but in that condition the arterial circulation is not impaired.

Prognosis. The outlook is serious, though deterioration is often slow. In progressive cases increasing ischaemia may lead eventually to gangrene of the foot. Peripheral vascular disease is often associated with cardiac disease; so the general prognosis must always be guarded.

Treatment. If the arterial obstruction is proximal, involving the aorta, iliac artery or common femoral artery, good results may be expected from prosthetic replacement of occluded vessels. In contrast, in peripheral disease the results of arterial reconstruction are often unsatisfactory, and if the viability of the foot is not in danger and rest pain is absent, operation is usually better avoided. It is important for the patient to give up smoking.

If the nutrition of the foot is threatened lumbar ganglionectomy is worth a trial as a means of improving the circulation in the skin, but it cannot be expected to have a significant effect on the symptoms of claudication.

DISORDERS OF THE ANKLE

PYOGENIC ARTHRITIS OF THE ANKLE
(General description of pyogenic arthritis, p. 109)

Pyogenic arthritis of the ankle is uncommon. The organisms reach the joint through the blood stream or through a penetrating wound; local spread from a focus of osteomyelitis of the tibia or fibula is rare because the bony metaphyses are entirely extra-capsular (see Fig. 51, p. 71).

RHEUMATOID ARTHRITIS OF THE ANKLE
(General description of rheumatoid arthritis, p. 111)

One or both ankles are often affected by rheumatoid arthritis in common with other joints.

Treatment. General treatment is along the lines suggested for the disease as a whole (p. 115). *Local treatment*: In the active phase rest in bed or in a plaster is sometimes required. But in most cases the patient should be encouraged to remain active as far as possible, with such help as may be gained from local support by a moulded polypropylene splint. Operation is advised mainly when destruction of articular cartilage has led to intractable pain with marked impairment of capacity for walking. Arthrodesis and replacement arthroplasty are the methods available. Arthrodesis is usually the operation of choice because it gives permanent relief of pain with good function. If the subtalar and midtarsal joints are also severely affected they should be included in the fusion. Replacement arthroplasty of the ankle is still on trial: its durability is open to question.

TUBERCULOUS ARTHRITIS OF THE ANKLE
(General description of tuberculous arthritis, p. 117)

Tuberculosis is much less common in the ankle than it is in the hip and knee. In Britain it is now seen very seldom.

The clinical features correspond to those of tuberculous arthritis of other superficial joints, with pain, swelling, increased warmth of the overlying skin, restriction of movement, and limp.

Treatment. Early conservative treatment (p. 120) may restore a mobile ankle, but if in a resistant case articular cartilage is badly eroded or destroyed arthrodesis may have to be undertaken.

OSTEOARTHRITIS OF THE ANKLE
(General description of osteoarthritis, p. 120)

Degenerative destruction of the articular cartilage is less common in the ankle than in the knee or hip. There is nearly always a known predisposing factor which causes the joint to wear out prematurely. The commonest is irregularity or mal-alignment of the joint surfaces after a fracture. Sometimes articular disease such as previous rheumatoid arthritis or osteochondromatosis is the primary factor.

Clinical features. The symptoms are pain which slowly increases over months and years, and limp. *On examination* the joint is a little thickened from hypertrophy of bone (osteophyte formation) at the joint margins. Movements are restricted slightly or severely according to the degree of arthritis.

Radiographs show the typical features of osteoarthritis—narrowing of the cartilage space, a tendency to sclerosis of the bone adjacent to the joint, and osteophyte formation at the joint margins (Fig. 339).

Fig. 339
Osteoarthritis of the ankle complicating fracture-subluxation ten years before. Note the marked narrowing of the cartilage space and the prominent osteophytes.

Treatment. In mild cases treatment is often unnecessary, because the patient may be willing to accept the disability when the nature of the trouble has been explained. When treatment is called for, conservative measures should be tried first if the disability is only moderate. Physiotherapy by short-wave diathermy, hot baths and active exercises is usually advised. Sometimes local splintage by a moulded polypropylene support will provide relief while allowing the patient to continue to walk. Such treatment, however, is only palliative, and if the disability increases to the extent of becoming a serious handicap operation should be undertaken. This should usually be by arthrodesis, which provides a painless stable joint. Replacement arthroplasty is a possible alternative, but the long-term results are so uncertain that it is not yet widely recommended.

GOUTY ARTHRITIS OF THE ANKLE

Although gout is commonest in the joints of the great toe it should be remembered that it can occur in the ankle and in other peripheral joints. The general features of gouty arthritis were described in Chapter 7 (p. 123).

HAEMOPHILIC ARTHRITIS OF THE ANKLE

(General description of haemophilic arthritis, p. 125)

Haemophilic arthritis is much less common in the ankle than in the knee or elbow, but it should be remembered as an occasional cause of a warm, swollen ankle in boys. Treatment is analogous to that for the knee (p. 341).

NEUROPATHIC ARTHRITIS OF THE ANKLE

(General description of neuropathic arthritis, p. 126)

Neuropathic arthritis is uncommon but nevertheless well recognised in the ankle. The underlying neurological disease is tabes dorsalis, diabetic neuropathy, syringomyelia, cauda equina lesion or, where it is prevalent, leprosy.

Treatment. In many cases protection by a firm surgical boot, reinforced if necessary by a below-knee brace, is all that is required. Occasionally arthrodesis of the ankle may have to be considered. Appropriate treatment must be given for the underlying neurological disorder.

RECURRENT SUBLUXATION OF THE ANKLE

When the lateral ligament of the ankle is torn and fails to heal there may be persistent instability with recurrent attacks of giving way in which the talus tilts medially in the ankle mortise. Anterior displacement relative to the tibial articular surface may also occur (Glasgow *et al.* 1980). The causative injury is always a severe inversion force.

Clinical features. The patient complains that the ankle 'goes over' at frequent intervals, often causing him to fall. Each incident is accompanied by pain at the lateral side of the ankle. There is always a history of previous severe injury, followed by much swelling and extensive bruising at the lateral side of the joint.

On examination there is often some oedema about the ankle. There is tenderness over the site of the lateral ligament. The normal ankle movements—dorsiflexion and plantarflexion—are unchanged, but abnormal mobility is present as shown by the fact that the heel can be inverted passively beyond the normal range permitted by the subtalar joint. Moreover, when the heel is fully inverted a dimple or depression of the skin may be visible in front of the lateral malleolus, where the soft tissues have been 'sucked' into the gap created between tibia and talus.

Radiographic features. Routine radiographs do not show any abnormality. Antero-posterior films must be taken while the heel is held fully inverted. If the lateral ligament is torn or lax the talus will be shown tilted away from the tibio-fibular mortise at the lateral side through 20 or 30 degrees or more (Fig. 340). Anterior displacement of the talus relative to the tibial articular surface may also be demonstrated in lateral radiographs taken while the foot is pushed forwards.

Fig. 340
Tilting of the talus in the ankle mortise under adduction stress; an indication of torn lateral ligament.

Diagnosis. Chronic strain of the lateral ligament may cause similar symptoms, but in that condition radiographs will not show the talus tilted significantly on forced inversion. (The talus may tilt up to 15 degrees in a normal ankle.)

Treatment. If the disability is slight it may be sufficient to strengthen the evertor muscles (mainly the peronei) by exercises, to enable them to control the ankle more efficiently. Stability may also be enhanced by broadening and 'floating out' the heel of the shoe. If the disability is severe operation is required. A new lateral ligament may be constructed either from the peroneus brevis tendon or from the peroneus tertius. Trials are also proceeding with the use of artificial ligaments, either as substitutes or as a means of promoting the growth of new ligamentous tissue.

DISORDERS OF THE FOOT

CONGENITAL CLUB FOOT
(Talipes equino-varus)

The rather vague term 'club foot' has come to be synonymous in the minds of most surgeons with the commonest and most important congenital deformity of the foot—talipes equino-varus (Fig. 341). The less common, and usually less serious, form of club foot, talipes calcaneo-valgus, will be considered later under that title.

Cause. This is still under debate. In most cases a defect of foetal development is responsible, with imbalance between the invertor-plantar-flexor muscles and the evertor-dorsiflexor muscles. A neuromuscular defect is possibly relevant. Minor degrees of the deformity may possibly be explained by prolonged mal-position of the foetal foot in the uterus, but this cannot be accepted as the usual cause.

Fig. 341
Bilateral club foot (talipes equino-varus) in an infant boy.
Note the poor development of the calf muscles.

Pathology. The crucial component of the deformity is subluxation of the talo-navicular joint, so that the navicular bone lies partly on the medial aspect of the head of the talus instead of on its distal aspect (Fig. 343). The soft tissues at the medial side of the foot are under-developed and shorter than normal. The foot is adducted and inverted at the subtalar, midtarsal, and anterior tarsal joints, and is held in equinus (plantarflexion) at the ankle. In most cases under-development of the calf and peroneal muscles is a striking feature. Thus if only one foot is affected there is a marked discrepancy in the girth of the calf between the two sides.

In the absence of early effective treatment the developing tarsal bones assume an abnormal shape as growth occurs, perpetuating the deformity.

Clinical features. The deformity is much commoner in boys than in girls. (Contrast congenital dislocation of the hip, which is much commoner in girls.) One or both feet may be affected. When the infant is born it is noticed that the foot is turned inwards so that the sole is directed medially (Fig. 341). The deformity, to be more precise, consists of three elements: 1) inversion (twisting inwards) of the foot; 2) adduction (inward deviation) of the forefoot relative to the hindfoot; and 3) equinus (plantarflexion). The foot cannot be pushed passively through the normal range of eversion and dorsiflexion. There may be obvious under-development of the muscles of the lower leg, especially noticeable when only one foot is affected.

Diagnosis. New-born infants should be examined routinely for evidence of club foot. It is not sufficient, for purposes of diagnosis, that the foot be found to rest in the position described, for often the feet of normal infants tend to lie naturally in a somewhat inverted position. The criterion for the diagnosis of club foot is that the deformity cannot readily be corrected and over-corrected to bring the foot into eversion and dorsiflexion. It should be remembered that in normal infants under one year old it is possible to evert and dorsiflex the foot far enough to bring the little toe into contact with the shin.

Fig. 342   **Fig. 343**

Figure 342—Normal alignment of the forefoot upon the long axis of the talus. Figure 343—Subluxation of the navicular bone medially on the head of the talus— the crucial component in the pathology of talipes equino-varus. Interrupted line shows forward projection of the long axis of the talus passing lateral to the first metatarsal—a useful radiological sign. In the normal state the line passes through or medial to the first metatarsal (Fig. 342).

Radiographic features. In the antero-posterior radiograph of a normal foot a line projecting the long axis of the talus forwards passes medial to the first metatarsal or coincides with it (Fig. 342). In uncorrected or incompletely corrected club foot the line passes lateral to the metatarsal (Fig. 343).

Prognosis. The prognosis depends largely upon the age at which primary treatment is begun, and upon the efficiency with which it is carried out. The longer the delay before treatment, the smaller is the prospect of complete cure. Yet even with prompt treatment the outcome is uncertain. In a proportion of cases, despite the greatest care from the time of birth, there is a tendency to relapse when treatment is discontinued. These are usually the cases that show marked hypoplasia of the muscles of the lower leg, especially of the peroneal group. Even in the most severe cases, however, it should always be possible to ensure a plantigrade foot, if not a normal foot, by operative means.

Treatment in a fresh case. Although it is seemingly a simple deformity talipes equino-varus presents difficult problems in treatment. In the past the most widely accepted practice was to rely upon conservative treatment by correction and splintage during the first year of life and often well beyond that; but in many cases the results were disappointing. All too often operation was needed later to correct recurrent deformity, and even then the foot was far from normal. Because of this the present trend is towards operative correction in early infancy if full and lasting correction is not obtained quickly by the traditional methods of conservative treatment.

Fig. 344
Correcting a club-foot deformity by manual pressure without anaesthesia. Note that pressure is applied under the midfoot, not under the forefoot.

Fig. 345
Plaster for maintaining correction in congenital club foot. It is essential to include the thigh, with the knee flexed to a right angle.

Primary conservative treatment. Ideally treatment should be begun immediately after birth—certainly not more than one week later. The principles of treatment are: 1) to correct and over-correct the deformity by repeated firm manual pressure; and 2) to hold the foot in the over-corrected position to counteract the natural tendency for the deformity to recur.

Correction of deformity. The deformity is corrected by firm manual pressure without anaesthesia (Fig. 344). The adduction and inversion are corrected first, and finally the equinus. Depending on the severity of the deformity, it may be possible to correct it fully by two or three manipulations, or as many as five or six manipulations at weekly intervals may be required.

Maintenance of correction. Three methods are available for holding the foot in the corrected position between manipulations: 1) a plaster of Paris case; 2) metal splints as advocated by Denis Browne (1956); and 3) adhesive strapping. Retention in a plaster is much to be preferred, because it holds the foot in the over-corrected position more efficiently and for a longer period than do metal splints or strapping. The plaster must extend to the upper thigh, with the knee flexed 90 degrees (Fig. 345); otherwise the infant is able to draw the foot up inside the plaster, with consequent loss of correction. The plaster must be changed every week at first, but the interval may be extended to two and then three weeks as the child grows larger.

Operative treatment. If at the end of three or four months the feet are not normal clinically and radiologically operation is undertaken. The idea behind early operation is to set the tarsal bones in normal relationship to one another and to remove deforming stresses, thus allowing the bones to develop in their normal shape from an early age. All taut ligaments at the medial side of the ankle and foot are divided and any tendon that is too tight to allow full correction is lengthened—including the calcaneal tendon. Finally the tarsal bones, thus released, are restored to their normal relationships, particular attention being paid to the talus and the navicular bone. After operation a plaster is worn for two or three months.

Treatment in neglected or relapsed cases. Repeated manipulation and retention in plaster can produce worthwhile improvement in children of up to 2 years of age. If significant deformity is still present after the age of 2, operative treatment is required. It should be appreciated that in these late cases no method of treatment—whether conservative or operative—is capable of restoring the foot to normal. The most that can be done is to restore a plantigrade foot.[1]

Types of operation. In children aged 2 to 12 years there is the option to employ any of six operations, depending upon the circumstances of each case: 1) division of the short soft tissues at the medial side of the foot, the foot thereafter being forced into a plantigrade position and immobilised in plaster for three months (Brockman 1930); 2) transfer of the tendon of the tibialis anterior to the outer side of the foot; 3) transfer of the tibialis posterior tendon through the interosseous membrane to the outer side of the foot, to supplement the action of the evertor muscles; 4) lengthening of a short calcaneal tendon; 5) arthrodesis of the calcaneo-cuboid joint, with excision of a wafer of bone to shorten the lateral border of the foot (Evans 1961); and 6) when inversion of the heel is a prominent feature, osteotomy of the calcaneus with insertion of a bone wedge in the medial side to correct the line of weight-bearing (Dwyer 1963).

In children over the age of 12 resort must be had to operation upon the

[1]Plantigrade = sole walking; with the sole on the ground.

bones: a wedge of bone of appropriate size (with base dorso-laterally) is removed from the tarsus so that when the resulting gap is closed the foot is plantigrade. This operation is not recommended for children under 12 because the growth of the foot is likely to be impaired.

COMMENT

Opinions vary on the correct duration of conservative treatment and on the timing of corrective operations in infants. If treatment by manipulation and retention fails, operation should usually be undertaken before the age of 9 months: some would say much earlier. As to secondary operative treatment for relapse in older children, the nature of the operation has to be decided according to the circumstances in each case—particularly the age of the patient and the site of the main deformity. In general, operations on bone should be avoided in children under 12 years old—that is, during the period of active growth: but after that age calcaneal osteotomy, or tarsal arthrodesis with removal of an appropriate wedge of bone, is often to be preferred.

CONGENITAL TALIPES CALCANEO-VALGUS

This is the opposite deformity to talipes equino-varus. The foot is everted and dorsiflexed. It is usually a less serious deformity than talipes equino-varus and with few exceptions, in which there is displacement at the talo-navicular joint (see congenital vertical talus, below), it responds readily to treatment.

Cause. The cause is unknown. In some cases it may simply be a postural deformity, from folding of the foot against the shin for a long time in intra-uterine life.

Fig. 346
Congenital talipes calcaneo-valgus. The typical deformity.

Clinical features. One foot or both feet may be affected. The foot rests in a position of eversion and dorsiflexion, so that its dorsum lies almost in contact with the shin (Fig. 346). Tightness of the dorso-lateral soft tissues prevents the foot from being brought down easily into inversion and equinus, though with steady pressure a fair degree of correction can usually be obtained.

Treatment. In most cases the deformity will respond readily to repeated manual stretching by the parents, who should be carefully instructed how to coax the foot into the over-corrected position of inversion and equinus by steady pressure upon the dorsum of the foot. The manipulations should be begun immediately after birth and should be carried out several times a day.

If calcaneo-valgus deformity still persists when the child is a month old more intensive supervision is required. The surgeon should gently over-correct the deformity as far as possible by manipulation without anaes-thesia, thereafter applying a plaster with the foot in the over-corrected position. The plaster is changed weekly until a full range of inversion and equinus is gained. At that stage the plaster may be discarded without fear of relapse.

CONGENITAL VERTICAL TALUS

In a small proportion of cases of talipes calcaneo-valgus there is an underlying skeletal deformity at the talo-navicular joint. The navicular bone is displaced onto the dorsal aspect of the head of the talus, which is thus pushed downwards so that the long axis of the talus becomes almost vertical. The condition may sometimes be associated with muscular imbalance consequent upon neurological deficit, as for instance in spina bifida. In some of these cases operative correction may be required.

ACCESSORY BONES IN THE FOOT

Many accessory bones have been described in the foot, but most are of little or no practical importance. The commonest is the **os trigonum**, which lies immediately behind the talus, on the upper surface of the tuberosity of the calcaneus (Fig. 347). It does not cause symptoms. It may be confused with a fracture of the talus.

Fig. 347   **Fig. 348**
Os trigonum.   Os tibiale externum.

The only tarsal accessory bone that is frequently responsible for symptoms is the **os tibiale externum**[1] (accessory navicular bone) (Fig. 348). This lies medial to the navicular bone, and forms a well marked prominence at the inner border of the foot which may become painful and tender from the pressure of the shoe. If the symptoms justify operation the accessory bone should be removed.

---

[1]The term *os tibiale externum* may seem confusing in so far as the ossicle is on the inner side of the foot. The title however relates to the embryonic position of the foot, in which the ossicle forms on the outer side.

PES CAVUS

In pes cavus or 'hollow foot' the longitudinal arch of the foot is accentuated.

Cause. In many cases the deformity has a congenital basis. It is sometimes familial. In other cases there is an underlying neurological disorder causing muscle imbalance. For instance, it is often associated with a minor degree of spinal dysraphism (p. 139), or it may follow poliomyelitis.

Fig. 349
Pes cavus. Typical deformity with high arch, clawed toes and prominence of the metatarsal heads in the sole. In such a case the spine should always be examined for evidence of dysraphism.

Pathology. The metatarsal heads are lowered in relation to the hind part of the foot, with consequent exaggeration of the longitudinal arch. The soft tissues in the sole are abnormally short, and eventually the bones themselves alter shape, perpetuating the deformity. There is always associated clawing of the toes, which are hyperextended at the metatarso-phalangeal joints and flexed at the proximal and distal interphalangeal joints (Fig. 349). This clawing seems to result from defective action of the intrinsic muscles— lumbricals and interossei. The effect is that the toes are almost functionless, and unable to take their normal share in weight-bearing. Consequently excessive weight falls upon the metatarsal heads on walking or standing, and hard callosities form in the underlying skin. The mal-alignment of the tarsal joints predisposes to the later development of osteoarthritis.

Clinical features. The deformity often becomes evident in childhood. It may affect one foot or both feet. In some cases the symptoms are negligible. When symptoms do arise they may take three forms: 1) painful callosities beneath the metatarsal heads; 2) tenderness over the deformed toes from pressure against the shoe; and 3) pain in the tarsal region from osteoarthritis of the tarsal joints.

On examination the deformity is characteristic and easily recognised (Fig. 349). The longitudinal arch is high; the forefoot is thick and splayed; the toes are clawed; the metatarsal heads are prominent in the sole. Callosities beneath the metatarsal heads indicate that they take excessive weight. The toes cannot be straightened at will by the patient, nor can they be pressed firmly upon the ground to take a share in weight-bearing. There may also be tender callosities where the tops of the toes have rubbed against the shoes.

The base of the spine should be examined for a congenital anomaly such as spina bifida, which may be suggested by the presence of a dimple, a tuft of hair or an area of pigmentation. If suspicion of spinal dysraphism exists radiographs of the spine should be obtained.

Treatment. In many cases treatment is not required. Mild symptoms can often be relieved by regular chiropody and by the provision of a resilient pad beneath the metatarsal heads to distribute the weight more widely. It is often helpful to prescribe surgical shoes, made to fit the altered shape of the feet.

If the symptoms are severe operation may be required. The nature of the operation should depend upon the cause of the main symptoms.

Operations on the toes. When local pressure upon the toes or beneath the metatarsal heads is the main complaint, adequate relief can often be afforded simply by straightening the clawed toes. This may be done by arthrodesing all the interphalangeal joints or, if the toes are still mobile, by transplanting the long flexor tendon into the extensor expansion to supplement the action of the intrinsic muscles.

Operations on the soft tissues of the sole. In appropriate cases arthrodesis of the toes may be supplemented by the Steindler muscle-slide operation, in which the taut ligamentous tissues in the sole of the foot are detached from the calcaneus and allowed to slide forwards as the height of the arch is reduced by strong manual force. After operation the correction is maintained by immobilising the foot in plaster for two months.

Operations on the tarsal joints. When osteoarthritis of the tarsal joints is the main cause of the symptoms arthrodesis of the affected joints—usually the subtalar, calcaneo-cuboid and talo-navicular joints (the so-called triple arthrodesis)—is required. At the same time the deformity is corrected by excising a wedge of bone, base upwards, from the metatarsus. When necessary, this operation may be combined with operations to straighten the toes.

PES PLANUS
(Flat foot; valgus foot)

In this common condition the longitudinal arch of the foot is reduced so that, on standing, its medial border is close to, or in contact with, the ground (Fig. 350). It is usually associated with some degree of twisting outwards of the foot on its longitudinal axis (eversion or valgus deformity).

Cause. In many cases it probably has a congenital basis, but it may be caused by selective muscle weakness or paralysis.

Pathology. All infants have flat feet for a year or two after they begin to stand. When the deformity persists into adult life it becomes a permanent structural defect, the tarsal bones being so shaped that when articulated they tend to form a straight line rather than an arch.

Fig. 350
Pes planus. Marked flattening of the longitudinal arch, with valgus deformity seen well from behind (inset).

Clinical features. In children, flat feet are usually symptomless, but the parents commonly complain that the uppers of the shoes persistently bulge inwards and that the heels wear down quickly at the inner sides.

In adults, too, flat feet are often free from symptoms, but they are more liable than are normal feet to suffer foot strain (p. 382), and when pain is complained of it is usually from that cause.

In later life pain may also arise from osteoarthritis of the tarsal joints consequent upon their mal-alignment.

Treatment. In children under 3 years old treatment is not required. In children over 3 the accepted method of treatment is to tilt the shoe slightly to the lateral side by inserting a wedge, base medially, between the layers of the heel (not the sole) (Fig. 351). This may help to overcome the valgus twist and to reduce the bulging-over of the uppers at the medial side, but it must be accepted that in most cases it is little more than a placebo. In older children it is better to insert a valgus insole (arch support) into the shoe, and this may be supplemented by a course of supervised exercises to strengthen the intrinsic muscles of the foot.

In cases of severe valgus deformity—which is usually the consequence of selective muscle imbalance, as after poliomyelitis—operation to restore the correct relationship between talus and calcaneus, and to fuse the two bones together (talo-calcaneal arthrodesis), may be considered. In children this operation may be done by placing bone grafts extra-articularly in the sinus tarsi, from the lateral side (Grice 1952).

Fig. 351
Shoes drawn from behind, to illustrate medial heel wedges.

In adults treatment is not needed unless symptoms are present, when the advisability of fitting an arch support should be considered. Supports are seldom of benefit when the foot is completely flat, but they often afford relief when the longitudinal arch is diminished but not lost.

If the symptoms in a case of long-established flat foot are ascribed to superimposed osteoarthritis of the tarsal joints, treatment should be directed against the arthritis (see below).

PERONEAL SPASTIC FLAT FOOT (Spasmodic painful flat foot) and TARSAL COALITION
Whereas in most cases flat foot is painless, in a small number the flattening may be associated with pain and intermittent spasm of the peroneal muscles, provoked by weight-bearing. Peroneal spastic flat foot is important because it is often associated with congenital tarsal coalitions which, if not treated by early surgical excision, may lead to secondary arthritic changes in the tarsal joints.

Pathology. Tarsal coalitions represent an inherited failure of bony development and are present in 1–2 per cent of the population. The characteristic feature is the existence of a cartilaginous or bony bar bridging two adjacent tarsal bones. The two commonest types are: 1) calcaneo-navicular coalition; and 2) talo-calcaneal coalition.

Clinical features. Symptoms usually begin in early adolescence, when the patient presents with a painful, rigid, valgus hindfoot. The symptoms are aggravated by prolonged standing or walking. Examination shows marked restriction of subtalar movement. Attempted eversion of the heel passively often provokes spasm of the peroneal muscles.

Diagnosis. Special oblique or axial radiographs may be required to show the abnormal bony bar. Later, secondary osteoarthritic changes may be seen in the tarsal joints.

Treatment. If coalition is diagnosed early, excision of the abnormal bar may relieve pain and restore some mobility. In the later stages, if degenerative arthritis causes severe disability arthrodesis of the affected joints may be required.

FOOT STRAIN

The term 'foot strain' implies a subacute or chronic strain of the tarsal ligaments, not an acute injury from sudden violence.

It may be caused in a normal foot by excessive standing or walking by a person unaccustomed to it: but it occurs mostly in those with a long established foot deformity such as pes planus (flat foot) or pes cavus, when the ligaments of the foot may be inadequately protected by muscles.

The main symptoms are prolonged aching in the feet, worse on standing or walking, often with aching also in the calves.

It is important to eliminate other causes of foot problems such as ischaemia, neurological deficit and, in boys, particularly muscular dystrophy.

Treatment should be by reducing the time spent in standing and walking, by the fitting of an arch support if indicated, by supervised foot and toe exercises, and sometimes by electrical stimulation to strengthen the muscles of the leg and foot.

OSTEOARTHRITIS OF THE TARSAL JOINTS

Osteoarthritis may affect any of the tarsal joints, but in practice it is seen most often in the subtalar and midtarsal joints. It seldom arises primarily: there is nearly always a predisposing cause such as previous fracture or disease involving the joint surfaces (especially fractures of the calcaneus), or mal-alignment of the tarsal bones (as in severe flat foot or severe pes cavus).

Clinical features. The main symptom is pain, which gradually increases over months or years and finally leads to a limp and impaired capacity for walking. Pain is localised fairly accurately to the particular joint or joints affected. A history will usually be obtained of previous injury, disease or deformity of the foot. *On examination* movement of the affected joint is impaired, and painful if forced.

Radiographs confirm the diagnosis and may give an indication of the primary underlying cause.

Treatment. In mild cases treatment is not required, especially if the patient can curtail his activities. When the disability is troublesome more active measures are needed. Conservative treatment is only palliative, but it is usually worth a trial. It should take the form of short-wave diathermy, muscle exercises, and support from an elastic bandage or moulded polypropylene heel seat. A trial may also be made of local injection of hydrocortisone into the affected joint; but repeated injections are not advised.

If conservative treatment fails to give adequate relief operation must be considered. The only effective method is by arthrodesis of the affected joint or joints.

OTHER FORMS OF ARTHRITIS OF THE TARSAL JOINTS

Like all true synovial joints, the tarsal joints are liable to any of the recognised forms of arthritis, including pyogenic arthritis, rheumatoid arthritis, tuberculous arthritis, gouty arthritis, and neuropathic arthritis. Of these, the only one that is at all common is rheumatoid arthritis, which affects particularly the subtalar joint.

OSTEOCHONDRITIS OF THE NAVICULAR BONE
(Köhler's disease)

The general subject of osteochondritis was discussed in Chapter 5 (p. 96). The growing navicular bone is one of its best recognised sites. The developing nucleus of the bone is temporarily softened and usually becomes compressed by the mechanical forces entailed in walking. A disturbance of blood supply is possibly a causative factor, but the pathogenesis is not fully understood.

Pathology. The pathology is believed to be like that of osteochondritis of other growing bony nuclei (see Fig. 85, p. 97). The bone, presumably necrotic from ischaemia, loses its normal trabecular structure and may become fragmented as it is gradually absorbed and

| Fig. 352 | Fig. 353 |

Köhler's osteochondritis of the navicular bone. Figure 352—Early stage. Bony nucleus dense and flattened antero-posteriorly. Figure 353—Two years later. Bone texture restored; slight residual flattening.

replaced by new living bone. After about two years the normal bone structure is restored and the bone may regain almost its normal size and shape. If slight deformation of the bone does remain, the growing foot seems to adapt itself to the altered shape and little or no disability persists.

Clinical features. Köhler's disease is confined to children aged about 3 to 5 years. The child complains of pain in the midtarsal part of the foot and is noticed to limp. *On examination* there may be slight swelling in the midtarsal region, with tenderness on firm palpation over the navicular bone and sometimes a slight increase in warmth. There may be some restriction of midtarsal movements with pain on forcing, but these signs are slight and sometimes absent.

Radiographic features. Radiographs are diagnostic. The ossifying nucleus of the navicular bone appears squashed antero-posteriorly (Fig. 352); it is denser than normal, and may have a fragmented appearance. Serial radiographs during the two-year span of the disease show the gradual evolution of the bone changes. After a stage of maximal density and deformation a few months after the onset there is gradual improvement until normal bone texture is restored (Fig. 353).

Treatment. Despite the slow evolution of the bone changes prolonged treatment is not required. Good results follow symptomatic treatment. Usually all that is necessary is to rest the foot for six to eight weeks in a walking plaster.

PAINFUL HEEL

The causes of painful heel are conveniently classified according to the site of the pain (Fig. 354).

Pain within the heel
Disease of the calcaneus
(osteomyelitis; tumour; Paget's
disease)
Arthritis of the subtalar joint

Pain behind the heel
Rupture of the calcaneal
tendon (p. 365)
Calcaneal paratendinitis
Post-calcaneal bursitis
Calcaneal apophysitis

Pain beneath the heel
Tender heel pad
Plantar fasciitis

DISEASE OF THE CALCANEUS

The calcaneus is subject, although rarely, to all types of infection of bone, the commonest being pyogenic infection (osteomyelitis). Occasionally it is the seat of a benign or malignant tumour. It may also be affected by other disorders of bone, such as Paget's disease.

ARTHRITIS OF THE SUBTALAR JOINT

The commonest type of arthritis in the subtalar joint is osteoarthritis secondary to fracture of the calcaneus (p. 383). The joint is occasionally subject to other forms of arthritis, such as pyogenic arthritis, rheumatoid arthritis, tuberculous arthritis, and gout.

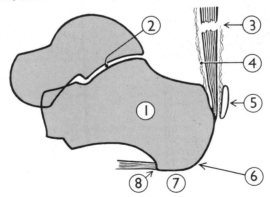

Fig. 354
Eight causes of painful heel, with site of pain. 1. Disease of the calcaneus. 2. Arthritis of the subtalar joint. 3. Ruptured calcaneal tendon. 4. Calcaneal paratendinitis. 5. Post-calcaneal bursitis. 6. Calcaneal apophysitis. 7. Tender heel pad. 8. Plantar fasciitis.

CALCANEAL PARATENDINITIS

(Calcaneal tenosynovitis)

The calcaneal tendon is surrounded by loose connective tissue, or paratenon, which allows gliding movements. Rarely, this becomes inflamed from excessive friction. The condition should be termed paratendinitis rather than tenosynovitis, because there is no true synovial sheath.

Clinical features. The patient is usually an active young adult. There is pain in the region of the calcaneal tendon, made worse by activities such as running or dancing. *On examination* there is tenderness on palpation between finger and thumb deep to the tendon (Fig. 354), and there is slight local thickening in this region. The tendon itself is of normal size and consistency.

Treatment. In many cases relief is afforded by local injection of hydrocortisone deep to the tendon. (The tendon itself must not on any account be injected lest it be weakened, with serious risk of rupture.) In a resistant case operation may be required: it consists in excising the loose connective tissue surrounding and deep to the tendon.

POST-CALCANEAL BURSITIS

This is the commonest cause of pain behind the heel. It is often a cause of troublesome disability in young women.

Pathology. An adventitious bursa forms at the back of the heel, between the tuberosity of the calcaneus and the skin. Repeated friction against the back of the shoe leads to chronic inflammation and thickening of the walls of the bursa, and the sac may be distended with fluid. Prominence of the underlying bone aggravates the bursitis.

Clinical features. There is troublesome tenderness where the swelling is in contact with the shoe (Fig. 354). The symptoms are aggravated by walking, and they tend to be worse in winter than in summer; hence the term 'winter heel'. *On examination* there is an obvious gristly prominence at the back of the heel; the overlying skin is thickened and may be red.

Treatment. In mild or recent cases the symptoms can be controlled by protecting the back of the heel with a double layer of elastic adhesive strapping and by wearing shoes with soft backs. If these measures fail the bursa should be excised: its recurrence must be prevented by excising the prominent upper posterior corner of the calcaneal tuberosity, immediately above the attachment of the calcaneal tendon.

CALCANEAL APOPHYSITIS
(Sever's disease)

This harmless condition occurs only in children, during the period of active growth of the calcaneal apophysis. It was formerly believed to be an example of osteochondritis (p. 96), but it is now generally agreed that it is nothing more than a chronic strain at the attachment of the posterior apophysis of the calcaneus to the main body of the bone, possibly from the pull of the calcaneal tendon. It may thus be regarded as analogous to Osgood-Schlatter's disease of the tibial tubercle (p. 355), and totally unrelated to osteochondritis.

Clinical features. The child is usually between 8 and 13 years old. He complains of pain behind the heel, and a slight limp may be noticed. *On examination* there is tenderness over the lower posterior part of the tuberosity of the calcaneus (Fig. 354). *Radiographs* usually fail to show any alternation from the normal. Importance has sometimes been attached to an appearance of fragmentation of the calcaneal apophysis, but this is a normal state, often seen in children without pain in the heel.

Treatment. In most cases treatment is not required, because the symptoms will gradually subside spontaneously. If the pain is troublesome, rest for a few weeks in a below-knee walking plaster will afford adequate relief.

TENDER HEEL PAD

This is a distinct clinical condition characterised by pain beneath the hind part of the heel on standing or walking.

Pathology. The site of the tenderness is the tough fibro-fatty tissue beneath the prominent weight-bearing part of the calcaneus. In some cases the lesion is probably no more than a simple contusion; but in most cases injury seems to play no part and it must be assumed that there is mild inflammation, of uncertain origin.

Clinical features. Pain beneath the heel on standing or walking is the only symptom. *On examination* there is well marked local tenderness on firm palpation over the heel pad (Fig. 354).

Treatment. There is a tendency to slow spontaneous improvement. Recovery may be hastened by the injection of hydrocortisone locally at the site of greatest tenderness, and by providing a sponge-rubber heel cushion on an insole. Short-wave diathermy or ultrasound to the tender area is also worth a trial if pain persists.

PLANTAR FASCIITIS

In this condition, which is believed to be inflammatory, there is pain beneath the anterior part of the calcaneus. It may be part of a more widespread inflammatory condition such as Reiter's disease.

Pathology. The lesion affects the soft tissues at the site of attachment of the plantar aponeurosis to the inferior aspect of the tuberosity of the calcaneus (Fig. 354).

Clinical features. The complaint is of pain beneath the heel on standing or walking; the pain extends medially and into the sole. The disability is sometimes severe. When the condition is part of a widespread inflammatory disorder both heels may be affected. *On examination* there is marked tenderness over the site of attachment of the plantar fascia to the calcaneus. The site of tenderness is further forward than it is in tender heel pad (Fig. 354). *Radiographs* usually do not show any abnormality. A sharp spur projecting forwards from the tuberosity of the calcaneus is sometimes found, but its significance is doubtful because such spurs may be present in patients without heel symptoms.

Treatment. Conservative treatment usually suffices if pursued energetically, though recovery may be slow. A course of non-steroidal anti-inflammatory drugs is usually prescribed. The heel should be protected by a resilient cushion on an insole. If these measures fail, local injection of hydrocortisone into the tender area may be tried. If the fasciitis is part of a widespread inflammatory disorder treatment appropriate to the underlying condition should be instituted.

PAIN IN THE FOREFOOT

(Metatarsalgia)

Pain in the forefoot is one of the commonest orthopaedic complaints. There are three main causes, of which the first is the most frequent: 1) anterior flat foot (dropped transverse arch); 2) stress fracture of a metatarsal bone (march fracture); 3) plantar digital neuritis (Morton's metatarsalgia).

ANTERIOR FLAT FOOT

(Dropped transverse arch)

Permanent flattening of the transverse arch of the foot, with excessive weight-bearing pressure beneath the metatarsal heads, is the commonest cause of metatarsalgia. In most cases the primary cause is inefficiency of the intrinsic muscles of the foot.

Fig. 355   **Fig. 356**

Figure 355—Diagram to show the normal action of the toes in raising the metatarsal heads from the ground, whereby they share the weight with the metatarsal heads. This action is controlled mainly by the intrinsic muscles, which, by producing flexion at the metatarso-phalangeal joints and extension at the interphalangeal joints, cause the toes to press upon the ground, lifting the metatarsal heads. Figure 356—If the intrinsic muscles are inefficient all the weight must be borne by the metatarsal heads.

Pathology. Even in normal feet the transverse arch is only a potential arch, not a constant one. But in the normal state the metatarsal heads can be raised from the ground at will by the action of the toes, held straight at the interphalangeal joints by the intrinsic muscles and flexed strongly at the metatarso-phalangeal joints by the intrinsic muscles in conjunction with the long and short flexors (Fig. 355). Thus the weight is shared between the metatarsal heads and the toes. If the intrinsic muscles are inefficient the toes are unable to fulfil their important weight-sharing function and all the pressure falls upon the metatarsal heads (Fig. 356). The excessive pressure leads to the formation of callosities.

Clinical features. The main complaint is of pain beneath the forefoot. There may be secondary symptoms from pressure of the shoes upon deformed toes. *On examination* the forefoot is often splayed, appearing broader than normal. There are callosities beneath some or all of the metatarsal heads. The toes are often curled. The patient is unable to raise the metatarsal heads from the ground by pressing downwards with the toes—an indication that the intrinsic muscles are inefficient.

Treatment. In patients under 50 worthwhile improvement can usually be gained by a prolonged course of physiotherapy, designed to strengthen the intrinsic muscles by special exercises aided by faradic stimulation. In older patients this treatment is seldom effective, and instead a trial may be made of a sponge-rubber support to distribute the weight-bearing pressure over a wide area of the metatarsus. If there is a prominent callosity it may be pared away, with temporary relief.

If disability is severe, pain from local prominence of an individual metatarsal head in the sole may be relieved by osteotomy of the neck of the metatarsal and dorsal displacement of the head (Helal 1975).

STRESS FRACTURE OF A METATARSAL BONE
(March fracture; fatigue fracture)

Stress or fatigue fractures are unusual in that there is no history of violence. The possibility of fracture may therefore be overlooked. A stress fracture of a metatarsal is not a common cause of pain in the forefoot but the possibility of its occurrence should be remembered.

Fig. 357	Fig. 358

Stress fracture of second metatarsal. Figure 357 shows the initial radiograph, taken a week after the onset of pain. The fracture is seen as a fine crack across the bone. Figure 358 shows the condition three weeks later, in the stage of healing. Abundant callus has formed about the site of fracture.

Cause. The fracture is ascribed to long-continued or oft-repeated stress; it has been likened to the fatigue fractures that sometimes occur in metals.

Pathology. The fracture usually affects the shaft of the second or third metatarsal bone, near its neck. It is no more than a hair-line crack, and there is no displacement of the fragments. In the process of healing a large mass of callus may form around the bone at the site of fracture. (This has occasionally been mistaken for a tumour.)

Clinical features. The complaint is of severe pain in the forefoot on walking. The onset is rapid but the patient is usually unable to ascribe it to an obvious cause. Enquiry may reveal, however, that he has recently done an unusual amount of walking or marching before the onset. *On examination* there is swelling at the dorsum of the forefoot, with marked and well localised tenderness over the affected metatarsal bone.

Radiographs at first show only a faint hair-line crack which is easily overlooked (Fig. 357), but after two or three weeks the callus surrounding the fracture is clearly visible and usually abundant (Fig. 358).

Treatment. The fracture heals spontaneously; so treatment is purely symptomatic. Indeed in some cases treatment is not needed; but if pain is severe immobilisation in a below-knee walking plaster for three or four weeks is advised.

PLANTAR DIGITAL NEURITIS
(Morton's metatarsalgia; interdigital neuroma)

This condition, which is primarily an affection of a digital nerve, is characterised typically by metatarsal pain combined with a radiating pain in the third and fourth toes.

Fig. 359
Fibrous thickening of an interdigital nerve, a characteristic feature of plantar digital neuritis (Morton's metatarsalgia). The 'neuroma' is usually in the 3–4 cleft.

Pathology. The underlying lesion is a fibrous thickening or 'neuroma' of the digital nerve of the 3–4 cleft just proximal to its point of division into terminal branches. It takes the form of a fusiform swelling, usually about a centimetre long, surrounding the nerve as it lies in the space between the heads of the third and fourth metatarsals (Fig. 359). Occasionally the nerve to the 2–3 cleft is the one affected. The cause of the fibrous thickening is uncertain.

Clinical features. The patient is often a woman of middle age. She complains of pain in the forefoot on standing or walking. A characteristic feature is that the pain, arising in the metatarsal region, radiates forwards into the contiguous sides of the third and fourth toes, or to the fourth toe alone. Rarely, the cleft between the second and third toes is affected. The pain, like nerve pain in general, is piercing and disabling. Patients often state that they can relieve the pain by taking the shoe off and squeezing or manipulating the forefoot.

On examination the forefoot is often splayed, as in anterior flat foot. Sometimes a painful click can be elicited by compressing the metatarsal heads together from side to side, and upward pressure on the sole between the third and fourth metatarsal heads is painful.

Treatment. The patient should try first the effect of wearing a sponge-rubber metatarsal pad to support the anterior arch. If this fails to relieve the symptoms operative excision of the thickened segment of the nerve is recommended.

PLANTAR WART
(Verruca pedis; verruca plantaris)

Plantar warts may occur in any part of the sole of the foot, including the under surface of the heel. They are like warts elsewhere, except that they do not project beyond the skin surface. They are distinct from plantar callosities, which are simply localised thickenings of the skin at points of excessive pressure.

Cause. A virus infection is thought to be responsible.

Pathology. A wart is a simple papilloma, growing outwards from the basal layers of the skin. It is prevented by the pressure of weight-bearing from projecting much beyond the skin surface, but the surrounding skin is thickened, so the wart may have a total depth of up to half a centimetre (Fig. 361). It slowly enlarges, but seldom reaches a diameter of as much as a centimetre.

Fig. 360
Plantar wart. Note the clearly circumscribed outline and the slight cleft when the skin is stretched away from the wart.

Clinical features. The chief complaint is of severe localised pain on walking. *On examination* the skin surrounding the wart is thickened and therefore raised. The wart, a little darker in colour and with a mosaic surface, is seen in the centre of the raised area (Fig. 360). Its edge is clearly demarcated from the surrounding skin: this can be discerned easily if the skin is stretched away from the wart, when a tiny cleft becomes apparent between wart and skin. There is always marked local tenderness on pressure over the wart.

Diagnosis. The main difficulty is to distinguish warts from callosities. Warts occur anywhere on the sole, callosities only over points of pressure. Warts are also much more tender than callosities. But the most reliable distinguishing feature is that a wart has a mosaic surface and a clearly defined margin with a potential cleft between it and the skin (Fig. 361), whereas a callosity blends imperceptibly with the surrounding normal skin (Fig. 362).

Treatment. The local application of appropriate caustics is often successful. If this treatment fails the wart should be curetted out and the base lightly cauterised.

CALLOSITIES

A callosity is simply a localised thickening of the skin in response to abnormal pressure. It is nearly always secondary to a pre-existing disorder of the foot.

Plantar callosities are callosities on the sole of the foot. They occur under a prominent bone. They are commonest beneath the metatarsal heads when deficient intrinsic muscles prevent the toes from taking their proper share in weight-bearing (anterior flat foot, p. 387). They are also common beneath the base of the fifth metatarsal in patients who for any reason walk with the foot inverted.

Fig. 361
Diagrammatic section of a plantar wart. It is clearly demarcated from the surrounding skin.

Fig. 362
Diagrammatic section of a callosity. It blends imperceptibly with the surrounding normal skin.

Callosities on the toes often take the form of localised thickenings, when they are termed *corns*. They are caused by pressure against the shoe, and they are especially common when the dorsum of a toe is made unduly prominent by a fixed flexion deformity, as in hammer toe (see Fig. 371, p. 396).

Treatment. The treatment is mainly that of the underlying condition. Palliative measures include paring of excess epidermis (preferably by a chiropodist, though simple instruments are available for use by the patient), and sponge-rubber padding to distribute the weight-bearing pressure over a wider area.

GANGLION

Ganglia are common on the dorsum of the foot and around the ankle. They are similar in all respects to the ganglia that occur at the back of the wrist and hand. They consist of thin-walled sacs filled with glairy viscous fluid, and the fibrous wall is usually connected deeply with a ligament, tendon sheath, or joint capsule. Clinically, a ganglion appears as a fluctuant subcutaneous swelling, which may be either soft or tense. If it causes trouble it should be excised.

DISORDERS OF THE TOES

HALLUX VALGUS

In hallux valgus the great toe is deviated laterally at the metatarso-phalangeal joint. It is common in women past middle age, and is not infrequent even in young women.

Cause. In a few cases hereditary factors are responsible. But in most the deformity is caused by the toe's being persistently forced laterally by enclosure in narrow pointed shoes. The wearing of high heels favours the development of hallux valgus because the forefoot is forced into the narrow pointed part of the shoe.

Fig. 363   **Fig. 364**

Figure 363—Hallux valgus of moderate degree in a woman of middle age.
Figure 364—After correction by displacement osteotomy of the neck of the first metatarsal. Normal appearance restored.

Pathology. Outward deviation of the great toe is the most obvious feature of the deformity, but a further, almost constant feature is that the first metatarsal is deviated medially, so that the gap between the heads of the first and second metatarsals is unduly wide (metatarsus primus varus). Indeed this may often be the primary defect. After several years two secondary changes occur. One is the formation of a thick-walled bursa (bunion) over the medial prominence of the metatarsal head; this may become inflamed, occasionally with suppuration. The second, a later development, is osteoarthritis of the metatarso-phalangeal joint consequent upon its mal-alignment (see Fig. 368).

Clinical features. The patient is nearly always a woman, who is often at or past middle age when she seeks advice but may sometimes be a young woman or even an adolescent girl. The early symptoms arise from tenderness over the bunion from pressure against the shoe. There is also difficulty in getting comfortable footwear. Later, additional symptoms arise from osteoarthritis of the metatarso-phalangeal joint, and from flattening of the transverse arch (anterior flat foot, p. 387), which is a common associated deformity.

On examination the deformity is obvious at a glance (Figs 363 and 365). The skin over the prominent joint is hard, reddened, and tender. Often a thick-walled bursa can be felt, and occasionally it is distended with fluid. In relatively early cases metatarso-phalangeal joint movements are free and painless, but in severe cases of many years' duration the secondary osteoarthritis makes movement limited and painful. In late cases the forefoot is often flat and splayed, and the toes may be severely curled (Fig. 365).

Fig. 365
Severe hallux valgus. The great toe
is over-riding the deformed second
toe.

Treatment. In mild cases treatment is not required, but footwear must be selected with care to obtain adequate width. It may also be worth-while to protect the bunion with pads of felt, and to wear a wedge of plastic foam between the great toe and the second toe to reduce the deformity.

If disability is troublesome operation is advisable. Mention will be made here of only four of the many methods that are available.

Trimming of 'exostosis'. When the deviation of the toe is slight, but troublesome symptoms arise from localised prominence or 'exostosis' of the first metatarsal head at the medial side of the foot, it may sometimes be sufficient simply to excise the bursa and chisel away the medial prominence of the metatarsal head without disturbing the joint itself. There is, however, a tendency for the symptoms to recur after this operation, and in general the results are so disappointing that the operation is now seldom recommended.

Displacement osteotomy of the neck of the first metatarsal bone. This is illustrated in Figures 366 and 367. After division of the neck of the metatarsal the head fragment is displaced markedly laterally (Fig. 367). (A spike of lateral cortex may be left on the shaft fragment to impale the head in its new position.) The outward shift of the metatarsal head eliminates the prominence of the 'exostosis' without the need for its removal. The soft

Fig. 366   **Fig. 367**

Displacement osteotomy of the neck of the first metatarsal. Figure 366—Before operation. Note the wide gap between the first and second metatarsals. Figure 367—After division of the first metatarsal through its neck the head fragment is displaced markedly laterally, so that its medial prominence (the 'exostosis') disappears. The metatarso-phalangeal subluxation is automatically reduced. Remodelling (interrupted line) alters the shape of the metatarsal and the intermetatarsal gap is narrowed.

tissues between the heads of the first and second metatarsals are also relaxed, allowing permanent reduction of the subluxation at the first metatarso-phalangeal joint. After operation the toe is immobilised in plaster for six weeks to ensure union at the site of osteotomy without loss of position.

By a process of remodelling, the alignment of the first metatarsal is gradually altered after operation so that it lies closer to the second metatarsal (Fig. 367).

In this operation the joint itself is left undisturbed, indeed unopened. The operation gives good results in patients with relatively slight deformity (Fig. 364): it does not shorten the toe appreciably or impair active movement, and it is therefore particularly suitable for young patients who wish to lead an energetic life.

Excision arthroplasty of the first metatarso-phalangeal joint by Keller's method is widely used in elderly patients. The object is to create a flail, freely movable false joint between the first metatarsal and the proximal phalanx, with correction of the mal-alignment. This is done by excising the proximal half of the proximal phalanx so that a gap is left between the two bones: at the same time the bursa is excised and the medial prominence of the metatarsal head is smoothed off with a chisel (Fig. 369).

The space created by excision of the base of the phalanx fills with rubbery fibrous tissue, and a false joint forms which allows a reasonable range of movement (Fig. 370).

| Fig. 368 | Fig. 369 | Fig. 370 |

Hallux valgus. Figure 368—Diagram showing the prominent metatarsal head with overlying bunion, and osteoarthritis from long-standing mal-alignment of the joint. Figure 369—Excision arthroplasty (Keller's operation): removal of the proximal half of the proximal phalanx. The resulting gap fills with flexible fibrous tissue. The bursa and the underlying prominence of the metatarsal head have also been removed. Figure 370—Radiograph ten years after Keller's operation for hallux valgus.

This operation leaves the great toe markedly shorter than normal and rather floppy, with poor active control over toe movements. The patient should be warned about this in advance. Nevertheless the main symptoms are relieved and the result is usually satisfactory in elderly patients who do not wish to walk long distances or to indulge in athletic pursuits.

Arthrodesis of the metatarso-phalangeal joint of the hallux in a position of slight extension allows full and permanent correction of the valgus deformity, even if it is very severe—but at the cost of loss of mobility.

COMMENT

There is much variation of opinion among different surgeons on the choice of treatment. The authors' preference is to advise displacement osteotomy of the neck of the metatarsal for the younger and more active patients and Keller's excision arthroplasty for patients over 65. Arthrodesis of the metatarso-phalangeal joint has a useful place for deformity of severe degree.

When severe hallux valgus in an elderly patient is associated with flattening of the transverse arch and marked clawing of the toes (Fig. 365), operation of any type may be disappointing and it may be wiser to rely upon well-made surgical shoes.

HAMMER TOE

The term hammer toe denotes a fixed flexion deformity of an inter-phalangeal joint.

Cause. Presumably an imbalance of the delicate arrangement of flexor and extensor tendons is responsible; but the precise explanation of its occurrence is unknown. Hammer deformity, especially of the second toe, is often associated with hallux valgus (Fig. 365).

Pathology. The proximal interphalangeal joint of the second toe is that most commonly affected. The affected joint is sharply angled into flexion. Secondary contracture of the plantar aspect of the joint capsule fixes the deformity, and a callosity usually forms over the dorsum of the flexed joint, from pressure against the shoe (Fig. 371).

Fig. 371   **Fig. 372**

Figure 371—Hammer toe: the typical deformity, with callosity over the prominent proximal joint. Figure 372—Peg arthrodesis, for correction of hammer toe.

Clinical features. Typically the deformity affects only one toe—usually the second. In the characteristic deformity the proximal interphalangeal joint is in fixed flexion, and the distal interphalangeal joint, though still mobile, rests in compensatory hyperextension (Fig. 371). The symptoms, if any, are caused by the overlying callosity or 'corn'.

Treatment. If symptoms are slight the deformity may be accepted, or conservative treatment by protective felt pads may be sufficient. In severe cases operation gives gratifying results. The joint surfaces are excised and the joint is arthrodesed in the straight position by the pegging technique shown in Figure 372.

UNDER-RIDING TOE
(Congenital curled toe)

Children are often brought for advice because one of the smaller toes, often the fourth, is curled inwards and lies beneath the adjacent toe. The condition does not cause any symptoms during childhood, and it should be left alone until adolescence or early adult life, when the toe can easily be straightened if it begins to cause symptoms. Similar principles apply to the management of over-riding toe.

RHEUMATOID ARTHRITIS OF THE TOE JOINTS

Deformity of the forefoot is a common cause of pain and disability in rheumatoid arthritis. Characteristically the metatarso-phalangeal joints are most affected, with destruction of articular cartilage, dorsal subluxation of the phalanges and clawing of the toes. Painful skin callosities then develop on the sole beneath the prominent metatarsal heads and on the dorsum of the flexed toes from the pressure of footwear.

In the early stages *radiographs* show only joint narrowing and marginal erosions. In the later stages there may be subluxation or dislocation of the metatarso-phalangeal joints with marked destruction of bone (Fig. 373).

Fig. 373
Severe toe deformities from long-established rheumatoid arthritis. Note the subluxation of the metatarso-phalangeal joint of the great toe, and dislocation of several of the lesser toes at the metatarso-phalangeal joints. Some of the metatarsal heads show erosion of bone.

Treatment. Minor deformity may be managed by the provision of moulded insoles and broad-fitting shoes with soft uppers. In advanced disease with fixed painful deformities forefoot reconstruction may be advised. This usually entails excision of the bases of the proximal phalanges and trimming of the metatarsal heads (excision arthroplasty) (Fowler 1959; Kates *et al.* 1967).

OSTEOARTHRITIS OF THE TOE JOINTS
In practice, osteoarthritis in the toes is seen commonly only in the metatarso-phalangeal joint of the great toe. This has been termed *hallux rigidus*. Occasionally the metatarso-phalangeal joint of one of the smaller toes is affected, usually as a late result of Freiberg's disease of the metatarsal head (p. 399).

HALLUX RIGIDUS
This is osteoarthritis of the metatarso-phalangeal joint of the great toe. Like osteoarthritis elsewhere, it is caused by wear and tear, but previous injury or disease of the joint is an important predisposing factor.

Pathology. The changes are like those of osteoarthritis in other joints. The articular cartilage is gradually worn away from both surfaces of the joint until eventually the subchondral bone is exposed. The exposed bone becomes hard and glossy (eburnation). The marginal bone hypertrophies to form osteophytes, which often cause obvious thickening, especially at the dorsum of the toe.

Clinical features. The complaint is of pain in the base of the great toe on walking. *On examination* the metatarso-phalangeal joint is palpably thickened from osteophyte formation. If an osteophyte is especially prominent on the dorsal or medial aspect of the joint a thick-walled bursa (bunion) may form over it; occasionally the bursa is distended with fluid. Flexion and extension of the toe at the metatarso-phalangeal joint are

Fig. 374 **Fig. 375**

Hallux rigidus. Figure 374 shows the marked impairment of dorsiflexion. Figure 375 shows the radiographic changes typical of osteoarthritis, namely narrowing of the cartilage space, subchondral sclerosis, and the formation of osteophytes.

restricted—usually markedly so by the time the patient seeks advice (Fig. 374). Forced dorsiflexion of the painful joint on walking is the main source of the disability. (It should be remembered that the normal range of dorsiflexion at the metatarso-phalangeal joint of the great toe is nearly 90 degrees).

Radiographs confirm the presence of osteoarthritis. The cartilage space is narrowed, the subchondral bone tends to be sclerotic, and there is osteophytic spurring of the joint margins (Fig. 375).

Treatment. In mild cases treatment is not required. When treatment is called for, conservative measures are usually worth a trial first. A metatarsal bar should be fitted beneath the sole of the shoe at the metatarso-phalangeal level. This acts as a rocker in walking, and so reduces the dorsiflexion required of the toes when weight is brought onto the forefoot from the heel.

When the disability is severe operation should be advised. One method is to create a flail joint by excision of the base of the proximal phalanx (Keller's arthroplasty), as for hallux valgus. Many surgeons find, however, that arthrodesis of the metatarso-phalangeal joint in a position of slight extension gives better results, with complete relief of pain.

OSTEOARTHRITIS OF OTHER TOE JOINTS

Osteoarthritis of the other metatarso-phalangeal joints is uncommon except as a sequel to Freiberg's disease of a metatarsal head (see below).

GOUTY ARTHRITIS OF THE GREAT TOE JOINTS
(General description of gouty arthritis, p. 123)

The joints of the great toe are those most often affected in gout, especially in the first attack.

Clinical features. The patient is usually over 40, and more commonly a man than a woman. There is a sudden onset of severe pain in the great toe, often during the night.

On examination the toe is swollen, red, and extremely tender. Joint movements are impossible because of pain. There is sometimes slight pyrexia. The patient will usually recall previous similar attacks lasting a few days, with freedom from pain in the intervals. *Radiographs* are normal in the early stages. *Investigations*: There is sometimes a mild leucocytosis. The plasma urate level is usually raised.

Chronic gout. In this form deposits of sodium biurate in and around the joints of the great toe lead to persistent nodular thickening. *Radiographs* show rounded areas of transradiance in the bone ends; these represent deposits of sodium biurate (which is transradiant) in the subchondral bone.

Diagnosis. Acute gout is easily mistaken for acute infective arthritis. Features suggestive of gout are: a raised plasma urate level; a history of previous attacks, with symptom-free intervals; and the presence of tophi in the ears or elsewhere.

Course. Gout usually occurs in recurrent attacks. In the early years, an acute attack subsides within a few days, leaving the joint clinically normal. In chronic gout the joint is gradually disorganised, causing permanent disability.

Treatment. Acute attacks respond to selected non-steroidal anti-inflammatory drugs such as indomethacin or naproxin, begun in high dosage which is reduced after two or three days, or to colchicum. Meanwhile the foot should be rested, and the toe should be protected from pressure by a bulky wool dressing. The treatment of recurrent and chronic gout was detailed on page 124.

FREIBERG'S DISEASE OF A METATARSAL HEAD
(Metatarsal osteochondritis)

Freiberg's disease of a metatarsal head is regarded by some as an example of osteochondritis juvenilis (p. 96) and by others as osteochondritis dissecans (p. 130). It may therefore be advisable to use the non-committal eponymous title for the present. The essential feature of Freiberg's disease is partial necrosis and fragmentation of a metatarsal head, which may become deformed under the pressure of weight-bearing. It is an uncommon condition.

Pathology. The epiphysis of one of the metatarsal heads—nearly always the second or third—is the part affected. The bony nucleus becomes necrotic and granular. Part of the articular surface separates, usually remaining attached only by a hinge of articular cartilage. While it is in this crumbly state the metatarsal head is crushed by the pressure against it of the base of the proximal phalanx of the toe. The articular surface of the metatarsal head thus loses its normal dome-shaped contour and becomes flat (Fig. 376). After about two years the texture of the bone returns to normal, but flattening of the articular surface remains. Later, the distortion of the joint surface often leads to osteoarthritis.

Fig. 376

Freiberg's disease of the second metatarsal head. Note the fragmentation and the square-cut deformity of the articular surface.

Clinical features. At the time of onset the patient is 14 to 17 years old. There is pain in the affected metatarso-phalangeal joint, worse on standing or walking. *On examination* there is slight thickening in the region of the head of the metatarsal, which is tender on pressure. Movements of the metatarso-phalangeal joint are slightly restricted and painful. *Radiographs* reveal the nature of the trouble, though at first the changes are very slight and may be overlooked. Later the head of the metatarsal appears fragmented, with patches of increased density. Finally, the articular surface is flattened, so that the end of the bone appears square-cut instead of round (Fig. 376).

Treatment. When the diagnosis can be made in the early stage—before marked radiographic changes are apparent—operation offers a hope of preventing permanent distortion of the joint surface. Through a window cut in the dorsal surface of the metatarsal neck the necrotic bone of the head is curetted out and replaced by cancellous chip bone grafts, packed firmly enough to restore the normal dome-shaped contour of the articular surface. Thereafter the toe is supported in a plaster cuff for six weeks.

When deformity of the metatarsal head is already well established at the time of diagnosis attempted restoration of the articular surface is of no avail. Expectant treatment is then recommended. If pain is troublesome rest in a walking plaster for two months may afford relief; but if disabling osteoarthritis develops later the head of the metatarsal should be excised.

INGROWING TOE NAIL

(Embedded toe nail)

Ingrowing toe nail is common only in the great toe.

Cause. Some persons have toes that are prone to develop ingrowing toe nail. But the main causative factors are incorrect cutting of the nail, pressure on the nail-wall (lateral skin fold) by the shoe or by the adjacent second toe, and accumulation of dirt and sweat.

When the nail is cut its sides should be left long enough to project beyond the terminal pulp (Fig. 377): if it is cut too short a sharp corner of nail lies in contact with the lateral skin fold (Fig. 378), and this corner may tend to embed itself in the skin, especially if there is local pressure at the side of the toe. In the presence of dirt and sweat, infection is then liable to arise.

Fig. 377   **Fig. 378**   **Fig. 379**   **Fig. 380**

Figure 377—Nail cut correctly. Figure 378—Nail cut too short: corners dig into pulp. Figure 379—Operation for ingrowing toe nail. A strip of nail is avulsed and its re-growth is prevented by excision of a segment of the germinal matrix. Figure 380—Operation for permanent ablation of the whole nail. After avulsion of the nail, only the germinal matrix need be excised to prevent re-growth. The raw area is covered by advancing the proximal skin flap.

Clinical features. The lesion may be at the medial or (more commonly) the lateral border of the nail, or both. There is pain at the affected anterior corner of the nail. *On examination* the skin fold is inflamed, and there may be local suppuration where the corner of the nail digs into the skin.

Treatment. In mild cases conservative treatment may suffice. Pledgets of gauze soaked in alcohol (surgical spirit) are tucked beneath the corner of the nail twice a day, and the nail is allowed to grow until its edges project beyond the skin folds (Fig. 377).

In long-standing cases operation is advisable. If only one side of the nail is involved it is sufficient to avulse a strip of nail at the affected side and then to prevent re-growth of this part. Since the nail is formed only from the germinal matrix—the proximal curved segment of the nail bed that corresponds to the lunula—and not from the nail bed as a whole, it is necessary to remove only an appropriate piece of the germinal matrix to prevent re-growth (Fig. 379).

In the worst cases, with infection at both sides of the nail, permanent ablation of the entire nail by excision of the whole of the germinal matrix is more satisfactory (Fig. 380). The small raw area that remains can be covered simply by advancing a dorsal skin flap, based proximally and with its free edge at the nail fold.

SUBUNGUAL EXOSTOSIS

A subungual exostosis is a bony outgrowth from the dorsal surface of the distal phalanx of a toe—usually the great toe. It projects upwards and forwards between the tip of the nail and the terminal pulp. The nail is raised and deformed, and the skin of the pulp overlying the outgrowth is thickened and hard. There is sharp pain when pressure is applied over the nail or terminal pulp. *Radiographs* show the exostosis, which is seen best in the lateral projection.

Treatment. The exostosis should be excised through a terminal incision just beyond the tip of the nail.

ONYCHOGRYPOSIS

Translated from the Greek, this means 'hooked nail'. The term is descriptive. The nail—usually of the great toe—is enormously thickened and curved, eventually resembling a miniature ox-horn (Fig. 381).

Fig. 381
Onychogryposis.

Treatment. Simple removal of the nail is an adequate temporary measure; but the new nail will become similarly deformed. For permanent cure the nail bed must be ablated by excision of the germinal matrix, as described in the section on ingrowing toe nail (p. 400).

References and bibliography, page 403.

References and bibliography

This list is not intended as a comprehensive guide even to the more recent literature on orthopaedic surgery: space does not permit the inclusion of more than a limited selection. The aim has been to choose books and papers that will be of the greatest service to those seeking detailed information on a given subject, and a paper has generally been selected for one or more of the following reasons: 1) it reports recent work; 2) it reports authoritative opinion; 3) it is of special intrinsic interest; 4) it contains a comprehensive list of references. An original description or a classic paper has not always been listed when reference to it is made in more recent works, because it can thereby be easily traced. In the main the references are to works in the English language which will be readily accessible to most readers.

The list is arranged in two parts, 'general' and 'specific'. The general list cites comprehensive works of reference on orthopaedic surgery as a whole or on branches of it. The specific list refers to papers or chapters on a particular topic.

Titles printed in italics refer to books or monographs; those in roman type refer to papers in journals.

GENERAL WORKS

ADAMS, J. C. & Stossel, C. A. (1992): *Standard Orthopaedic Operations*, 4th edn. Edinburgh: Churchill Livingstone.

ADAMS, R. D. (1975): *Diseases of Muscle*, 3rd edn. London: Henry Kimpton.

AMERICAN ACADEMY OF ORTHOPAEDIC SURGEONS (1987): *Instructional Course Lectures*, vol. 36 (ed. Griffin). Chicago: AAOS.

AMERICAN ACADEMY OF ORTHOPAEDIC SURGEONS (1988): *Instructional Course Lectures*, vol. 37 (ed. Bassett). Chicago: AAOS.

APLEY, A. G. & SOLOMON, L. (1993): *A System of Orthopaedics and Fractures*, 7th edn. London: Butterworth.

BIRCH, R. (1987): The place of microsurgery in orthopaedics. In *Recent Advances in Orthopaedics* (5) (ed. Catterall). Edinburgh: Churchill Livingstone.

BURNETT, W. (1981): *Clinical Science for Surgeons*. London: Butterworth.

CAMPBELL, W. C. (1992): *Operative Orthopaedics*, 8th edn., (ed. Crenshaw). London: Henry Kimpton.

CAMPION, G. V. & Dixon, A. St J. (1989): *Rheumatology*. Oxford: Blackwell.

CATTERALL, A. (ed.) (1987): *Recent Advances in Orthopaedics (5)*. Edinburgh: Churchill Livingstone.

CATTERALL, A. (ed.) (1992): *Recent Advances in Orthopaedics (6)*. Edinburgh: Churchill Livingstone.

CURREY, H. L. F. (1988): *Essentials of Rheumatology*, 2nd edn. Edinburgh: Churchill Livingstone.

DUTHIE, R. B. & Bentley, G. (eds.) (1983): *Mercer's Orthopaedic Surgery*, 8th edn. London: Edward Arnold.

EASTCOTT, H. H. G. (1994): *Arterial Surgery*, 3rd edn. London: Pitman.

GALASKO, C. S. B. (ed.) (1987): *Neuromuscular Problems in Orthopaedics*. Oxford: Blackwell.

GALASKO, C. S. B. & Noble, J. (eds.) (1988): *Current Trends in Orthopaedic Surgery*. Manchester: Manchester University Press.

GARTLAND, J. J. (1988): Orthopaedic clinical research. Journal of Bone and Joint Surgery, **70A**, 1357.

HUGHES, S., BENSON, M. K. D. & COLTON, C. L. (1987): *The Principles and Practice of Musculo-skeletal Surgery*. Edinburgh: Churchill Livingstone.

JONES, J. P. (1993): Fat embolism, intravascular coagulation, and osteonecrosis. Clinical Orthopaedics, **292**, 294.

McKIBBIN, B. (ed.) (1983): *Recent Advances in Orthopaedics* (4). Edinburgh: Churchill Livingstone.

McNALLY, M. A., & MOLLAN, R. A. B. (1993): Venous thrombo-embolism and orthopaedic surgery. Journal of Bone and Joint Surgery, **75B**, 517.

MOLL, J. M. H. (1992): *Rheumatology*. Edinburgh: Churchill Livingstone.

NICKEL, V. L., & Botte, M. J. (1992): *Orthopaedic Rehabilitation*, 2nd edn. Edinburgh: Churchill Livingstone.

NOBLE, J. & GALASKO, C. S. B. (1987): *Recent Developments in Orthopaedic Surgery*. Manchester: Manchester University Press.

RANG, M. (ed.) (1969): The *Growth Plate and its Disorders*. Edinburgh: Livingstone.

RATLIFF, A. H. C., Atkins, R. M., & Eastwood, D. M. (1991): *Selected References in Elective Orthopaedics*. London: Springer-Verlag.

RENSHAW, T. S. (1987): *Paediatric Orthopaedics*. Philadelphia: Saunders.

ROACH, H. I., SHEARER, J. R. & ARCHER, C. (1989): The choice of an experimental model: a guide for research workers. Journal of Bone and Joint Surgery, **71B**, 549.

SCOTT, J. T. (ed) (1986): *Copeman's Textbook of the Rheumatic Diseases*, 6th edn. Edinburgh: Churchill Livingstone.

SHARRARD, W. J. W. (1993): *Paediatric Orthopaedics and Fractures*, 3rd edn. Oxford: Blackwell.

STEWART, J. D. M. & HALLETT, J. P. (1983): *Traction and Orthopaedic Appliances*. Edinburgh: Churchill Livingstone.

SPECIFIC WORKS

INTRODUCTION

ANDRY, N. (1743, reprod. 1961): *Orthopaedia*. Philadelphia: Lippincott.

BIGELOW, H. J. (1846): Insensibility during surgical operations produced by inhalation. Boston Medical and Surgical Journal, **35**, 309.

COOPER, A. (1823): *Treatise on Dislocations and Fractures of the Joints*, 2nd edn., London: Longmans [etc.].

DUBOS, R. J. (1951): *Louis Pasteur: Freelance of Science*. London: Gollancz.

JONES, A. ROCYN (1956): A review of orthopaedic surgery in Britain. Journal of Bone and Joint Surgery, **38B**, 27.

JONES, A. ROCYN (1948): Hugh Owen Thomas. Journal of Bone and Joint Surgery, **30B**, 547.

JONES, A. ROCYN (1948): Lister. Journal of Bone and Joint Surgery, **30B**, 196.

JONES, A. ROCYN (1948): John Hunter. Journal of Bone and Joint Surgery, **30B**, 357.

LISTER, J. (1867): On the antiseptic principle in the practice of surgery. Lancet, **2**, 353.

LONG, C. W. (1849): An account of the first use of sulphuric ether by inhalation as an anaesthetic in surgical operations. Southern Medical and Surgical Journal, **5**, 705.

MAYER, L. (1950): Orthopaedic surgery in the United States of America. Journal of Bone and Joint Surgery, **32B**, 461.

MORTON, W. T. G. (Quoted by Bigelow; see above).

MORTON, W. T. G: Letheon [a circular]. Boston: Dutton & Wentworth.

OSMOND-CLARKE, H. (1950): Half a century of orthopaedic progress in Great Britain: Journal of Bone and Joint Surgery, **32B**, 620.

PLATT, H. (1950): Orthopaedics in Continental Europe, 1900–50. Journal of Bone and Joint Surgery, **32B**, 570.

RÖNTGEN, W. C. (1896): On a new kind of rays. Nature, **53**, 274, 377.

CHAPTER ONE

Clinical Methods
Joint Movement: Method of Recording

AMERICAN ACADEMY OF ORTHOPAEDIC SURGEONS (1966): *Joint Motion: Method of Measuring and Recording.* Edinburgh: Livingstone.

Diagnostic Imaging

BASSETT, L. W. & GOLD, R. H. (1989): Magnetic resonance imaging of the musculo-skeletal system: an overview. Clinical Orthopaedics, **244**, 17.

BERQUIST, T. H. (1989): Magnetic resonance imaging of musculo-skeletal neo-plasms. Clinical Orthopaedics, **244**, 101.

BLOEM, J. & SARTORIS, D. J. (1994): *MRI and CT of the Musculo-Skeletal system.* Baltimore: Williams and Wilkins.

CAVANAGH, S., STEVENS, J., & JOHNSON, J. R. (1993): High resolution MRI in the investigation of recurrent pain after lumbar discectomy. Journal of Bone Surgery, **75B**, 524.

GALASKO, C. S. B. & WEBER, D. A. (1984): *Radionuclide Scintigraphy in Orthopaedics.* Edinburgh: Churchill Livingstone.

GREENSPAN, A. (ed.) (1988): Orthopaedic Radiology: *A Practical Approach.* Philadelphia: Lippincott.

JOHNSTONE, A. J., & BEGGS, L. (1994): Ultrasound imaging of soft tissue masses in the extremities. Journal of Bone and Joint Surgery, **76B**, 688.

LAREDO, J-D (1993): Gadolinium-enhanced MRI in orthopaedic surgery. Journal of Bone and Joint Surgery, **75B**, 521.

MURRAY, R. O. & JACOBSON, H. G. (1994): *The Radiology of Skeletal Disorders*, 3rd revised edn. Edinburgh: Churchill Livingstone.

O'KEEFE, D., & MAMTORA, H. (1992): Ultrasound in clinical orthopaedics. Journal of Bone and Joint Surgery, **74B**, 488.

PATERSON, D. C., FOSTER, B. K. & SAVAGE, J. P. (1987): The present status of bone scanning in clinical orthopaedic diagnosis. In *Recent Advances in Orthopaedics (5)* (ed. Catterall). Edinburgh: Churchill Livingstone.

RESNICK, D. & NIWAYAMA, G. (1994): *Diagnosis of Bone and Joint Disorders*, 3rd revised edn. Philadelphia: Saunders.

ROGERS, L. F. (ed.) (1994): *Radiology of Skeletal Trauma (2 vols)*, 3rd revised edn. Edinburgh: Churchill Livingstone.

SARTORIS, D. J. (ed.) (1994): Advances in Musculo-Skeletal Imaging. The Radiologic Clinics of North America, **32**. Philadelphia: Saunders.

SISSONS, H. A., MURRAY, R. O. & KEMP, H. B. S. (1984): *Orthopaedic Diagnosis*: *Clinical, Radiological and Pathological Coordinates*. Berlin: Springer-Verlag.
WATT, I. (1991): Magnetic resonance imaging in orthopaedics. Journal of Bone and Joint Surgery, **73B**, 539–50.
WILSON, D. J. (1988): Diagnostic ultrasound in the musculo-skeletal system. Current Orthopaedics, **2**, 41.

Pathology
BULLOUGH, P. G. & VIGORITA, V. J. (1994): *Atlas of Orthopaedic Pathology with Clinical and Radiological Correlations*, 2nd revised edn. Philadelphia: Lippincott.
GARDNER, D. L. (1992): *Pathology of the Connective Tissue Diseases*. London: Edward Arnold.
SALISBURY, J. R., WOODS, C. G. & BYERS, P. D. (eds) (1994): *Diseases of Bones and Joints. Cell biology, mechanisms, pathology*. London: Chapman and Hall Medical.

Electrodiagnosis
BROWN, W. F. & BOLTON, C. F. (eds) (1987): *Clinical Electromyography*. Boston: Butterworth.
DAVIDSON, D. M., HALLETT, M. & MILLENDER, L. H. (eds) (1990): *Entrapment Neuropathies*, 2nd edn. Boston: Little, Brown.
KIMURA, J. (ed) (1989): *Electrodiagnosis of Diseases of Nerve & Muscle: Principles and Practice*, 2nd edn. Philadelphia: F. A. Davis.
MUMENTHALER, M., SCHLIAK, H. (eds) (1990): *Peripheral Nerve Lesions, Diagnosis and Therapy*. Stuttgart: Thieme.
PARRY, C. B. WYNN (1961): Electrodiagnosis. Journal of Bone and Joint Surgery, **43B**, 222.

Treatment of Orthopaedic Disorders
ADAMS, J. C. & STOSSEL, C. A. (1992): *Standard Orthopaedic Operations*, 4th edn. Edinburgh: Churchill Livingstone.
ALLISON, D. J. (1982): Therapeutic embolisation. Journal of Bone and Joint Surgery, **64B**, 151.
AMERICAN ACADEMY OF ORTHOPAEDIC SURGEONS (1985): *Atlas of Orthotics: Biomechanical Principles and Application*. St Louis: Mosby.
AMSTUTZ, H. C. & SAKAI, D. N. (1978): Equalisation of leg length (editorial). Clinical Orthopaedics and Related Research, **136**, 2.
BERGER, R. G. (1994): Non-steroidal anti-inflammatory drugs: Making the right choices. Journal of American Academy of Orthopaedic Surgeons, **2**, 255.
BRIGDEN, R. J. (1980): *Operating Theatre Technique*, 4th edn. Edinburgh: Churchill Livingstone.
BROUGHTON, N. S., DICKENS, D. R. V., COLE, W. G. & MENELAUS, M. B. (1989): Epiphyseolysis for partial growth plate arrest. Journal of Bone and Joint Surgery, **71B**, 13.
BROUGHTON, N. S., OLNEY, B. W. & MENELAUS, M. B. (1989): Tibial shortening for leg length discrepancy. Journal of Bone and Joint Surgery, **71B**, 242.
CAMPBELL, W. C. (1980): *Operative Orthopaedics*, 6th edn., (ed. Edmonson and Crenshaw). London: Henry Kimpton.
CORLETT, R. J. (1988): Principles of skin cover. Surgery, **54**, 1276.
CYRIAX, J. (1983): *Text-book of Orthopaedic Medicine*, 8th edn. London: Baillière Tindall.
FADALE, P. D., & WIGGINS, M. E. (1994): Corticosteroid injections: their use and abuse. Journal of the American Academy of Orthopaedic Surgeons, **2**, 133.

GAZDAG, A. R., LANE, J. M., GLASER, D., & FORSTER, R. A. (1995): Alternatives to autogenous bone graft. Journal of the American Academy of Orthopaedic Surgeons, **3**, 1.

GOLDBERG, V. M. & STEVENSON, S. (1987): Natural history of autografts and allografts. Clinical Orthopaedics, **225**, 7.

GOULET, J. A. *et al.* (1989): Intra-operative autologous transfusion in orthopaedic patients. Journal of Bone and Joint Surgery, **71A**, 3.

GRAY, R. G. & GOTTLIEB, N. L. (1983): Intra-articular corticosteroids: an updated assessment. Clinical Orthopaedics, **177**, 235.

HERNIGON, P. *et al.* (1993): Massive allografts sterilised by irradiation. Journal of Bone and Joint Surgery, **75B**, 904.

HEYDEMANN, J. S. & NELSON, C. L. (1986): Short-term preventive antibiotics. Clinical Orthopaedics, **205**, 184.

IVORY, J. P., & THOMAS, I. H. (1993): Audit of a bone bank. Journal of Bone and Joint Surgery, **75B**, 355.

KENWRIGHT, J. (1989): Leg length inequality. Current Orthopaedics, **3**, 176.

KENWRIGHT, J., & ALBINANA (1991): Problems encountered in leg shortening. Journal of Bone and Joint Surgery, **73B**, 671.

LUCAS, G. (1978): Microvascular surgery and limb replantation (editorial). Clinical Orthopaedics, **133**, 2.

MCGREGOR, I. A. (1980): *Fundamental Techniques of Plastic Surgery and their Surgical Application*, 7th edn. Edinburgh: Churchill Livingstone.

MCNALLY, M. A., & MOLLAN, R. A. B. (1993): Venous thrombo-embolism and orthopaedic surgery. Journal of Bone and Joint Surgery, **75B**, 517.

Macnicol, M. F. & Catto, A. M. (1982): Twenty-year review of tibial lengthening for poliomyelitis. Journal of Bone and Joint Surgery, **64B**, 607.

MOSELEY, C. F. (1989): Leg lengthening. Clinical Orthopaedics, **247**, 38.

PARRY, C. B. WYNN (1980): *Rehabilitation of the Hand*, 4th edn. London: Butterworth.

PERKINS, G. (1953): Rest and movement. Journal of Bone and Joint Surgery, **35B**, 521.

RATLIFF, A. H. C., ATKINS, R. M., & EASTWOOD, D. M. (1991): *Selected References in Elective Orthopaedics*. London: Springer-Verlag.

STEWART, J. D. M. & HALLETT, J. P. (1983): *Traction and Orthopaedic Appliances*. Edinburgh: Churchill Livingstone.

THOMAS, H. O. (1875, reprod. 1962): *Diseases of the Hip, Knee and Ankle Joints*. Boston: Little, Brown.

CHAPTER TWO

General Survey of Orthopaedic Disorders

Injuries

ADAMS, J. C. & HAMBLEN, D. L. (1992): *Outline of Fractures*, 10th edn. Edinburgh: Churchill Livingstone.

WILSON, J. N. (ed.) (1982): *Watson-Jones's Fractures and Joint Injuries*, 6th edn. Edinburgh: Churchill Livingstone.

Deformities and Malformations

BEIGHTON, P. (1988): *Inherited Disorders of the Skeleton*, 2nd edn. Edinburgh: Churchill Livingstone.

BRUCE, C. & COWELL, H. R. (1987): The prevention of genetically determined orthopaedic defects. Clinical Orthopaedics, **222**, 85.

Crossan, J. F. & Wynne-Davies, R. (1986): Research for genetic and environmental factors in orthopaedic diseases. Clinical Orthopaedics, **210**, 97.

DUTHIE, R. B. & YOUNG, A. (eds.): (1987): Pathophysiology of joint contractures and their correction (symposium). Clinical Orthopaedics, **219**, 2.
HENKEL, L. & WILLERT, H.-G. (1969): Dysmelia. Journal of Bone and Joint Surgery, **51B**, 399.
McKENZIE, D. S. (1957): The prosthetic management of congenital deformities of the extremities. Journal of Bone and Joint Surgery, **39B**, 233.
ZIONTS, L. E. *et al.* (1984): Congenital annular bands in identical twins. Journal of Bone and Joint Surgery, **66A**, 450.

General Affections of the Skeleton

ALDEGHERI, R., TRIVELLA, G., RENZI-BRIVICO, L. *et al.* (1988): Lengthening of the lower limbs in achondroplastic patients: a comparative study of four techniques. Journal of Bone and Joint Surgery, **70B**, 69–73.
BARTH, R. W. & LANE, J. M. (1988): Osteoporosis. Orthopaedic Clinics of North America, **19**: 845–858.
BEIGHTON, P. (1988): *Inherited Disorders of the Skeleton*, 2nd edn. Edinburgh: Churchill Livingstone.
BLACK, B., *et al.* (1993): Multiple hereditary exostoses. Clinical Orthopaedics, **287**, 212.
BRILL, C. B. (1989): Neurofibromatosis: Clinical overview. Clinical Orthopaedics, **245**, 10.
BUCHANAN, J. R., MYERS, C. A. & GREER, R. B. (1988): A comparison of the risk of vertebral fracture in menopausal osteopenia and other metabolic disturbances. Journal of Bone and Joint Surgery, **70A**, 704.
CAMPBELL, G. A., COMPSTON, J. E., & CRISP, A. J. (1993): *The Management of Common Metabolic Bone Disorders*. Cambridge: Cambridge University Press.
CHALMERS, J., CONACHER, W. D. H., GARDNER, D. L. & SCOTT, P. J. (1967): Osteomalacia: a common disease in elderly women. Journal of Bone and Joint Surgery, **49B**, 403.
CONNOR, J. M. & EVANS, D. A. P. (1982): Fibrodysplasia ossificans progressive. Journal of Bone and Joint Surgery, **64B**, 76.
COOPER C. (1989): Osteoporosis: a review. Journal of the Royal Society of Medicine, **82**, 753.
FELSON, D. T., *et al.* (1993): The effect of postmenopausal estrogen therapy on osteoporosis. New England Journal of Medicine, **329**, 1141–1146.
HARINCK, H. I. J. *et al* (1987): Efficacious management with aminobisphosphonate (APD) in Paget's disease. Clinical Orthopaedics, **217**, 79.
HARRIS, W. H., DUDLEY, H. R. & BARRY, R. J. (1962): The natural history of fibrous dysplasia: an orthopaedic pathological and roentgenographic study. Journal of Bone and Joint Surgery, **44A**, 207–233.
HORAN, F. & BEIGHTON, P. (1982): *Orthopaedic Problems in Inherited Skeletal Disorders*. Berlin: Springer-Verlag.
KANIS, J. A. & GRAY, R. E. S (1987): Long-term follow-up observations on treatment in Paget's disease of bone. Clinical Orthopaedics, **217**, 99.
MACINTYRE, I., ALEVIZAK, M., BEVIS, P. J. R. & ZAIDI, M. (1987): Calcitonin and the peptides from the calcitonin gene. Clinical Orthopaedics, **217**, 45.
MACKIE, I. G. *et al.* (1989): Treatment of bone weakness in patients with femoral neck fracture by fluoride, calcium and vitamin D. Journal of Bone and Joint Surgery, **71B**, 111.
MANKIN, H. J. (1990): Rickets, osteomalacia and renal osteodystrophy: an update. Orthopaedic Clinics of North America, **21**: 81–96.
MANKIN, H. J. (1993): Gaucher's disease: A novel treatment and an important breakthrough. Journal of Bone and Joint Surgery, **75B**, 2.

McKusick, V. A. (1993): *Heritable Disorders of Connective Tissue*, 5th edn, (ed. P. Beighton). St Louis: C. V. Mosby.

Mills, B. G. & Singer, F. R. (1987): Clinical evaluation of viral antigen data in Paget's disease of bone. Clinical Orthopaedics, **217**, 16.

Mirra, J. M. (1987): Pathogenesis of Paget's disease based on viral etiology. Clinical Orthopaedics, **217**, 162.

Nordin, B. E. C. (ed.): (1993): *Metabolic Bone and Stone Disease*, 3rd edn. Edinburgh: Churchill Livingstone.

Nordin, B. E. C., Needs, A. G. & Horowitz, M. (1985): New approaches to the problems of osteoporosis. Clinical Orthopaedics, **200**, 181.

O'Doherty, D. P., Bickerstaff, D. R., Kanis, J. A. & Russell, R. G. G. (1989): Paget's disease of bone. Current Orthopaedics, **3**, 262.

Peterson, H. A. (1989): Multiple hereditary osteochondromata. Clinical Orthopaedics, **239**, 222.

Rebel, A. (Ed) (1987): Paget's disease (symposium). Clinical Orthopaedics, **217**, 2.

Riggs, B. L. & Melton, L. J. (1992): The prevention and treatment of osteoporosis. New England Journal of Medicine, **327**, 620–627.

Rogers, J. G. & Geho, W. B. (1979): Fibrodysplasia ossificans progressiva. Journal of Bone and Joint Surgery, **61A**, 909.

Shapiro, F., Simon, S. & Glimcher, M. J. (1979): Hereditary multiple exostoses. Journal of Bone and Joint Surgery, **61A**, 815.

Smith, R., Francis, M. J. O. & Houghton, G. R. (1983): *The Brittle Bone Syndrome: Osteogenesis Imperfecta*. London: Butterworth.

Sofield, H. A. (1959): Fragmentation, realignment and intramedullary rod fixation of deformities of the long bones in children. Journal of Bone and Joint Surgery, **41A**, 1371.

Stockley, I., Bell, M. J. & Sharrard, W. J. W. (1989): The role of expanding intramedullary rods in osteogenesis imperfecta. Journal of Bone and Joint Surgery, **71B**, 422–427.

Stoltz, M. R., Dietrich, S. L. & Marshall, G. J. (1989): Osteogenesis imperfecta. Clinical Orthopaedics, **242**, 120.

Wolf, A. & Dixon, A. St. J. (1988): *Osteoporosis*. London: Martin Dunitz.

Wynne-Davies, R. & Fairbank, T. J. (1976): *Fairbank's Atlas of General Affections of the Skeleton*. Edinburgh: Churchill Livingstone.

Wynne-Davies, R., Hall, C. M. & Apley, A. G. (1994): *Atlas of Skeletal Dysplasias*. Edinburgh: Churchill Livingstone.

Wynne Davies, R., Walsh, W. K. & Gormley, J. (1981): Achondroplasia and hypochondroplasia: clinical variation and spinal stenosis. Journal of Bone and Joint Surgery, **63B**, 508–515.

Infections of Bone

Craigen, M. A. C., Watters, J. & Hackett, J. S. (1992): The changing epidemiology of osteomyelitis in children. Journal of Bone and Joint Surgery, **74B**, 541.

Davies, P. D. O., Humphries, M. J., Byfield, S. P. *et al.* (1984): Bone and joint tuberculosis. Journal of Bone and Joint Surgery, **66B**, 326.

Dormans, J. P., & Drummond, D. S. (1994): Pediatric hematogenous osteomyelitis: New trends in presentation, diagnosis and treatment. Journal of American Academy of Orthopaedic Surgeons, **2**, 333.

Evans, E. M. & Davies, D. M. (1969): Treatment of chronic osteomyelitis by saucerisation and secondary skin grafting. Journal of Bone and Joint Surgery, **51B**, 454.

Knudsen, C. J. M. & Hoffman, E. B. (1990): Neonatal osteomyelitis. Journal of Bone and Joint Surgery, **72B**, 846–851.

LEONG, J. C. (1988): Bone and joint infection: Treatment of tuberculous infection. Current Orthopaedics, 2, 86.

LETTS, R. M. (1988): Bone and joint infection: Treatment of pyogenic infection. Current Orthopaedics, 2, 80.

LINDENBAUM, S. & ALEXANDER, H. (1984): Infections simulating bone tumors: a review of subacute osteomyelitis. Clinical Orthopaedics, 184, 193.

MARTINI, M. (ed.) (1988): *Tuberculosis of the Bones and Joints.* Berlin: Springer-Verlag.

MCNALLY, M. A. et al. (1993): Two-stage management of chronic osteomyelitis of the long bones. Journal of Bone and Joint Surgery, 75B, 375.

NADE, S. (1983): Acute haematogenous osteomyelitis in infancy and childhood. Journal of Bone and Joint Surgery, 65B, 109.

RASOOL, M. N. & GOVENDER, S. (1989): The skeletal manifestations of congenital syphilis. Journal of Bone and Joint Surgery, 71B, 752.

ROSS, E. R. S. & COLE, W. G. (1985): Treatment of subacute osteomyelitis in childhood. Journal of Bone and Joint Surgery, 67B, 443.

SCOLES, P. V. & ARONOFF, S. C. (1984): Antimicrobial therapy in childhood skeletal infections. Journal of Bone and Joint Surgery, 66A, 1487.

TUSON, C. E., HOFFMAN, E. B., & MANN, M. D. (1994): Isotope bone scanning for acute osteomyelitis and septic arthritis in children. Journal of Bone and Joint Surgery, 76B, 281.

WEDGE, J. H. (1988): Bone and joint infection: clinical presentation. Current Orthopaedics, 2, 65.

WOODS, C. G. (1988): Bone and joint infection: pathology. Current Orthopaedics, 2, 76.

Tumours of Bone

BERTONI, F., BORIANI, S., LAUS, M. & CAMPANACCI, M. (1982): Periosteal chondrosarcoma and periosteal osteosarcoma. Journal of Bone and Joint Surgery, 64B, 370.

BERTONI, F., PRESENT, D. & ENNEKING, W. F. (1985): Giant-cell tumour of bone with pulmonary metastases. Journal of Bone and Joint Surgery, 67A, 890.

BRAGE, M. E. & SIMON, M. A. (1992): Metastatic bone disease: evaluation, prognosis, and medical treatment considerations of metastatic bone tumours. Orthopaedics, 15, 589.

DOLLAHITE, B. A. et al (1989): Aspiration biopsy of primary neoplasms of bone. Journal of Bone and Joint Surgery, 71A, 1166.

ENNEKING, W. F. (1986): A system of staging musculoskeletal neoplasms. Clinical Orthopaedics, 204, 9.

GALASKO, C. S. B. (1986): Skeletal metastases. Clinical Orthopaedics, 210, 18.

GRIFFITHS, D. LL. (1966): Orthopaedic aspects of myelomatosis. Journal of Bone and Joint Surgery, 48B, 703.

HARRINGTON, K. D. (1986): Metastatic disease of the spine. Journal of Bone and Joint Surgery, 68A, 1110.

HURSON, B. J. (1995): Limb-sparing surgery for patients with sarcomas. Journal of Bone and Joint Surgery, 77B, 173.

HUVOS, A. G., BUTLER, A., & BRETSKY, S. S. (1983): Osteogenic sarcoma associated with Paget's disease of bone. Cancer, 52, 1489.

LARSSON, S.-E., LORENTZON, R. & BOQUIST, L. (1975): Giant-cell tumour of bone. Journal of Bone and Joint Surgery, 57A, 167.

MILLER, F. & WHITEHILL, R. (1984): Carcinoma of the breast metastatic to the skeleton. Clinical Orthopaedics, 184, 121.

PORTER, D. E. et al. (1992): A significant proportion of patients with osteosarcoma may belong to Li-Fraument cancer families. Journal of Bone and Joint Surgery, 74B, 883.

Rosen, G. *et al.* (1981): Ewing's sarcoma: ten year experience with adjuvant chemotherapy. Cancer, **47**, 2204.

Ruggieri, P., *et al.* (1993): Complications and surgical indications in 144 cases of non-metastatic osteosarcoma of the extremities treated with neoadjuvant chemotherapy. Clinical Orthopaedics, **295**, 226.

Schajowicz, F. (ed) (1994): *Tumors and Tumorlike Lesions of Bone. Pathology, Radiology and Treatment*, 2nd edn. Berlin: Springer-Verlag.

Schajowicz, F., Araujo, E. S. & Berenstein, M. (1985): Sarcoma complicating Paget's disease of bone. Journal of Bone and Joint Surgery, **65B**, 299.

Simon, M. A. (1988): Limb salvage for osteosarcoma. Journal of Bone and Joint Surgery, **70A**, 307.

Simon, M. A. & Biermann, J. S. (1993): Biopsy of bone and soft tissue tumours. Journal of Bone and Joint Surgery, **75A**, 616–621.

Simon, M. A. & Finn, H. A. (1993): Diagnostic strategy for bone and soft tissue tumours. Journal of Bone and Joint Surgery, **75A**, 622–631.

Souhami, R. & Craft, A. (1988): Progress in management of malignant bone tumours. Journal of Bone and Joint Surgery, **70B**, 345.

Springfield, D. S. *et al.* (1988): Surgical treatment for osteosarcoma. Journal of Bone and Joint Surgery, **70A**, 1124.

Sweetnam, R. (1989): Malignant bone tumour management. Clinical Orthopaedics, **247**, 67.

Other Local Affections of Bone

Bennett, O. M., & Namnyak, S. S. (1990): Bone and joint manifestations of sickle cell anaemia. Journal of Bone and Joint Surgery, **72B**, 494.

Boseker, E. H., Bickel, W. H. & Dahlin, D. C. (1968): Clinico-pathologic study of simple unicameral bone cysts. Surgery, Gynecology and Obstetrics, **127**, 550.

Chigira, M., Maehara, S., Arita, S. & Udagawa, E. (1983): The aetiology and treatment of simple bone cysts. Journal of Bone and Joint Surgery, **65B**, 633.

Clough, J. R. & Price, C. H. G. (1968); Aneurysmal bone cysts. Journal of Bone and Joint Surgery, **50B**, 116.

Dabska, M. & Buraczewski, J. (1969): Aneurysmal bone cyst. Cancer, **23**, 371.

Ennis, J. T., Whitehouse, G., Ross, F. G. M. & Middlemiss, J. H. (1973): Radiology of bone changes in histiocytosis X. Clinical Radiology, **24**, 212.

Fahey, J. J. (1973): Subtotal resection and grafting in selected cases of solitary unicameral bone cyst. Journal of Bone and Joint Surgery, **55A**, 59.

Fowles, J. V. & Bobechko, W. P. (1970): Solitary eosinophilic granuloma in bone. Journal of Bone and Joint Surgery, **52B**, 238.

Henry, A. (1969): Monostotic fibrous dysplasia. Journal of Bone and Joint Surgery, **51B**, 300.

McQueen, M M., Chalmers, J. & Smith, G. D. (1985): Spontaneous healing of aneurysmal bone cysts. Journal of Bone and Joint Surgery, **67B**, 310.

Poulsen, J. O. (1969): Osteoid osteoma. Acta Orthopaedica Scandinavica, **40**, 198.

Resnick, D., & Greenaway, G. (1982): Distal femoral cortical defects, irregularities and excavations. Radiology, **143NN**, 345.

Schajowicz, F., Sainz, M. C. & Slullitel, J. A. (1979): Juxta-articular bone cysts (intra-osseous ganglia). Journal of Bone and Joint Surgery, **61B**, 107.

Schajowicz, F. & Slullitel, J. (1973): Eosinophilic granuloma of bone and its relationship to Hand-Schüller-Christian and Letterer-Siwe syndromes. Journal of Bone and Joint Surgery, **55B**, 545.

Tumours of Soft Tissue

Bell, R. S. *et al.* (1989): The surgical margin in soft tissue sarcoma. Journal of Bone and Joint Surgery, **71A**, 370.

ELIAS, A. D. (1993): Chemotherapy for soft-tissue sarcomas. Clinical Orthopaedics, **289**, 94.

HAYS, D. M. (1993): Rhabdomyosarcoma. Clinical Orthopaedics, **289**, 36.

NINFO, V., CHUNG, E. B. & CAVAZZANA, A. O. (1994): *Tumors and Tumorlike Lesions of Soft Tissue*. Edinburgh: Churchill Livingstone.

ROSENTHAL, H. G., TEREK, R. M., & LANE, J. M. (1993): Management of extremity soft-tissue sarcomas. Clinical Orthopaedics, **289**, 66.

RYDHOLM, A. (1983): Management of patients with soft tissue tumours. Acta Orthopaedica Scandinavica, supplement **203**.

SADDEGH, M. K., *et al.* (1992): Staging of soft tissue sarcomas: Prognostic analysis of clinical and pathological features. Journal of Bone and Joint Surgery, **74B**, 495–500.

SIM, F. H., FRASSICA, F. J., & FRASSICA, D. A. (1994): Soft tissue tumours: Diagnosis, evaluation and management. Journal of the American Academy of Orthopaedic Surgeons, **2**, 202

SPRINGFIELD, D. (1993): Liposarcoma. Clinical Orthopaedics, **289**, 50.

WESTBURY, G. (1989): The management of soft tissue sarcomas. Journal of Bone and Joint Surgery, **71B**, 2.

WESTBURY, G. (1992): Prognostic factors in soft-tissue sarcoma. Journal of Bone and Joint Surgery, **74B**, 486.

Arthritis

ANSELL, B. M. & SWANN, M. (1983): The management of chronic arthritis in children. Journal of Bone and Joint Surgery, **65B**, 536.

BYERS, P. D., *et al* (1968): The diagnosis and treatment of pigmented villonodular synovitis. Journal of Bone and Joint Surgery, **50B**, 290.

CURREY, H. L. F. & MASON, R. M. (1969): Gout and chondrocalcinosis (pseudogout). In *Recent Advances in Orthopaedics* (ed. Apley). London: Churchill.

DAVIES, P. D. O., HUMPHRIES, M. J., BYFIELD, S. P., *et al* (1984): Bone and joint tuberculosis. Journal of Bone and Joint Surgery, **66B**, 326.

DIEPPE, P. (1993): Drug treatment of osteoarthritis. Journal of Bone and Joint Surgery, **75B**, 673.

EHRLICH, M. G. (ed.) (1986): Osteoarthritis (symposium). Clinical Orthopaedics, **213**, 2.

FLANDRY, F., *et al.* (1994): Diagnostic features of diffuse pigmented villonodular synovitis of the knee. Clinical Orthopaedics, **298**, 212.

ISHIKAWA, K. *et al.* (1989): A histological study of calcium pyrophosphate dihydrate crystal deposition disease. Journal of Bone and Joint Surgery, **71A**, 875.

KELLGREN, J. H. (1964): The epidemiology of rheumatic diseases. Annals of the Rheumatic Diseases, **23**, 109.

LEVY, R. N. *et al.* (1985): Progress in arthritis surgery. Clinical Orthopaedics, **200**, 299.

LUCK, J. V. & KASPER, C. K. (1989): Surgical management of advanced haemophilic arthropathy. Clinical Orthopaedics, **242**, 60.

PATERSON, D. C. (1970): Acute suppurative arthritis in infancy and childhood. Journal of Bone and Joint Surgery, **52B**, 424.

SCHWARTZ, H. S., UNNI, K. K. & PRITCHARD, D. J. (1989): Pigmented villonodular synovitis. Clinical Orthopaedics, **247**, 243.

SLEDGE, C. B. (1989): Surgery for rheumatoid arthritis. Current Orthopaedics, **3**, 1.

SWANN, M. (1987): Juvenile chronic arthritis. Clinical Orthopaedics, **219**, 38.

SWEETNAM, R. (1969): Corticosteroid arthropathy and tendon rupture. Journal of Bone and Joint Surgery, **51B**, 397.

WATT, I. (1989): Imaging for rheumatoid arthritis. Current Orthopaedics, **3**, 141.

Osteochondritis Dissecans; Loose Bodies

JEFFREYS, T. E. (1967): Synovial chondromatosis. Journal of Bone and Joint Surgery, **49B**, 530.

MAURICE, H., CRONE, M. & WATT, I. (1988): Synovial chrondromatosis. Journal of Bone and Joint Surgery, **70B**, 807.

Poliomyelitis

BROOKS, D. (1989): Surgery for poliomyelitis. Current Orthopaedics, **3**, 101.

CLARK, J. M. P. (1956): Muscle and tendon transposition in poliomyelitis. In *Modern Trends in Orthopaedics* (2). London: Butterworth.

SHARRARD, W. J. W. (1967): Paralytic deformity of the lower limb. Journal of Bone and Joint Surgery, **49B**, 731.

Cerebral Palsy

COOKE, P. H., COLE, W. G. & CAREY, R. P. L. (1989): Dislocation of the hip in cerebral palsy. Journal of Bone and Joint Surgery, **71B**, 441.

HOFFER, M., KNOEBEL, R. T. & ROBERTS, R. (1987): Contractures in cerebral palsy. Clinical Orthopaedics, **219**, 70.

POLLOCK, G. A. & ENGLISH, T. A. (1967): Transplantation of the hamstring muscles in cerebral palsy. Journal of Bone and Joint Surgery, **49B**, 80.

SAMILSON, R. L. (1976): Tendon transfers in cerebral palsy. Journal of Bone and Joint Surgery, **58B**, 153.

SAMILSON, R. L., TSOU, P., AAMOTH, G. & GREEN, W. M. (1972): Dislocation and subluxation of the hip in cerebral palsy. Journal of Bone and Joint Surgery, **54A**, 863.

SHARRARD, W. J. W. (1969): The orthopaedic surgery of cerebral palsy and spina bifida. In *Recent Advances in Orthopaedics* (ed. Apley). London: Churchill.

SKOFF, H. & WOODBURY, D. F. (1985): The management of the upper extremity in cerebral palsy. Journal of Bone and Joint Surgery, **67A**, 500.

Myelomeningocele; Spina Bifida

DRUMMOND, D. S., MOREAU, M. & CRUESS, R. L. (1980): The results and complications of surgery for the paralytic hip and spine in myelomeningocele. Journal of Bone and Joint Surgery, **62B**, 49.

HUFF, C. W. & RAMSEY, P. (1978): Myelodysplasia. Journal of Bone and Joint Surgery, **60A**, 432.

JAMES, C. C. M. & LASSMAN, L. P. (1981): *Spina Bifida Occulta*. London: Academic Press. New York: Grune & Stratton.

MAZUR, J. M. et al. (1989): Orthopaedic management of high level spina bifida. Journal of Bone and Joint Surgery, **71A**, 56.

MENELAUS, M. B. (1980): *The Orthopaedic Management of Spina Bifida Cystica*. Edinburgh: Churchill Livingstone.

SCHAFER, M. F. & DIAS, L. S. (1983): *Myelomeningocele: Orthopaedic Treatment*. Baltimore: Williams & Wilkins.

Sharrard, W. J. W. & GROSFIELD, I. (1968): The management of deformity and paralysis of the foot in myelomeningocele. Journal of Bone and Joint Surgery, **50B**, 456.

Peripheral Nerve Injuries

BIRCH, R. (1993): Surgery for brachial plexus injuries. Journal of Bone and Joint Surgery, **75B**, 346.

BOOME, R. S. & KAYE, J. C. (1988): Obstetric traction injuries of the brachial plexus. Journal of Bone and Joint Surgery, **70B**, 571.

GALASKO, C. S. B. (ed.) (1985): *Neurological Problems in Orthopaedics*. Oxford: Blackwell.

0

0

0

GODDARD, N. J. & FIXSEN, J. A. (1984): Rotation osteotomy of the humerus for birth injuries of the brachial plexus. Journal of Bone and Joint Surgery, **66B**, 257.

GUPTA, S. K., HELAL, B. H. & KIELY, P. (1969): The prognosis in zoster paralysis. Journal of Bone and Joint Surgery, **51B**, 593.

JACKSON, S. T., HOFFER, M. M. & PARRISH, N. (1988): Brachial plexus palsy in the newborn. Journal of Bone and Joint Surgery, **70A**, 1217.

LEFFERT, R. D. (1986): *Brachial Plexus Injuries*. Edinburgh: Churchill Livingstone.

MARSHALL, R. W., WILLIAMS, D. H., BIRCH, R. & BONNEY, G. (1988): Operations to restore elbow flexion after brachial plexus injuries. Journal of Bone and Joint Surgery, **70B**, 577.

MEDICAL RESEARCH COUNCIL (1943): Aids to the investigation of peripheral nerve injuries. War Memorandum No. 7. London: H.M.S.O.

NARAKAS, A. (1978): Surgical treatment of traction injuries of the brachial plexus. Clinical Orthopaedics, **133**, 71.

NORRIS, R. W. *et al.* (1988): Peripheral nerve repair in humans using muscle autografts. Journal of Bone and Joint Surgery, **70B**, 530.

SCHUTZER, S. & GOSSLING, H. R. (1984): Treatment of reflex sympathetic dystrophy syndrome. Journal of Bone and Joint Surgery, **66A**, 625.

SEDDON, H. J. (1942): Classification of nerve injuries. British Medical Journal, **2**, 237.

SEDDON, H. J. (1976): *Surgical Disorders of the Peripheral Nerves*, 2nd edn. Edinburgh: Churchill Livingstone.

SEDEL, L. (1982): The results of surgical repair of brachial plexus injuries. Journal of Bone and Joint Surgery, **64B**, 54:

SUNDERLAND, S. (1991): Nerve Injuries and their repair. Edinburgh: Churchill Livingstone.

CHAPTER THREE

Neck and Cervical Spine

Deformities

BROUGHAM, D. I., COLE, W. G., DICKENS, D. R. V. & MENELAUS, M. B. (1989): Torticollis due to a combination of sternomastoid contracture and congenital vertebral anomalies. Journal of Bone and Joint Surgery, **71B**, 404.

GARBER, N. (1964): Abnormalities of the atlas and axis vertebrae. (Instructional Course Lecture, American Academy of Orthopaedic Surgeons.) Journal of Bone and Joint Surgery, **46A**, 1782.

GRAY, S. W., ROMAINE, C. B. & SKANDALAKIS, J. E. (1964): Congenital fusion of the cervical vertebrae. Surgery, Gynecology and Obstetrics, **118**, 373.

GROGAN, D. P., STANLEY, E. A. & BOBECHKO, W. P. (1983): The congenital undescended scapula. Journal of Bone and Joint Surgery, **65B**, 598.

HENSINGER, R. N., LANG, J. E. & MacEWEN, G. D. (1974): Klippel-Feil syndrome. Journal of Bone and Joint Surgery, **56A**, 1246.

IPPOLITO, E., TUDISCO, C. & MASSOBRIO, M. (1985): Long-term results of open sternocleidomastoid tenotomy for idiopathic muscular torticollis. Journal of Bone and Joint Surgery, **67A**, 30.

JEFFREYS, E. (ed.) (2nd edn.) (1993): *Disorders of the Cervical Spine*. Oxford: Butterworth-Heninemann.

MACDONALD, D. (1969): Sternomastoid tumour and muscular torticollis. Journal of Bone and Joint Surgery, **51B**, 432.

WOODWARD, J. W. (1961): Congenital elevation of the scapula. Journal of Bone and Joint Surgery, **43A**, 219.

Infections

HODGSON, A. R., STOCK, F. E., FANG, H. S. Y. & ONG, G. B. (1960): Anterior spinal fusion [for tuberculosis]. British Journal of Surgery, **48**, 172.

HSU, L. C. S. & LEONG, J. C. Y. (1984): Tuberculosis of the lower cervical spine. Journal of Bone and Joint Surgery, **66B**, 1.

Arthritis, Disc Lesions and Instability

BERNARD, T. N. & WHITECLOUD, T. S. (1987): Cervical spondylotic myelopathy and myeloradiculopathy. Clinical Orthopaedics, **221**, 149.

CAPEN, D. A., GARLAND, D. E. & WATERS, R. L. (1985): Surgical stabilisation of the cervical spine: a comparative analysis of anterior and posterior spine fusions. Clinical Orthopaedics, **196**, 229.

FEHRING, T. K. & BROOKS, A. L. (1987): Upper cervical instability in rheumatoid arthritis. Clinical Orthopaedics, **221**, 137.

FIELDING, J. W. (1988): The status of arthrodesis of the cervical spine. Journal of Bone and Joint Surgery, **70A**, 1571.

FLOYD, A. S. et al. (1989): Atlanto-axial instability and neurologic indicators in rheumatoid arthritis. Clinical Orthopaedics, **241**, 177.

FRIED, J. A., ATHREYA, B., GREGG, J. R., et al. (1983): The cervical spine in juvenile rheumatoid arthritis. Clinical Orthopaedics, **179**, 102.

GLYNN, M. K. & SHEEHAN, J. M. (1983): Fusion of the cervical spine for instability. Clinical Orthopaedics, **179**, 97.

HEYWOOD, A. W. B., LEARMONTH, I. D. & THOMAS, M. (1988): Cervical spine instability in rheumatoid arthritis. Journal of Bone and Joint Surgery, **70B**, 702.

JOHNSON, R. M., OWEN, J. R., HART, D. L. & CALLAHAN, R. A. (1981): Cervical orthoses: A guide to their selection and use. Clinical Orthopaedics, **154**, 34.

KELSEY, J. L., GITHENS, P. B., WALTER, S. D., et al. (1984): An epidemiological study of acute prolapsed cervical intervertebral disc. Journal of Bone and Joint Surgery, **66A**, 907.

KONTTINEN, Y. T. et al. (1989): Atlanto-axial laxity in rheumatoid arthritis. Acta Orthopaedica Scandinavica, **60**, 379.

LIPSON, S. J. (1989): Rheumatoid arthritis in the cervical spine. Clinical Orthopaedics, **239**, 121.

MCAFEE, P. C. & BOHLMAN, H. H. (1989): One-stage anterior cervical decompression and posterior stabilisation with circumferential arthrodesis. Journal of Bone and Joint Surgery, **71A**, 78.

SANTAVIRTA, S. et al. (1988): Treatment of the cervical spine in rheumatoid arthritis. Journal of Bone and Joint Surgery, **70A**, 658.

SAUNDERS, R. L. & WILSON, D. H. (1980): The surgery of cervical disk disease. Clinical Orthopaedics, **146**. 119.

STIRRAT, A. N., & FYFE, I. S. (1993): Surgery of the rheumatoid cervical spine. Clinical Orthopaedics, **293**, 135.

WETZEL, F. T. & LA ROCCA, H. (1989): Grisel's syndrome. Clinical Orthopaedics, **240**, 141.

Cervical Rib and Outlet Syndrome

BONNEY, G. (1965): The scalenus medius band. Journal of Bone and Joint Surgery, **47B**, 268.

BRANNON, E. W. (1963): Cervical rib syndrome. Journal of Bone and Joint Surgery, **45A**, 977.

EASTCOTT, H. H. G. (1962): Reconstruction of the subclavian artery for complications of cervical rib and thoracic outlet syndrome. Lancet, **2**, 1243.

LEFFERT, R. D. (1994): Thoracic outlet syndrome. Journal of American Academy of Orthopaedic Surgeons, **2**, 317.

MOORE, M. (ed.) (1986): Thoracic outlet syndrome (symposium). Clinical Orthopaedics, **207**, 2.

Apical Lung Tumour

SPENGLER, D. M., KIRSH, M. N. & KAUFER, H. (1973): Orthopaedic aspects and early diagnosis of superior sulcus tumour of the lung (Pancoast). Journal of Bone and Joint Surgery, **55A**, 1645.

CHAPTER FOUR

Trunk and Spine

General

JAYSON, M. I. V. (1987): *The Lumbar Spine and Back Pain*. Edinburgh: Churchill Livingstone.

MORRISH, G. & WHITTLE, M. W. (1989): Spinal orthoses. Current Orthopaedics, **3**, 122.

Uhthoff, H. K. & Armstrong, G. (eds.) (1988): New horizons in spinal surgery (symposium). Clinical Orthopaedics, **227**, 2.

Deformities and Anomalies

BARRETT, D. S., *et al.* (1993): Costoplasty in adolescent idiopathic scoliosis. Journal of Bone and Joint Surgery, **75B**, 881.

BIRCH, J. G. *et al* (1988): Cotrel-Dubousset instrumentation in idiopathic scoliosis. Clinical Orthopaedics, **227**, 24.

BRADFORD, D. S. (1986); Instrumentation of the lumbar spine: An overview. Clinical Orthopaedics, **203**, 209.

BROOM, M. J., BANTA, J. V. & RENSHAW, T. S. (1989): Spinal fusion augmented by Luque rod segmental instrumentation for neuromuscular scoliosis. Journal of Bone and Joint Surgery, **71A**, 32.

BUNNELL, W. P. (1988): The natural history of idiopathic scoliosis. Clinical Orthopaedics, **229**, 20–25.

CALVERT, P. T., EDGAR, M. A. & WEBB, P. J. (1989): Scoliosis in neurofibromatosis. Journal of Bone and Joint Surgery, **71B**, 246.

CAPANNA, R., ALBISINNI, U., PICCI, P. *et al.* (1985): Aneurysmal bone cyst of the spine. Journal of Bone and Joint Surgery, **67A**, 527.

COLLIS, D. K. & PONSETI, I. V. (1969): Long-term follow-up of patients with idiopathic scoliosis not treated surgically. Journal of Bone and Joint Surgery, **51A**, 425.

COTREL, Y., DUBOUSSET, J. & GUILLAUMAT, M. (1988): New universal instrumentation in spinal surgery. Clinical Orthopaedics, **227**, 10.

CRUIKSHANK, J. L., KOIKE, M. & DICKSON, R. A. (1989): Curve patterns in idiopathic scoliosis. Journal of Bone and Joint Surgery, **71B**, 259.

DENIS, F. (1994): Anterior surgery in scoliosis. Clinical Orthopaedics, **300**, 38.

DICKSON, R. A. (1985): Conservative treatment for idiopathic scoliosis. Journal of Bone and Joint Surgery, **67B**, 176.

DICKSON, R. A. (1989): Idiopathic spinal deformities. Current Orthopaedics, **3**, 86.

DICKSON, R. A., LAWTON, J. O., ARCHER, I. A. & BUTT, W. P. (1984): The pathogenesis of idiopathic scoliosis. Journal of Bone and Joint Surgery, **66B**, 8.

EDGAR, M. A. & MEHTA, M. H. (1988): Long-term follow-up of fused and unfused idiopathic scoliosis. Journal of Bone and Joint Surgery, **70B**, 712.

GAINES, R. W. (1989): Congenital spinal deformities. Current Orthopaedics, **3**, 86.

HALL, J. E. (1989): Spinal deformities. Current Orthopaedics, **3**, 69.

HOWELL, F. R. & DICKSON, R. A. (1989): The deformity of idiopathic scoliosis made visible by computer graphics. Journal of Bone and Joint Surgery, **71B**, 399.

KALKMAN, C. J., BEEN, H. D. & ONGERBOER DE VISSER, B. W. (1993): Intra-operative monitoring of spinal cord function: a review. Acta Orthopaedica Scandinavica, **64**, 114.

KRISTIMUNDSDOTTIR, F., BURWELL, R. G. & JAMES, J. I. P. (1985): The rib-vertebra angles on the convexity and concavity of the spinal curve in infantile idiopathic scoliosis. Clinical Orthopaedics, **201**, 205.

LAWTON, J. O. & DICKSON, R. A. (1986): The experimental basis of idiopathic scoliosis. Clinical Orthopaedics, **210**, 9.

LENKE, L. G., BRIDWELL, K. H., BALDUS, C., BLANK, K. & SCHOENECKER, P. L. (1992): Cotrel-Dubousset instrumentation for adolescent idiopathic scoliosis. Journal of Bone and Joint Surgery, **74A**, 1056–1067.

LUQUE, E. R. (1986): Interpeduncular segmental fixation. Clinical Orthopaedics, **203**, 54.

McMASTER, M. J. (1983): Infantile idiopathic scoliosis: Can it be prevented? Journal of Bone and Joint Surgery, **65B**, 612.

MIELKE, C. H. et al. (1989): Surgical treatment of adolescent idiopathic scoliosis. Journal of Bone and Joint Surgery, **71A**, 1170.

MURRAY, P. M., WEINSTEIN, S. L. & SPRATT, K. F. (1993): The natural history and long-term follow-up of Scheuermann kyphosis. Journal of Bone and Joint Surgery, **75A**, 236–248.

NASH, C. L. & BROWN, R. H. (1989): Spinal cord monitoring. Journal of Bone and Joint Surgery, **71A**, 627.

PEHRSSON, K., LARSSON, S., ODEN, A. & NACHEMSON, A. (1992): Long term follow-up of patients with untreated scoliosis: a study of mortality, causes of death, and symptoms. Spine, **17**, 1091–1096.

RAJASEKARAN, S. & SOUNDARAPANDIAN, M. S. (1989): Progression of kyphophis in tuberculosis of the spine treated by anterior arthrodesis. Journal of Bone and Joint Surgery, **71A**, 1314.

THULBOURNE, T. & GILLESPIE, R. (1976): The rib hump in idiopathic scoliosis. Journal of Bone and Joint Surgery, **58B**, 64.

WILLIAMSON, J. B., & GALASKO, C. S. B. (1992): Spinal cord monitoring during operative correction of neuromuscular scoliosis. Journal of Bone and Joint Surgery, **74B**, 870.

WILTSE, L. L. (ed.) (1986): Internal fixation of the lumbar spine (symposium). Clinical Orthopaedics, **203**, 2.

Infections and Inflammatory Lesions

BABHULKAR, S. S., TAYADE, W. B. & BABHULKAR, S. K. (1984): Atypical spinal tuberculosis. Journal of Bone and Joint Surgery, **66B**, 239.

DESAI, S. S. (1994): Early diagnosis of spinal tuberculosis by MRI. Journal of Bone and Joint Surgery, **76B**, 863.

EISMONT, F. J., BOHLMAN, H .H, PRASANNA, L. S., et al. (1983): Pyogenic and fungal vertebral osteomyelitis with paralysis. Journal of Bone and Joint Surgery, **65A**, 19.

FREDERICKSON, B., YUAN, H. & OLANS, R. (1978): Management and outcome of pyogenic vertebral osteomyelitis. Clinical Orthopaedics, **131**, 160.

GARCIA, A. & GRANTHAM, S. A. (1960): Haematogenous pyogenic vertebral osteomyelitis. Journal of Bone and Joint Surgery, 42A, 429.

HODGSON, A. R., & STOCK F. E. (1956): Anterior spinal fusion: A preliminary communication in the radical treatment of Pott's disease and Pott's paraplegia. British Journal of Surgery, **44**, 266.

Hsu, L. C. S., Cheng, C. L. & Leong, J. C. Y. (1988): Pott's paraplegia of late onset. Journal of Bone and Joint Surgery, **70B**, 534.

Knudsen, C. J. M. & Hoffman, E. B. (1990): Neonatal osteomyelitis. Journal of Bone and Joint Surgery, **72B**, 846–851.

Leong, J. C. Y (1993): Tuberculosis of the spine. Journal of Bone and Joint Surgery, **75B**, 173.

Upadhyay, S. S., et al. (1994): Surgical management of spinal tuberculosis in adults. Clinical Orthopaedics, **302**, 173.

Osteoarthritis and Disc Lesions

Alexander, A. H. et al. (1989): Chymopapain chemonucleolysis versus surgical discectomy in a military population. Clinical Orthopaedics, **244**, 158.

Børgesen, S. E. & Wang, P. S. (1974): Herniation of lumbar intervertebral disc in children and adolescents. Acta Orthopaedica Scandinavica, **45**, 540.

Cavanagh, S., Stevens, J., & Johnson, J. R. (1993): High-resolution MRI in the investigation of recurrent pain after lumbar discectomy. Journal of Bone & Joint Surgery, **75B**, 524

Crawshaw, C., Kean, D. M., Mulholland, R. C., et al. (1984): The use of nuclear magnetic resonance in the diagnosis of lateral canal entrapment. Journal of Bone and Joint Surgery, **66B**, 711.

Cuckler, J. M., Bernini, P. A., Wiesel, S. W., et al. (1985): The use of epidural steroids in the treatment of lumbar radicular pain. Journal of Bone and Joint Surgery, **67A**, 63.

Eismont, F. J. & Currier, B. (1989): Surgical management of lumbar intervertebral disc disease. Journal of Bone and Joint Surgery, **71A**, 1266.

Hill, G. M. & Ellis, E. A. (1987): Chemonucleolysis as an alternative to laminectomy for herniated lumbar disc. Clinical Orthopaedics, **225**, 229.

Jepson, K., Nada, A & Rymaszewski (1982): The role of radiculography in the management of lesions of the lumbar disc. Journal of Bone and Joint Surgery, **64B**, 405.

Kitchel, S. H., & Brown, M. D. (1992): Complications of chemonucleolysis. Clinical Orthopaedics, **284**, 63

Kopp, J. R. et al. (1986): The use of lumbar extension in the evaluation and treatment of patients with acute herniated nucleus pulposus. Clinical Orthopaedics, **202**, 211.

Lewinneck, G. E. & Warfield, C. A. (1986): Facet joint degeneration as a cause of low back pain. Clinical Orthopaedics, **213**, 216.

Nordby, E. J. (1985): A comparison of discectomy and chemonucleolysis. Clinical Orthopaedics, **200**, 279.

Nordby, E. J. (ed.) (1986): Long-term results in chemonucleolysis (symposium). Clinical Orthopaedics, **206**, 2.

Nordby, E. J., et al. (1993): Safety of chemonucleolysis: Adverse effects reported in the United States 1982–1991. Clinical Orthopaedics, **293**,

Parry, C. B. Wynn, Girgis, F., Moffat, B. & Bhalla, A. K. (1989): The failed back: a review. Journal of the Royal Society of Medicine, **81**, 348.

Smith, L. (1993): Chemonucleolysis. Clinical Orthopaedics, **287**, 117.

Szypryt, E. P. et al. (1988): Diagnosis of lumbar disc protrusion. Journal of Bone and Joint Surgery, **70B**, 717.

Tay, E. C. K. & Chacha, P. B. (1979): Midline prolapse of a lumbar intervertebral disc with compression of the cauda equina. Journal of Bone and Joint Surgery, **61B**, 43.

Spinal Fusion

Freebody, D., Bendall, R. & Taylor, R. D. (1971): Anterior transperitoneal lumbar fusion. Journal of Bone and Joint Surgery, **53B**, 617.

McMurray, G. N. (1982): The evaluation of Kiel bone in spinal fusions. Journal of Bone and Joint Surgery, **64B**, 101.

Mehdian, H., Jaffray, D. & Eisenstein, S. M. (1989): Dwyer-Hartshill transpedicular fixation for spinal fusion. Journal of Bone and Joint Surgery, **71B**, 689.

Ankylosing Spondylitis

Adams, J. C. (1952): Technique dangers and safeguards in osteotomy of the spine. Journal of Bone and Joint Surgery, **34B**, 226.

Graham, D. C. (1960): Leukaemia following X-ray therapy for ankylosing spondylitis. American Medical Association Archives of Internal Medicine, **105**, 51.

Wright, V. & Moll, J. M. H. (1973): Ankylosing spondylitis. British Journal of
ᶜ Hospital Medicine, **9**, 331.

Calvé's disease; Scheuermann's disease

Compere, E. L., Johnson, W. E. & Coventry, M. B. (1954): Vetrebra plana (Calvé's disease) due to eosinophilic granuloma. Journal of Bone and Joint Surgery, **36A**, 969.

Ippolito, E., et al. (1984): Vertebra plana. Journal of Bone and Joint Surgery, **66A**, 1364.

Stoddard, A. & Osborn, J. F. (1979): Scheuermann's disease or spinal osteochondrosis. Journal of Bone and Joint Surgery, **61B**, 56.

Spondylolysis and Spondylolisthesis

Boxall, D., Bradford, D. S., Winter, R. B. & Moe, J. H. (1979): Management of severe spondylolisthesis in children and adolescents. Journal of Bone and Joint Surgery, **61A**, 479.

Buck, J. E. (1970): Direct repair of the defect in spondylolisthesis. Journal of Bone and Joint Surgery, **52B**, 432.

Cheng, C. L., Fang, D., Lee, P. C. & Leong, J. C. Y. Anterior spinal fusion for spondylolysis and isthmic spondylolisthesis. Journal of Bone and Joint Surgery, **71B**, 264.

Fredrickson, B. E., Baker, D., McHolick, W. J., et al. (1984): The natural history of spondylolysis and spondylolisthesis. Journal of Bone and Joint Surgery, **66A**, 699.

Freeman, B. L. & Donati, N. L. (1989): Spinal arthrodesis for severe spondylolisthesis in children and adolescents. Journal of Bone and Joint Surgery, **71A**, 594.

Hensinger, R. N. (1989): Spondylolysis and spondylolisthesis in children and adolescents. Journal of Bone and Joint Surgery, **71A**, 1098.

Yamane, T., Yoshida, T., & Mimatsu, K. (1993): Early diagnosis of lumbar spondylolysis by MRI. Journal of Bone and Joint Surgery, **75B**, 764.

Spinal Stenosis

Naylor, A. (1979): Factors in the development of the spinal stenosis syndrome. Journal of Bone and Joint Surgery, **61B**, 352.

Postacchini, F., Pezzeri, G., Montanaro, A. & Natali, G. (1980): Computerised tomography in lumbar stenosis. Journal of Bone and Joint Surgery, **62B**, 78.

Sanderson, P. L., & Wood, P. L. R. (1993): Surgery for lumbar spinal stenosis in old people. Journal of Bone and Joint Surgery.

Non-specific Back Pain

Bernard, T. N. & Kirkaldy-Willis, W. H. (1987): Recognising specific characteristics of non-specific low back pain. Clinical Orthopaedics, **217**, 266.

Getty, C. J. M. (1987): Management of the problem back. In *Recent Advances in Orthopaedics (5)* (ed. Catterall). Edinburgh: Churchill Livingstone.

Tumours

KER, N. B. & JONES, C. B. (1985): Tumours of the cauda equina. Journal of Bone and Joint Surgery, **67B**, 358.

KIRWAN, E. O'G., HUTTON, P. A. N., POZO, J. L. & RANSFORD, A. O. (1984): Osteoid osteoma and benign osteoblastoma of the spine. Journal of Bone and Joint Surgery, **66B**, 21.

ROZA, A. C. DA (1964): Primary intraspinal tumours. Journal of Bone and Joint Surgery, **46B**, 8.

SISSONS, H. A. (1959): Tumours of the vertebral column. In *Modern Trends in Diseases of the Vertebral Column*. London: Butterworth.

CHAPTER FIVE

The Shoulder Region

General

KELLY, I. G. (ed.) (1993): *The Practice of Shoulder Surgery*. Oxford: Butterworth-Heinemann.

KESSEL, L. (1986): *Clinical Disorders of the Shoulder*, 2nd edn. Edinburgh, London: Churchill Livingstone.

POST, M. (ed.) (1988): *The Shoulder*. Philadelphia: Lea & Febiger.

WATSON, M. S. (ed.) (1991): *Surgical Disorders of the Shoulder*. Edinburgh: Churchill Livingstone.

Deformities

FIDDIAN, N. J. & KING, R. J. (1984): The winged scapula. Clinical Orthopaedics, **185**, 228.

LAMB, D. W. & LAW, H. T. (1987): *Upper Limb Deficiencies in Children: Prosthetic, Orthotic & Surgical Management*. Edinburgh: Churchill Livingstone.

See also bibliography for Chapter Nine.

Arthritis

AMERICAN ACADEMY OF ORTHOPAEDIC SURGEONS (1982): *Symposium on Total Joint Replacement of the Upper Extremity*. St Louis: C. V. Mosby.

BROWNE, A. O. & MCCANN, P. D. (1988): The current status of shoulder arthroplasty. Clinical Orthopaedics, **2**, 94.

COFIELD, R. H. (1984): Total shoulder arthroplasty with the Neer prosthesis. Journal of Bone and Joint Surgery, **66A**, 899.

COFIELD, R. H. (1994); Uncemented total shoulder arthroplasty. Clinical Orthopaedics, **307**, 86.

KELLY, I. G., Foster, R. S. & Fisher, W. D. (1987): Neer total shoulder replacement in rheumatoid arthritis. Journal of Bone and Joint Surgery, **69B**, 723.

LETTIN, A. W. F., COPELAND, S. A. & SCALES, J. T. (1982): The Stanmore total shoulder replacement. Journal of Bone and Joint Surgery, **64B**, 47.

MACDONALD, P. B., *et al.* (1990): Haemophilic arthropathy of the shoulder. Journal of Bone and Joint Surgery, **72B**, 470.

NEWMAN, R. J. (1989): Surgery for rheumatoid arthritis: the shoulder. Current Orthopaedics, **3**, 4.

ROCKWOOD, C. A. (1988): Shoulder arthroplasty. Journal of Bone and Joint Surgery, **70A**, 639.

See also bibliography for Chapter Seven.

Dislocation

MOWERY, C. A., GARFIN, S. R., BOOTH, R. E. & ROTHMAN, R. H. (1985): Recurrent posterior dislocation of the shoulder. Journal of Bone and Joint Surgery, **67A**, 777.

OSMOND-CLARK, H. (1948): Habitual dislocation of the shoulder: the Putti-Platt operation. Journal of Bone and Joint Surgery, **30B**, 19.

REEVES, B. (1966): Arthrography of the shoulder. Journal of Bone and Joint Surgery, **48B**, 424.

ROWE, C. R. (1962): Acute and recurrent dislocations of the shoulder. (Instructional Course Lecture, American Academy of Orthopaedic Surgeons.) Journal of Bone and Joint Surgery, **44A**, 998.

Lesions of the Tendinous Cuff and Biceps Tendon

BASSETT, R. W. & COFIELD, R. H. (1983): Acute tears of the rotator cuff: the timing of surgical repair. Clinical Orthopaedics, **175**, 18.

BURNS, W. C., & WHIPPLE, T. L. (1993): Anatomic relationships in the shoulder impingement syndrome. Clinical Orthopaedics, **294**, 96.

COFIELD, R. H. (1985): Rotator cuff disease of the shoulder. Journal of Bone and Joint Surgery, **67A**, 974.

DEBEYRE, J., PATTE, D. & ELMELIK, E. (1965): Repair of ruptures of the rotator cuff of the shoulder. Journal of Bone and Joint Surgery, **47B**, 36.

HAWKINS, R. J. et al. (1988): Acromioplasty for impingement with an intact rotator cuff. Journal of Bone and Joint Surgery, **70B**, 795.

IANNOTTI, J. P. (1994): Full-thickness rotator cuff tears: Factors affecting surgical outcome. Journal of American Academy of Orthopaedic Surgeons, **2**, 87.

NORWOOD, L. A., BARRACK, R. & JACOBSON, K. E. (1989): Clinical presentation of complete tears of the rotator cuff. Journal of Bone and Joint Surgery, **71A**, 499.

PACKER, N. P., CALVERT, P. T., BAYLEY, J. I. L. & KESSEL, L. (1983): Operative treatment of chronic ruptures of the rotator cuff of the shoulder. Journal of Bone and Joint Surgery, **65B**, 171.

POST, M. & BENCA, P. (1989): Primary tendinitis of the long head of the biceps. Clinical Orthopaedics, **246**, 117.

POST, M. & COHEN, J. (1986): Impingement syndrome. Clinical Orthopaedics, **207**, 126.

WATSON, M. (1989): Rotator cuff function in the impingement syndrome. Journal of Bone and Joint Surgery, **71B**, 361.

Frozen Shoulder

LUNDBERG, B. J. (1969): The frozen shoulder. Acta Orthopaedica Scandinavica Supplementum No. 119.

NEVIASER, R. J. & NEVIASER T. J. (1987): The frozen shoulder: diagnosis and management. Clinical Orthopaedics, **223**, 59.

Sterno-clavicular and Acromio-clavicular Joints

AMERICAN ACADEMY OF ORTHOPAEDIC SURGEONS (1962): Treatment of complete acromio-clavicular dislocation. (Instructional Course Lecture.) Journal of Bone and Joint Surgery, **44A**, 1008.

BANNISTER, G. C., WALLACE, W. A., STABLEFORTH, P. G. & HUTSON, M. A. (1989): The management of acute acromioclavicular dislocation. Journal of Bone and Joint Surgery, **71B**, 848.

BURROWS, H. J. (1951): Tenodesis of subclavius in the treatment of recurrent dislocation of the sterno-clavicular joint. Journal of Bone and Joint Surgery, **33B**, 240.

ESKOLA, A. et al. (1989): Operation for old sternoclavicular dislocation. Journal of Bone and Joint Surgery, **71B**, 63.

ROCKWOOD, C. A. & ODOR, J. M. (1989): Spontaneous atraumatic subluxation of the sternoclavicular joint. Journal of Bone and Joint Surgery, **71A**, 1280.

ROPER, B. A. & LEVACK, B. (1982): The surgical treatment of acromioclavicular dislocations. Journal of Bone and Joint Surgery, **64B**, 597.

CHAPTER SIX

The Upper Arm and Elbow

General

WADSWORTH, T. G. (ed.) (1982): *The Elbow*. Edinburgh: Churchill Livingstone.

Infections of Bone

See bibliography for Chapter Five.

Tumours of Bone

See bibliography for Chapter Five.

Arthritis

DICKSON, R. A., HAIM, S. & BENTLEY, G. (1976): Excision arthroplasty of the elbow in rheumatoid disease. Journal of Bone and Joint Surgery, **58B**, 227.

FERLIC, D. C. *et al.* (1987): Elbow synovectomy in rheumatoid arthritis. Clinical Orthopaedics, **220**, 119.

GOLDBERG, V. M., FIGGIE, H. E., INGLIS, A. E. & FIGGIE, M. P. (1988): Total elbow arthroplasty. Journal of Bone and Joint Surgery, **70A**, 778.

RYMASZEWSKI, L. A., MACKAY, I., AMIS, A. A. & MILLER, J. H. (1984): Long-term effects of excision of the radial head in rheumatoid arthritis. Journal of Bone and Joint Surgery, **66B**, 109.

SOUTER, W. A. (1989): Surgery for rheumatoid arthritis: the elbow. Current Orthopaedics, **3**, 9.

TULP, N. J. A. & WINIA, W. P. C. A. (1989): Synovectomy of the elbow in rheumatoid arthritis: Long-term results. Journal of Bone and Joint Surgery, **71B**, 664.

See also bibliography for Chapter Seven.

Osteochondritis Dissecans

BAUER, M., *et al.* (1992): Osteochondritis of the elbow. Clinical Orthopaedics, **284**, 156.

ROBERTS, N. W. (1957): Osteochondritis dissecans. Journal of Bone and Joint Surgery, **39B**, 219.

Tennis Elbow

BOSWORTH, D. M. (1955): The role of the orbicular ligament in tennis elbow. Journal of Bone and Joint Surgery, **37A**, 527.

CYRIAX, J. (1983): *Text-book of Orthopaedic Medicine*. London: Baillière-Tindall.

SPENCER, G. E. & HERNDON, C. H. (1953): Surgical treatment of epicondylitis. Journal of Bone and Joint Surgery, **35A**, 421.

Ulnar Neuritis

MACNICOL, M. F. (1979): The results of operation for ulnar neuritis. Journal of Bone and Joint Surgery, **61B**, 159.

VANDERPOOL, D. W., CHALMERS, J., LAMB, D. W. & WHISTON, T. B. (1968): Peripheral compression lesions of the ulnar nerve. Journal of Bone and Joint Surgery, **50B**, 792.

CHAPTER SEVEN

The Forearm, Wrist and Hand
General

AMERICAN SOCIETY FOR SURGERY OF THE HAND (1983): *The Hand: Examination and Diagnosis*. New York, Edinburgh: Churchill Livingstone.

CARTER, P. R. (1983): *Common Hand Injuries and Infections*: Philadelphia: W. B. Saunders.

FISK, G. R. (1984): The wrist. Journal of Bone and Joint Surgery, **66B**, 396.

LAMB, D. W., HOPPER, G. & KUCZYNSKI, K. (1989): *The Practice of Hand Surgery*, 2nd edn. Oxford: Blackwell.

LISTER, G. (1984): *The Hand*, 2nd edn. New York: Churchill Livingstone.

MACNICOL, M. F. & LAMB, D. W. (1983): *Basic Care of the Injured Hand*. Edinburgh: Churchill Livingstone.

PARRY, C. B. WYNN (1980): *Rehabilitation of the Hand*, 4th edn. London: Butterworth.

RAZEMON, J. P. & FISK, G. R. (eds.) (1988): *The Wrist*. Edinburgh: Churchill Livingstone.

Infections of Bone
See bibliography for Chapter Five.

Tumours of Bone

LACKMAN, R. D. *et al.* (1987): Fibular reconstruction for giant cell tumour of the distal radius. Clinical Orthopaedics, **218**, 232.

Volkmann's Ischaemic Contracture

GELBERMAN, R. H., ZAKAIB, G. S., MUBARAK, S. J., HARGENS, A. R. & AKESON, W. H. (1978): Decompression of forearm compartment syndromes. Clinical Orthopaedics, **134**, 225.

HOLDEN, C. E. A. (1979): The pathology and prevention of Volkmann's ischaemic contracture. Journal of Bone and Joint Surgery, **61B**, 296.

MUBARAK, S. J. & CARROLL, N. C. (1979): Volkmann's contracture in children. Journal of Bone and Joint Surgery, **61B**, 285.

MUBARAK, S. J., PEDOWITZ, R. A. & HARGENS, A. R. (1989): Compartment syndromes. Current Orthopaedics, **3**, 36.

SEDDON, H. J. (1956): Volkmann's contracture: Treatment by excision of the infarct. Journal of Bone and Joint Surgery, **38B**, 152.

Deformities

BARSKY, A. J. (1951): Congenital anomalies of the hand. Journal of Bone and Joint Surgery, **33A**, 35.

ENTIN, M. A. (1958): Reconstruction of congenital abnormalities of the upper extremities. Journal of Bone and Joint Surgery, **41A**, 681.

MASADA, K. *et al.* (1989): Operations for forearm deformity caused by multiple osteochondromas. Journal of Bone and Joint Surgery, **71B**, 24.

RANAWAT, C. S., DeFIORE, J. & STRAUB, L. R. (1975): Madelung's deformity. Journal of Bone and Joint Surgery, **57A**, 772.

Arthritis

BLAIR, W. F., SHURR, D. G. & BUCKWALTER, J. A. (1984): Metacarpophalangeal joint implant arthroplasty with a silastic spacer. Journal of Bone and Joint Surgery, **66A**, 365.

DRYER, R. F., BLAIR, W. F., SHURR, D. G. & BUCKWALTER, J. A. (1984): Proximal interphalangeal joint arthroplasty. Clinical Orthopaedics, **185**, 187.

HARALDSSON, S. (1972): Extirpation of the trapezium for osteoarthritis of the first carpo-metacarpal joint. Acta Orthopaedica Scandinavica, 43, 347.

KESSLER, I. (1966): Posterior synovectomy for rheumatoid involvement of the hand and wrist. Journal of Bone and Joint Surgery, 48A, 1085.

KLEINERT, J. M., STERN, P. J., LISTER, G. D. & KLEINHANS, R. J. (1985): Complications of scaphoid silicone arthroplasty. Journal of Bone and Joint Surgery, 67A, 422.

MACK, G. R., et al. (1984): The natural history of scaphoid non-union. Journal of Bone and Joint Surgery, 66A, 504.

MENON, J. (1983): The problem of trapeziometacarpal degenerative arthritis. Clinical Orthopaedics, 175, 155.

NALEBUFF, E. A. (1969): Metacarpo-phalangeal surgery in rheumatoid arthritis. Surgical Clinics of North America, 49, 823.

NALEBUFF, E. A. (1989): Surgery for rheumatoid arthritis: the wrist and hand. Current Orthopaedics, 3, 14.

RASHKOFF, E. S., BURKHALTER, W. E. & MANN, R. J. (1983): Septic arthritis of the wrist. Journal of Bone and Joint Surgery, 65A, 824.

VARLEY, G. W. et al. (1994): Excision of the trapezium for osteoarthritis at the base of the thumb. Journal of Bone and Joint Surgery, 76B, 964.

WILSON, J. N. & BOSSLEY, C. J. (1983): Osteotomy in the treatment of osteoarthritis of the first carpo-metacarpal joint. Journal of Bone and Joint Surgery, 65B, 179.

Kienböck's Disease
ALMQUIST, E. E. (1986): Kienbock's disease. Clinical Orthopaedics, 202, 68.

LEE, M. L. H. (1963): The intra-osseous arterial pattern of the carpal lunate bone and its relation to avascular necrosis. Acta Orthopaedica Scandinavica, 33, 43.

LIGHTMAN, D. M., MACK, G. R., MACDONALD, R. I., et al. (1978): Kienböck's disease: the role of silicone replacement arthroplasty. Journal of Bone and Joint Surgery, 59A, 899.

RAMAKRISHNA, B., D'NETTO, C. & SETHU, A. U. (1982): Long-term results of silicone rubber implants for Kienbock's disease. Journal of Bone and Joint Surgery, 64B, 361.

SUNDBERG, S. B. & LINSCHEID, R. L. (1984): Kienbock's disease: Results of treatment with ulnar lengthening. Clinical Orthopaedics, 187, 43.

Infections of the Hand
PIMM, L. H. & WAUGH, W. (1957): Tuberculous tenosynovitis. Journal of Bone and Joint Surgery, 39B, 91.

Tumours
BUTLER, E. D., HAMILL, J. P., SEIPEL, R. S. & de LORIMIER, A. A. (1960): Tumours of the hand. American Journal of Surgery, 100, 293.

IOIA, J. V., SUMNER, J. M. & GALLAGHER, T. (1984): Presentation of malignancy by metastases to the carpal navicular bone. Clinical Orthopaedics, 188, 230.

PHO, R. W. H. (1979): Free vascularised fibular transplant for replacement of the lower radius. Journal of Bone and Joint Surgery, 61B, 362.

Carpal Tunnel Syndrome
BUCHTHAL, F., ROSENFALCK, A. & TROJABORG, W. (1974): Electrophysiological findings in entrapment of the median nerve at the wrist and elbow. Journal of Neurology, Neurosurgery and Psychiatry, 37, 340.

HARRIS, C. M., TANNER, E., GOLDSTEIN, M. N. & PETTEE, D. S. (1979): The surgical treatment of the carpal tunnel syndrome correlated with preoperative nerve conduction studies. Journal of Bone and Joint Surgery, 61A, 93.

PHALEN, G. S. (1966): The carpal tunnel syndrome. Journal of Bone and Joint Surgery, **48A**, 211.

SZABO, R. M., & STEINBERG, D. R. (1994): Nerve entrapment syndromes in the wrist. Journal of American Academy of Orthopaedic Surgeons, **2**, 115.

Ganglion

MCEVEDY, B. V. (1962): Simple ganglia. British Journal of Surgery, **49**, 585.

Dupuytren's Contracture

HONNER, R., LAMB, D. W. & JAMES, J. I. P. (1971): Dupuytren's contracture. Journal of Bone and Joint Surgery, **53B**, 240.

HUESTON, J. T. (1975): Dupuytren's contracture: Selection for surgery. British Journal of Hospital Medicine, **13**, 361.

HUESTON, J. T. & TUBIANA, R. (1985): *Dupuytren's Disease*, 2nd edn. Edinburgh: Churchill Livingstone.

MURRELL, G. A. C., FRANCIS, M. J. O. & HOWLETT, C. R. (1989): Dupuytren's contracture. Journal of Bone and Joint Surgery, **71B**, 367.

Tendon Lesions

BROOKS, D. M. (1970): Problems of restoration of tendon movements after repair and grafts. Proceedings of the Royal Society of Medicine, **63**, 67.

HALLBERG, D. & LINDHOLM, A. (1960): Subcutaneous rupture of extensor tendon of distal phalanx of finger (mallet finger). Acta Chirurgica Scandinavica, **119**, 260.

MATTHEWS, P. (1979): Biological factors in the management of flexor tendon injuries. In *Recent Advances in Orthopaedics* (3) (ed. McKibbin). Edinburgh: Churchill Livingstone.

MEALS, R. A. (1985): Flexor tendon injuries. Journal of Bone and Joint Surgery, **67A**, 817.

PULVERTAFT, R. G. (1973): Twenty-five years of hand surgery. Journal of Bone and Joint Surgery, **55B**, 32.

RICHARDS, H. J. (1979): The role of primary suture in injuries to the flexor tendon. In *Recent Advances in Orthopaedics* (3) (ed. McKibbin). Edinburgh: Churchill Livingstone.

SEMPLE, J. C. (1991): Tenosynovitis, repetitive strain injury, cumulative trauma disorder, and over-use syndrome et cetera. Journal of Bone and Joint Surgery, **73B**, 536.

SCHMITZ, P. W. & Stromberg, W. B. (1978): Two-stage flexor tendon reconstruction in the hand. Clinical Orthopaedics, **131**, 185.

STRICKLAND, J. W. (1989): Flexor tendon surgery. Journal of Hand Surgery, **14B**, 368.

STRICKLAND, J. W. (1995): Flexor tendon injuries: I. Foundations of treatment. Journal of American Academy of Orthopaedic Surgeons, **3**, 44.

STRICKLAND, J. W. (1995): Flexor tendon injuries: II. Operative technique. Journal of American Academy of Orthopaedic Surgeons, **3**, 55.

STARK, H. H. & WILSON, J. N. (1962): Mallet finger. Journal of Bone and Joint Surgery, **44A**, 1061.

URBANIAK, J. R. & GOLDNER, L. (1973): Laceration of the flexor pollicis longus tendon: delayed repair by advancement, free graft or direct suture. Journal of Bone and Joint Surgery, **55A**, 1123.

VERDAN, C. (ed.) (1979): *Tendon Surgery in the Hand*. Edinburgh: Churchill Livingstone.

WOOD, V. E., & SICILIA, M. (1992): Congenital trigger digit. Clinical Orthopaedics, **285**, 205.

The Thumb
BRAUN, R. M. (1985): The thumbs (symposium). Clinical Orthopaedics, **195**, 2.

CHAPTER EIGHT

The Hip Region
Congenital Dislocation
BARLOW, T. G. (1968): Congenital dislocations of the hip. Hospital Medicine, 2, 571.
BENNET, G. C. (1992): Screening for congenital dislocation of the hip. Journal of Bone and Joint Surgery, **74B**, 643.
BENNETT, J. T. & MACEWEN, G. D. (1989): Congenital dislocation of the hip: recent advances and current problems. Clinical Orthopaedics, **247**, 15.
BENSON, M. K. D. & EVANS, D. C. J. (1976): The pelvic osteotomy of Chiari. Journal of Bone and Joint Surgery, **58B**, 164.
BERKELEY, M. E., DICKSON, J. E. CAIN, T. E. & DONOVAN, M. M. (1984): Surgical therapy for congenital dislocation of the hip in patients who are twelve to thirty-six months old. Journal of Bone and Joint Surgery, **66A**, 412.
BLOCKEY, N. J. (1984): Derotation osteotomy in the management of congenital dislocation of the hip. Journal of Bone and Joint Surgery, **66B**, 485.
BOERCE, N. R., & CLARKE, N. M. P. (1994): Ultrasound imaging and secondary screening for congenital dislocation of the hip. Journal of Bone and Joint Surgery, **76B**, 525.
CARTER, C. O. & WILKINSON, J. A. (1964): Genetic and environmental factors in the etiology of congenital dislocation of the hip. Clinical Orthopaedics, **33**, 119.
CATTERALL, A. (1994): The early diagnosis of congenital dislocation of the hip. Journal of Bone and Joint Surgery, **76B**, 515.
CLARKE, N. M. P., HARCKE, H. T., MCHUGH, P., et al. (1985): Real-time ultrasound in the diagnosis of congenital dislocation and dysplasia of the hip. Journal of Bone and Joint Surgery, **67B**, 407.
CLARKE, N. M. P., CLEGG, J. & AL-CHALABI, A. N. (1989): Ultrasound screening of hips at risk for congenital dislocation. Journal of Bone and Joint Surgery, **71B**, 9.
DEROSA, G. P. & FELLER, N. (1987): Treatment of congenital dislocation of the hip: management before walking age. Clinical Orthopaedics, **225**, 77.
DIAS, J. J., et al. (1993): The reliability of ultrasonographic assessment of neonatal hip. Journal of Bone and Joint Surgery, **75B**, 479.
EYRE-BROOK, A. L., JONES, D. A. & HARRIS, F. C. (1978): Pemberton's acetabuloplasty for congenital dislocation or subluxation of the hip. Journal of Bone and Joint Surgery, **60B**, 18.
GAGE, J. R. & WINTER, R. B. (1972): Avascular necrosis of the capital femoral epiphysis as a complication of closed reduction of congenital dislocation of the hip. Journal of Bone and Joint Surgery, **54A**, 373.
GALPIN, R. D. et al. (1989): One-stage treatment of congenital dislocation of the hip in older children. Journal of Bone and Joint Surgery, **71A**, 734.
GRAHAM, S. et al (1986): The Chiari osteotomy. Clinical Orthopaedics, **208**, 249.
HADLOW, V. (1988): Neonatal screening for congenital dislocation of the hip. Journal of Bone and Joint Surgery, **70B**, 740.
HANSSON, G. (1988): Congenital dislocation of the hip joint: problems in diagnosis and treatment. Current Orthopaedics, **2**, 104.
HEIKKILA, E., RYOPPY, S. & LOUHIMO, I. (1985): The management of primary acetabular dysplasia. Journal of Bone and Joint Surgery, **67B**, 25.
HENDERSON, R. S. (1970): Osteotomy for unreduced congenital dislocation of the hip in adults. Journal of Bone and Joint Surgery, **52B**, 468.

HERNANDEZ, R. S., CORNELL, R. G., & HENSINGER, R. N. (1994): Ultrasound diagnosis of neonatal congenital dislocation of the hip. Journal of Bone and Joint Surgery, 76B, 539.

LOVE, B. R. T., STEVENS, P. M. & WILLIAMS, P. F. (1980): A long-term review of shelf arthroplasty. Journal of Bone and Joint Surgery, 62B, 321.

MACEWEN, G. D. (1987): Treatment of congenital dislocation of the hip in older children. Clinical Orthopaedics, 225, 86.

MARKS, D. S., CLEGG, J., & AL-CHALABI, A. (1994): Routine ultrasound screening for neonatal hip instability. Journal of Bone and Joint Surgery, 76B, 534.

MCKIBBIN B. (1970): Anatomical factors in the stability of the hip joint in the newborn. Journal of Bone and Joint Surgery, 52B, 148.

MOORE, F. H. (1989): Examining infants' hips: Can it do harm? Journal of Bone and Joint Surgery, 71B, 4.

POUL, J. et al. (1992): Early diagnosis of congenital dislocation of the hip. Journal of Bone and Joint Surgery, 74B, 695.

SHERLOCK, D. A., GIBSON P. H. & BENSON, M. K. D. (1985): Congenital subluxation of the hip. Journal of Bone and Joint Surgery, 67B, 390.

SMITH, W. S., PONSETI, I. V., RYDER, C. T. & SALTER, R. B. (1966): Congenital dislocation of the hip in the older child (Symposium) (Instructional Course Lectures, American Academy of Orthopaedic Surgeons). Journal of Bone and Joint Surgery, 48A, 1390.

SOMERVILLE, E. W. (1978): A long-term follow-up of congenital dislocation of the hip. Journal of Bone and Joint Surgery, 60B, 25.

SUSUKI, S et al. (1987): Diagnosis by ultrasound of congenital dislocation of the hip joint. Clinical Orthopaedics, 217, 171.

TERGESEN, T., BREDLAND, T. & BERG, V. (1989): Ultrasound for hip assessment in the newborn. Journal of Bone and Joint Surgery, 71B, 767.

WAINWRIGHT, D. (1976): The shelf operation for hip dysplasia in adolescence. Journal of Bone and Joint Surgery, 58B, 159.

WILLIAMSON, D. M., GLOVER, S. D. & BENSON, M. K. D'A. (1989): Congenital dislocation of the hip presenting after the age of three years. Journal of Bone and Joint Surgery, 71B, 745.

WYNNE-DAVIES, R. (1970): Acetabular dysplasia and familial joint laxity: two etiological factors in congenital dislocation of the hip. Journal of Bone and Joint Surgery, 52B, 704.

Arthritis

BRADLEY, G. W. et al. (1987): Resurfacing arthroplasty: femoral head viability. Clinical Orthopaedics, 220, 137.

CAMPBELL, J. A. B., & HOFFMAN, E. B. (1995): Tuberculosis of the hip in children. Journal of Bone and Joint Surgery, 77B, 319.

CHARNLEY, J. (1970): Total hip replacement by low-friction arthroplasty. Clinical Orthopaedics and Related Research, 72, 7.

DOBBS, H. S. (1980): Survivorship of total hip replacements. Journal of Bone and Joint Surgery, 62B, 168.

EFTEKHAR, N. S. (ed.): Low friction arthroplasty (symposium). Clinical Orthopaedics, 211, 2.

EYRE-BROOK, A. (1960): Septic arthritis of the hip and osteomyelitis of the upper end of the femur in infants. Journal of Bone and Joint Surgery, 42B, 11.

GRAUER, J. D. et al. (1989): Resection arthroplasty of the hip. Journal of Bone and Joint Surgery, 71A, 669.

HARDINGE, K. (1970): The etiology of transient synovitis of the hip in childhood. Journal of Bone and Joint Surgery, 52B, 100.

HARRIS, C. M. & BAUM, J. (1988): Involvement of the hip in juvenile rheumatoid arthritis. Journal of Bone and Joint Surgery, **70A**, 821.

HARRIS, W. H. (1986): Etiology of osteoarthritis of the hip. Clinical Orthopaedics, **213**, 20.

JONES, D. A. (1989): Irritable hip and Campylobacter infection. Journal of Bone and Joint Surgery, **71B**, 227.

LLOYD-ROBERTS, G. C. (1960): Suppurative arthritis in infancy. Journal of Bone and Joint Surgery, **42B**, 706.

LYNCH, A. F. (1982): Tuberculosis of the greater trochanter. Journal of Bone and Joint Surgery, **64B**, 185.

McKEE, G. K. (1970): Development of total prosthetic replacement of the hip. Clinical Orthopaedics, **72**, 85.

NUNN, D. (1988): The Ring uncemented plastic-on-metal total hip replacement. Journal of Bone and Joint Surgery, **70B**, 40.

RANAWAT, C. S. (1989): Surgery for rheumatoid arthritis: the hip. Current Orthopaedics, **3**, 146.

RING, P. A. (1968): Complete replacement arthroplasty of the hip by the Ring prosthesis. Journal of Bone and Joint Surgery, **50B**, 720.

RUSSOTTI, G. M., COVENTRY, M. B. & STAUFFER, R. N. (1988): Cemented total hip arthroplasty with contemporary techniques. Clinical Orthopaedics, **235**, 141.

TOLAT, V., et al. (1993): Evidence for a viral aetiology of transient synovitis of the hip. Journal of Bone and Joint Surgery, **75B**, 973.

WEISL, H. (1980): Intertrochanteric osteotomy for osteoarthritis. Journal of Bone and Joint Surgery, **62B**, 37.

WROBLEWSKI, B. M., & SINEY, P. D. (1993): Charnley low friction arthroplasty of the hip: Long term results. Clinical Orthopaedics, **292**, 191.

Perthes' Disease

BOWEN, J. R., FOSTER, B. K. & HARTZELL, C. (1984): Legg-Calvé-Perthes' disease. Clinical Orthopaedics, **185**, 97.

BURWELL, R. G. & HARRISON, M. H. M. (eds.) (1986): Perthes' disease (symposium). Clinical Orthopaedics, **209**, 2.

CATTERALL, A. (1971): The natural history of Perthes's disease (symposium). Journal of Bone and Joint Surgery, **53B**, 37.

COOPERMAN, D. R. & STULBERG, S. D. (1986): Ambulatory containment treatment in Perthes' disease. Clinical Orthopaedics, **203**, 289.

HALL, A. J. (1987): Perthes' disease: progression in aetiological research. In *Recent Advances in Orthopaedics* (5) (ed. Catterall). Edinburgh: Churchill Livingstone.

KERET, D., HARRISON, M. H. M., CLARKE, N. M. P., et al. (1984): Coxa plana: the fate of the physis. Journal of Bone and Joint Surgery, **66A**, 870.

McANDREW, M. P. & WEINSTEIN, S. L. (1984): A long-term follow-up of Legg-Calvé-Perthes' disease. Journal of Bone and Joint Surgery, **66A**, 860.

MAXTED, M. J. & JACKSON, R. K. (1985): Innominate osteotomy in Perthes' disease. Journal of Bone and Joint Surgery, **67B**, 399.

MENELAUS, M. B. (1986): Lessons learned in the management of Legg-Calvé-Perthes' disease. Clinical Orthopaedics, **209**, 41.

MUIRHEAD-ALLWOOD, W. & CATTERALL, A. (1982): The treatment of Perthes' disease. Journal of Bone and Joint Surgery, **64B**, 282.

PATERSON, D. & SALVAGE, J. P. (1986): The nuclide bone scan in the diagnosis of Perthes' disease. Clinical Orthopaedics, **209**, 23.

POUSSA, M., et al. (1993): Prognosis after conservative and operative treatment in Perthes' disease. Clinical Orthopaedics, **297**, 82.

RATLIFF, A. H. C. (1967): Perthes' disease: A study of thirty-four hips observed for thirty years. Journal of Bone and Joint Surgery, **49B**, 102.

Slipped Upper Femoral Epiphysis and Coxa Vara

BLOCKEY, N. J. (1969): Observations on infantile coxa vara. Journal of Bone and Joint Surgery 51B, 106.

BRENKEL, I. J. et al. (1989): Hormone status in patients with slipped capital femoral epiphysis. Journal of Bone and Joint Surgery, 71B, 33.

CAREY, R. P. L., MORAN, P. L. & COLE, W. G. (1987): The place of threaded pin fixation in the treatment of slipped upper femoral epiphysis. Clinical Orthopaedics, 224, 45.

COLTON, C. L. (1987): Slipped upper femoral epiphysis. In Recent Advances in Orthopaedics (5) (ed. Catterall). Edinburgh: Churchill Livingstone.

CRAWFORD, A. H. (1988): Slipped capital femoral epiphysis. Journal of Bone and Joint Surgery, 70A, 1422.

DIETZ, F. R. (1994): Traction reduction of acute and acute-on-chronic slipped capital femoral epiphysis. Clinical Orthopaedics, 302, 101.

DUNN, D. M. & ANGEL, J. C. (1978): Replacement of the femoral head by open operation in severe adolescent slipping of the upper femoral epiphysis. Journal of Bone and Joint Surgery, 60B, 394.

GRIFFITH, M. J. (1976): Slipping of the capital femoral epiphysis. Annals of the Royal College of Surgeons of England, 58, 34.

HAGGLUND, G. et al. (1986): Slipped capital femoral epiphysis in southern Sweden. Clinical Orthopaedics, 210, 152.

JERRE, R., et al. (1994): The contralateral hip in patients primarily treated for unilateral slipped upper femoral epiphysis. Journal of Bone and Joint Surgery, 76B, 563.

KOVAL, K. J. et al. (1989): Treatment of slipped capital femoral epiphysis with cannulated screw technique. Journal of Bone and Joint Surgery, 71A, 1370.

LYNCH, G. J. & STEVENS, D. B. (1987): Slipped capital femoral epiphysis: Treatment by pinning in situ. Clinical Orthopaedics, 221, 260.

STANITSKI, C. L. (1994): Acute slipped capital femoral epiphysis: Treatment alternatives. Journal of American Academy of Orthopaedic Surgeons, 2, 96.

VRETTOS, B. C., & HOFFMAN, E. B. (1993): Chondrolysis in slipped upper femoral epiphysis. Journal of Bone and Joint Surgery, 75B, 956.

CHAPTER NINE

The Thigh and Knee

General; Arthroscopy

BUCKLEY, J. R., HOOD, G. M. & MACRAE, W. (1989): Arthroscopy under local anaesthesia. Journal of Bone and Joint Surgery, 71B, 126.

DANDY, D. J. (1984): Arthroscopic surgery. Journal of Bone and Joint Surgery, 66B, 627.

DANDY, D. J. (1987): Arthroscopic Management of the Knee, 2nd edn. Edinburgh: Churchill Livingstone.

ENGEN, T. J. & LEHMKUHL, L. D. (1989): Lower extremity orthoses. Current Orthopaedics, 3, 194.

FRANK, C. (1986): Accurate interpretation of the Lachman test. Clinical Orthopaedics, 213, 163.

GURTLER, R. A., STINE, R. & TORG, J. S. (1987): Lachman test evaluated. Clinical Orthopaedics, 216, 141.

IRELAND, J., TRICKEY, E. L. & STOKER, D. J. (1980): Arthroscopy and arthrography of the knee. Journal of Bone and Joint Surgery, 62B, 3.

STOKER, D. J. (1980): *Knee Arthrography*. London: Chapman & Hall.
STROBEL, M., EICHHORN, J., & SCHIESSLER, W. (1992): *Basic Principles of Knee Arthroscopy*. Berlin: Springer-Verlag.

Infections of Bone
See bibliography for Chapter Five.

Bone Tumours
See bibliography for Chapter Five.

Arthritis
ABERNETHY, P. J. (1989): Surgery for rheumatoid arthritis: the knee. Current Orthopaedics, **3**, 150.
ACKROYD, C. E. & POLYZOIDES, A. J. (1978): Patellectomy for osteoarthritis. Journal of Bone and Joint Surgery, **60B**, 353.
ESKOLA, A. *et al.* (1988): Arthroplasty for old tuberculosis of the knee. Journal of Bone and Joint Surgery, **70B**, 767.
FERN, E. D., STEWART, H. D. & NEWTON, G. (1989): Curved Kuntscher nail arthrodesis after failure of knee replacement. Journal of Bone and Joint Surgery, **71B**, 588.
FREEMAN, M. A. R. & LEVACK, B. (1986): British contribution to knee arthroplasty. Clinical Orthopaedics, **210**, 69.
GOODFELLOW, J. W. *et al.* (1988): The Oxford knee for unicompartmental osteoarthritis. Journal of Bone and Joint Surgery, **79B**, 692.
GRAHAM, J. & CHECKETTS, R. G. (1973): Synovectomy of the knee joint in rheumatoid arthritis. Journal of Bone and Joint Surgery, **55B**, 786.
HEALY, W. L. & RILEY, L. H. (1986): High tibial valgus osteotomy. Clinical Orthopaedics, **209**, 227.
HUNGERFORD, D. S. & KRACKOW, K. A. (1985): Total joint arthroplasty of the knee. Clinical Orthopaedics, **192**, 23.
INSALL, J. N. (1988): Choices and compromises in total knee arthroplasty. Clinical Orthopaedics, **226**, 43.
INSALL, J. N., JOSEPH, D. M. & MSIKA, C. (1985): High tibial osteotomy for varus gonarthrosis. Journal of Bone and Joint Surgery, **67A**, 1040.
ISHIKAWA, H., *et al.* (1994): Painful bipartite patella in young athletes. Clinical Orthopaedics, **305**, 223.
KARPINSKI, R. K. & GRIMER, R. J. (1987): Hinged knee replacement in revision arthroplasty. Clinical Orthopaedics, **220**, 185.
KNUTSON, K., LINDSTRAND, A. & LIDGREN, L. (1985): Arthrodesis for failed knee arthroplasty. Journal of Bone and Joint Surgery, **67B**, 47.
LEE, S. S., CAMPBELL, J. A. B., & HOFFMAN, E. B. (1995): Tuberculosis of the knee in children. Journal of Bone and Joint Surgery, **77B**, 313.
LETTIN, A. W. F., KAVANAGH, T. G. & SCALES, J. T. (1984): The long-term results of Stanmore total knee replacements. Journal of Bone and Joint Surgery, **66B**, 349.
MORREY, R. (1989): Upper tibial osteotomy for secondary osteoarthritis of the knee. Journal of Bone and Joint Surgery, **71B**, 554.
OGLESBY, J. W. & WILSON, F. C. (1984): The evolution of knee arthroplasty. Clinical Orthopaedics, **186**, 96.
SCOTT, W. N. (ed.) (1986): Total knee arthroplasty: the state of the art (symposium). Clinical Orthopaedics, **205**, 2.
SCUDERI, G. R., INSALL, J. N., WINDSOR, R. E. & MORAN, M. C. (1989): Survivorship of cemented knee replacements. Journal of Bone and Joint Surgery, **71B**, 798.
VERDECK, W. N. & McBEATH, A. A. (1978): Knee synovectomy for rheumatoid arthritis. Clinical Orthopaedics, **134**, 168.

VINCE, K. G., INSALL, J. N. & KELLY, M. A. (1989): The total condylar prosthesis. Journal of Bone and Joint Surgery, 71B, 793.

WAUGH, W. (1986): Tibial osteotomy in the management of osteoarthritis of the knee. Clinical Orthopaedics, 210, 55.

Also see bibliography for Chapter Seven.

Chondromalacia of Patella

BENTLEY, G. & DOWD, G. (1984): Current concepts of etiology and treatment of chondromalacia patellae. Clinical Orthopaedics, 189, 209.

FULKERSON, J. P. (1994): Patello-femoral pain disorders: Evaluation and management. Journal of American Academy of Orthopaedic Surgeons, 2, 124.

GOODFELLOW, J. et al. (1976): Patello-femoral joint mechanics and pathology. Journal of Bone and Joint Surgery, 58B, 270.

McCARROLL, J. R., O'DONOGHUE, D. H. & GRANA, W. A., (1983): The surgical treatment of chondromalacia of the patella. Clinical Orthopaedics, 175, 130.

OGILVIE-HARRIS, D. J. & JACKSON, R. W. (1984): The arthroscopic treatment of chondromalacia patellae. Journal of Bone and Joint Surgery, 66B, 660.

OHNO, O. et al. (1988): An electron microscopic study of early pathology in chondromalacia of the patella. Journal of Bone and Joint Surgery, 70A, 883.

SANDOW, M. J. & GOODFELLOW, J. W. (1985): The natural history of anterior knee pain in adolescents. Journal of Bone and Joint Surgery, 67B, 36.

Injuries of the Menisci and Ligaments

AMIS, A. A. (1989): Anterior cruciate ligament replacement. Journal of Bone and Joint Surgery, 71B, 819.

GLASGOW, M. M. S., ALLEN, P. W., & BLAKEWAY, C. (1993): Arthroscopic treatment of cysts of the lateral meniscus. Journal of Bone and Joint Surgery, 75B, 299.

GOODFELLOW, J. (1980): Meniscal lesions (editorial). Journal of Bone and Joint Surgery, 62B, 1.

HAMBERG, P., GILLQUIST, J. & LYSHOLM, J. (1984): A comparison between arthroscopic meniscectomy and modified open meniscectomy. Journal of Bone and Joint Surgery, 66B, 189.

McGINTY, J. B., GEUSS, L. F. & MARVIN, R. A. (1977): Partial or total meniscectomy? Journal of Bone and Joint Surgery, 59A, 763.

MUCKLE, D. (1984): Open meniscectomy: enhanced recovery after synovial prostaglandin inhibition. Journal of Bone and Joint Surgery, 66B, 193.

NOBLE, J. & ERAT, J. (1980): In defence of the meniscus: a prospective study of 200 meniscectomy patients. Journal of Bone and Joint Surgery, 62B, 7.

OGILVIE-HARRIS, D. J., BAUER, M. & COREY, P. (1985): Prostaglandin inhibition and the rate of recovery after arthroscopic meniscectomy. Journal of Bone and Joint Surgery, 67B, 567.

SHAKESPEARE, D. J. & RIGBY, H. S. (1983): The bucket-handle tear of the meniscus. Journal of Bone and Joint Surgery, 65B, 383.

Osteochondritis Dissecans; Loose Bodies

BRADLEY, J. & DANDY, D. J. (1989): Results of drilling osteochondritis dissecans before skeletal maturity. Journal of Bone and Joint Surgery, 71B, 642.

COOLIGAN, M. R. & DANDY, D. J. (1989): Arthroscopic management of synovial chondromatosis of the knee. Journal of Bone and Joint Surgery, 71B, 498.

MURPHY, F. P., DAHLIN, D. C. & SULLIVAN, C. R. (1962): Articular synovial chondromatosis. Journal of Bone and Joint Surgery, 44A, 77.

SMILLIE, I. S. (1957): Treatment of osteochondritis dissecans. Journal of Bone and Joint Surgery, 39B, 248.

STOUGAARD, J. (1964): Familial occurrence of osteochondritis dissecans. Journal of Bone and Joint Surgery, **46B**, 542.
THOMSON, J. L. (1987): Osteochondritis dissecans and osteochondral fragments managed by Herbert compression screw fixation. Clinical Orthopaedics, **224**, 71.

Recurrent Dislocation of Patella
CARTER, C. & SWEETNAM, R. (1960): Recurrent dislocation of the patella and of the shoulder. Journal of Bone and Joint Surgery, **42B**, 721.
JACKSON, A. M. (1992): Recurrent dislocation of the patella. Journal of Bone and Joint Surgery, **74B**, 2.
RIEGLER, H. F. (1988): Recurrent dislocation and subluxation of the patella. Clinical Orthopaedics, **227**, 201.
SCUDERI, G., CUOMO, F. & SCOTT, N. (1988): Lateral release and proximal re-alignment for patellar subluxation and dislocation. Journal of Bone and Joint Surgery, **70A**, 856.

CHAPTER TEN

The Leg, Ankle and Foot
General
FIXSEN, J. A. & LLOYD-ROBERTS, G. C. (1988): *The Foot in Childhood*. Edinburgh: Churchill Livingstone.
HELAL, B. & WILSON, D. (1988): *The Foot*. Edinburgh: Churchill Livingstone.
JONES, F. WOOD (1949): *Structure and Function as Seen in the Foot*. London: Baillière, Tindall and Cox.
KLENERMAN, L. (ed.) (1982): *The Foot and its Disorders*, 2nd edn. Oxford: Blackwell.
MANN, R. A. (ed.) (1986): *Surgery of the Foot*. St Louis: Mosby.
NEALE, D. & ADAMS, I. M. (eds) (1989): *Common Foot Disorders*, 3rd edn. Edinburgh: Churchill Livingstone.
WILLIAMS, P. F. (1976): Restoration of muscle balance of the foot by transfer of the tibialis posterior. Journal of Bone and Joint Surgery, **58B**, 217.

Rupture of Calcaneal Tendon
GILLIES, H. & CHALMERS, J. (1970): The management of fresh ruptures of the tendo achillis. Journal of Bone and Joint Surgery, **52A**, 337.
KELLAM, J. F., HUNTER, G. A. & McELWAIN, J. P. (1985): Review of the operative treatment of Achilles tendon rupture. Clinical Orthopaedics, **201**, 80.
LEA, R. B. & SMITH, L. (1972): Non-surgical treatment of tendo achillis rupture. Journal of Bone and Joint Surgery, **54A**, 1398.
WILLS, C. A et al. (1986): Achilles tendon rupture. Clinical Orthopaedics, **207**, 156.

Osteomyelitis
MAY, J. W. et al. (1989): Clinical classification of post-traumatic tibial osteomyelitis. Journal of Bone and Joint Surgery, **71A**, 1422.
See bibliography for Chapter Five.

Tumours
See bibliography for Chapter Five.

Vascular lesions
CONSUMERS' ASSOCIATION (1990): Do drugs help intermittent claudication? Drug & Therapeutics Bulletin, **28**, 1.
DUNCAN, J. A. T. (1985): Chemical lumbar sympathectomy. Journal of Bone and Joint Surgery, **67B**, 174.

KIKUCHI, S., HASUE, M. & WATANABE, M. (1978): Ischemic contracture in the lower limb. Clinical Orthopaedics, **134**, 185.

MANOLI, A., *et al.* (1993): Scarred muscle excision for the treatment of established ischaemic contracture of the lower extremity. Clinical Orthopaedics, **292**, 309.

MOZES, M., RAMON, Y. & JAHR, J. (1962): The anterior tibial syndrome. Journal of Bone and Joint Surgery, **44A**, 730.

SEDDON, H. J. (1966): Volkmann's ischaemia in the lower limb. Journal of Bone and Joint Surgery, **48B**, 627.

Arthritis

ABDO, R. V., & IORIO, L-J. (1994): Rheumatoid arthritis of the foot and ankle. Journal of American Academy of Orthopaedic Surgeons, **2**, 326.

DEMOTTAZ, J. D., MAZUR, J. M., THOMAS, W. H., SLEDGE, C. B. & SIMON, S. R. (1979): Clinical study of total ankle replacement with gait analysis. Journal of Bone and Joint Surgery, **61A**, 976.

FIGGIE, M. P., *et al.* (1993): Triple arthrodesis in rheumatoid arthritis. Clinical Orthopaedics, **292**, 250.

HELAL, B. (1989): Surgery for rheumatoid arthritis: the foot and ankle. Current Orthopaedics, **3**, 157.

HEYWOOD, A. W. BROOKES (1983): Supramalleolar osteotomy in the management of the rheumatoid hindfoot. Clinical Orthopaedics, **177**, 76.

MANN, R. A. & THOMPSON, F. M. (1984): Arthrodesis of the first metatarso-phalangeal joint for hallux valgus in rheumatoid arthritis. Journal of Bone and Joint Surgery, **66A**, 687.

McGUIRE, M. R. *et al.* (1988): Comparative analysis of ankle arthroplasty versus ankle arthrodesis. Clinical Orthopaedics, **226**, 174.

Also see bibliography for Chapter Seven.

Recurrent Subluxation of Ankle

AHLGREN, O. & LARSSON S. (1989): Reconstruction for lateral ligament injuries of the ankle. Journal of Bone and Joint Surgery, **71B**, 300.

GLASGOW, M., JACKSON, A. & JAMIESON, A. M. (1980): Instability of the ankle after injury to the lateral ligament. Journal of Bone and Joint Surgery, **62B**, 196.

RIEGLER, H. F. (1984): Reconstruction for lateral instability of the ankle. Journal of Bone and Joint Surgery, **66A**, 336.

SEFTON, K. K., GEORGE, J., FITTON, J. M. & McMULLEN, H. (1979): Reconstruction of the anterior talofibular ligament for the treatment of the unstable ankle. Journal of Bone and Joint Surgery, **61B**, 352.

Osteochondritis Dissecans

ZINMAN, C., WOLFSON, N. & REIS, N. D. (1988): Osteochondritis dissecans of the dome of the talus. Journal of Bone and Joint Surgery, **70A**, 1017.

Foot Deformities

ADDISON, A., FIXSEN, J. A. & LLOYD-ROBERTS G. C. (1983): A review of the Dillwyn Evans type collateral operation in severe club feet. Journal of Bone and Joint Surgery, **65B**, 12.

BEATSON, T. R. & PEARSON, J. R. (1966): A method of assessing correction in club feet. Journal of Bone and Joint Surgery, **48B**, 40.

CLARK, J. M. P. (1968): Surgical treatment of club foot. Proceedings of the Royal Society of Medicine, **61**, 779.

CUMMINGS, R. J. & LOVELL, W. W. (1988): Operative treatment of congenital idiopathic club foot. Journal of Bone and Joint Surgery, **70A**, 1108.

DWYER, F. C. & MAISELS, D. O. (1976): Lobster-claw deformities of the feet. Proceedings of the Royal Society of Medicine, **69**, 178.

FUKUHARA, K, SCHOLLMEIER, G., & UHTHOFF, H. K. (1994): The pathogenesis of club foot. Journal of Bone and Joint Surgery, **76B**, 450.

GRAHAM, G. P., & DENT, C. M. (1992): Dillwyn Evans operation for relapsed club foot. Journal of Bone and Joint Surgery, **74B**, 445.

HARROLD, A. J. & WALKER, C. J. (1983): Treatment and prognosis in congenital club foot. Journal of Bone and Joint Surgery, **65B**, 8.

HUDSON, L., & CATTERALL, A. (1994): Postero-lateral release for resistant club foot. Journal of Bone and Joint Surgery, **76B**, 281.

ISAACS, H., HANDELSMAN, J. E., BADENHORST, M. & PICKERING, A. (1977): The muscles in club foot: a histological, histochemical and electron microscope study. Journal of Bone and Joint Surgery, **59B**, 465.

KUMAR, P. N. H., LAING, P. W., & KLENERMAN, L. (1993): Medial calcaneal osteotomy for relapsed equinovarus deformity. Journal of Bone and Joint Surgery, **75B**, 967.

MAIN, B. J., CRIDER, R. J., POLK, M. & LLOYD-ROBERTS, G. C. (1977): The results of early operation in talipes equino-varus. Journal of Bone and Joint Surgery, **59B**, 337.

MAIN, B. J. & CRIDER, R. J. (1978): An analysis of residual deformity in club feet submitted to early operation. Journal of Bone and Joint Surgery, **60B**, 536.

MCCLUSKEY, W. P., LOVELL, W. W. & CUMMINGS, R. J. (1989): The cavo-varus foot deformity. Clinical Orthopaedics, **247**, 27.

MOSIER, K. M. & ASHER, M. (1984): Tarsal coalitions and peroneal spastic flat foot. Journal of Bone and Joint Surgery, **66A**, 976.

RICHARD, B. M. (1989): Interosseous transfer of tibialis posterior for common peroneal nerve palsy. Journal of Bone and Joint Surgery, **71B**, 834.

ROPER, B. & TIBREWAL, S. B. (1989): Soft tissue surgery in Charcot-Marie-Tooth disease. Journal of Bone and Joint Surgery, **71B**, 17.

SAMILSON, A. L. & DILLIN, W. (1983): Cavus, cavovarus and calcaneocavus. Clinical Orthopaedics, **177**, 125.

SANGEORZAN, B. J., et al. (1993): Triple arthrodesis using internal fixation in treatment of adult foot disorders. Clinical Orthopaedics, **294**, 299.

SINGER, M. (1961): Tibialis posterior transfer in congenital club foot. Journal of Bone and Joint Surgery, **43B**, 717.

SWANN, M., LLOYD-ROBERTS, G. C. & CATTERALL, A. (1969): The anatomy of uncorrected club feet. Journal of Bone and Joint Surgery, **51B**, 263.

TIBREWAL, S. B. et al. (1992): The Oxford club-foot programme. Journal of Bone and Joint Surgery, **74B**, 528.

WILDE, P. H., et al. (1994): Resection for symptomatic talocalcaneal coalition. Journal of Bone and Joint Surgery, **76B**, 797.

Accessory Bones
O'RAHILLY, R. (1953): A survey of carpal and tarsal anomalies. Journal of Bone and Joint Surgery, **35A**, 626.

Pes Planus
BARRY, R. J. & SCRANTON, P. E. (1983): Flat feet in children. Clinical Orthopaedics, **181**, 68.

GRICE, D. S. (1952): An extra-articular arthrodesis of the subastragalar joint for correction of paralytic flat feet in children. Journal of Bone and Joint Surgery, **34A**, 927.

MANN, R. A. (1983): Acquired flat foot in adults. Clinical Orthopaedics, **181**, 46.

POWELL, H. D. W. (1983): Pes planovalgus in children. Clinical Orthopaedics, **177**, 133.

ROSE, G. K., WELTON, E. A. & MARSHALL, T. (1985): The diagnosis of flat foot in the child. Journal of Bone and Joint Surgery, **67B**, 71.

Walker, A. P., Ghali, N. N. & Silk, F. F. (1985): Congenital vertical talus. Journal of Bone and Joint Surgery, **67B**, 117.

Wenger, D R. *et al.* (1989): Corrective shoes and inserts as treatment for flexible flat foot in infants and children. Journal of Bone and Surgery, **71A**, 800.

Zachariae, L. (1963): The Grice operation for paralytic flat feet in children. Acta Orthopaedica Scandinavica, **33**, 80.

Painful Heel

Bordelon, R. L. (1983): Subcalcaneal pain. Clinical Orthopaedics, **177**, 49.

Cracchiolo, A. (1983): Heel and hindfoot pain. Clinical Orthopaedics, **177**, 2.

Duckworth, T. (1983): The hindfoot and its relation to rotational deformities of the forefoot. Clinical Orthopaedics, **177**, 39.

Furey, J. G. (1975): Plantar fasciitis. Journal of Bone and Joint Surgery, **57A**, 672.

Lapidus, P. W. & Guidotti, F. P. (1965): Management of painful heel. Clinical Orthopaedics, **39**, 178.

Lester, D. K. & Buchanan, J. R. (1984): Surgical treatment of plantar fasciitis. Clinical Orthopaedics, **186**, 202.

Forefoot and Toes

Adams, J. C. & Stossel, C. A. (1992): Hallux valgus. In *Standard Orthopaedic Operations* 4th edn. Edinburgh: Churchill Livingstone.

Antrobus, J. N. (1984): The primary deformity in hallux valgus and metatarsus primus varus. Clinical Orthopaedics, **184**, 251.

Cholmeley, J. A. (1958): Hallux valgus in adolescents. Proceedings of the Royal Society of Medicine, **51**, 903.

Cockin, J. (1968): Butler's operation for over-riding fifth toe. Journal of Bone and Joint Surgery, **50B**, 78.

Fowler, A. W. (1958): Excision of the germinal matrix: A unified treatment for embedded toe-nail and onychogryposis. British Journal of Surgery, **45**, 382.

Fowler, A. W. (1959): A method of forefoot reconstruction [for claw toes]. Journal of Bone and Joint Surgery, **41B**, 507.

Gibson, J. & Piggott, H. (1962): osteotomy of the neck of the first metatarsal in the treatment of hallux valgus. Journal of Bone and Joint Surgery, **44B**, 349.

Greig, J. D. (1989): Results of surgery for ingrowing toe-nails. Journal of Bone and Joint Surgery, **71B**, 859.

Guiloff, R. J., Scadding, J. W. & Klenerman, L. (1984): Morton's metatarsalgia. Journal of Bone and Joint Surgery, **66B**, 586.

Johnson, J. E., Johnson, K. A. & Unni, K. K. (1988): Persistent pain after excision of an interdigital neuroma. Journal of Bone and Joint Surgery, **70A**, 651.

Helal, B. & Greiss, M. (1984): Telescoping osteotomy for pressure metatarsalgia. Journal of Bone and Joint Surgery, **66B**, 213.

Kessel, L. & Bonney, G. (1958): Hallux rigidus in the adolescent. Journal of Bone and Joint Surgery, **40B**, 668.

Mann, R. A. (1955): Disorders of the first metatarso-phalangeal joint. Journal of American Academy of Orthopaedic Surgeons, **3**, 34.

Morris, E. W., Scullion, J. E. & Mann, T. S. (1982): Varus fifth toe. Journal of Bone and Joint Surgery, **64B**, 99.

Scranton, P. E. (1983): Principles in bunion surgery. Journal of Bone and Joint Surgery, **65A**, 1026.

Sullivan, D., Warren, R. F., Pavlov, H. & Kelman, G. (1984): Stress fractures in 51 runners. Clinical Orthopaedics, **187**, 188.

Taylor, R. G. (1951): The treatment of claw toes by multiple transfers of flexor into extensor tendons. Journal of Bone and Joint Surgery, **33B**, 539.

Index

(Where bold type is used it indicates the main reference)